Allergy in ENT Practice
A Basic Guide

Allergy in ENT Practice
A Basic Guide

Hueston C. King, M.D., F.A.C.S., F.A.A.O.A., F.A.C.A.A.I.
Clinical Professor, Department of Otorhinolaryngology
University of Texas Southwestern Medical Center
Dallas, Texas
Clinical Professor, Department of Otolaryngology
University of Florida College of Medicine
Gainesville, Florida

Richard L. Mabry, M.D., F.A.C.S., F.A.A.O.A., Sc.F.A.C.A.A.I.
Professor, Department of Otorhinolaryngology
University of Texas Southwestern Medical Center
Dallas, Texas

Cynthia S. Mabry, R.N., B.S.N., C.O.R.L.N.
Staff Nurse III (Otolaryngic Allergy)
Department of Otorhinolaryngology
University of Texas Southwestern Medical Center
Dallas, Texas

1998
Thieme
New York • Stuttgart

Thieme New York
333 Seventh Avenue
New York, NY 10001

Allergy in ENT Practice: A Basic Guide
Hueston C. King, M.D.
Richard L. Mabry, M.D.
Cynthia S. Mabry, R.N.

Library of Congress Cataloging-in-Publication Data
King, Hueston C.
    Allergy in ENT practice : a basic guide / Hueston C. King, Richard L. Mabry,
    Cynthia S. Mabry
        p. cm.
    Includes bibliographical references and index.
    ISBN 0-86577-798-5. — ISBN 3-13-112761-9
    1. Allergy.   2. Respiratory allergy.   3. Otolaryngology.
    I. Mabry, Richard L.   II. Mabry, Cynthia S.   III. Title.
    [DNLM: 1. Hypersensitivity.   WD 300 K52a 1998]
    RC564.K549   1998
    616.97—dc21
    DNLM/DLC   98-9595
        For Library of Congress   CIP

Important note: Medical knowledge is ever-changing. As new research and clinical
experience broaden our knowledge, changes in treatment and drug therapy may be required.
The authors and the editors of the material herein have consulted sources believed to be
reliable in their efforts to provide infomration that is complete and in accord with the standards
accepted at the time of publication. However, in view of the possibility of human error by the
authors, editors, or publisher of the the work herein, or changes in medical knowledge, neither
the authors, editors, publisher, nor any other party who has been involved in the preparation of
this work, warrants that the information contained herein is in every respect accurate or
complete, and they are not responsible for any errors or omissions or for the results obtained
from use of such information. Readers are encouraged to confirm the information contained
herein with other sources. For example, readers are advised to check the product information
sheet included in the package of each drug they plan to administer to be certain that the
information contained in this publication is accurate and that changes have not been made in
the recommended dose or in the contraindications for administration. This recommendation is
of particular importance in connection with new or infrequently used drugs.

Some of the product names, patents, and registered designs referred to in this book are
in fact registered trademarks or proprietary names even though specific reference to
this fact is not always made in the text. Therefore, the appearance of a name without
designation as proprietary is not to be construed as a representation by the publisher
that it is in the public domain.

Printed in the United States of America
Composition by Maryland Composition Company, Inc.; Printed by Hamilton Printing
Company

5 4 3 2

TNY ISBN 0-86577-798-5
GTV ISBN 3-13-112761-9

It has been our privilege to contribute to the education of numerous individuals in otolaryngic allergy through the years. In this sense, we have been permitted to create a legacy in the specialty that will survive us. However, we are even prouder of the individual accomplishments of our children, who comprise the most important legacy we, or anyone, can leave. In this spirit, we fondly dedicate this work to Brian and Mindy, and to Allen, Brian, and Ann.

HCK, RLM, CSM

Contents

Foreword

Scholars, teachers, friends—Doctors Hueston King and Richard Mabry are all these. They are also scientists who, in this book, contribute essential knowledge to the present and future generations of otolaryngic allergists. Mrs. Cynthia Mabry, an experienced otolaryngic allergy nurse, adds a very special aspect, not previously available, to this textbook. *Allergy in ENT Practice*, subtitled *A Basic Guide*, encompasses all aspects of basic allergy and will be a remarkable resource for physicians in any field of medicine who are preparing to add allergy to their practices. It answers questions that invariably arise in the course of a practice, and provides references to advanced data that a physician may wish to investigate to understand better the basic science of the practice of allergy. In addition, it should become the companion of allergy assistants in every office. These authors possess a wealth of knowledge and, in an easy-to-understand way, offer it both to beginning students and to those beyond the basic stage who need answers to fill gaps in their practical knowledge. I value their willingness to teach, and their friendship.

Helen Fox Krause, M.D., F.A.C.S., F.A.A.O.A.
Clinical Associate Professor of Surgery
Department of Otolaryngology
University of Pittsburgh School of Medicine
Pittsburgh, Pennsylvania

Preface

This book's predecessor, *An Otolaryngologist's Guide to Allergy*, was prepared under the assumption that the vast majority of readers would be otolaryngologists becoming aware of the role of allergy in their practices. This assumption was largely, but by no means entirely, correct. Otolaryngologists did welcome the book. So did many primary care physicians and ancillary personnel. The book served its purpose by providing an introduction, not elsewhere available, for the novice in any field of medicine to the importance, recognition and integration of allergy evaluation and treatment to any aspect of primary care.

Those accepting the challenge of treating allergy are now faced with the hurdle of actually performing the integration: adding the necessary space, selecting and training personnel, procuring the necessary equipment and coping with the inevitable problems involved, in the presence of less peripheral support than they would like to have available.

This book is directed to these people. We hope that it will serve as a guide to all those determined souls, through all the difficult stages of undergoing the transition, and do so in as practical and rewarding a manner as possible.

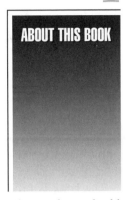

ABOUT THIS BOOK

Before purchasing a book, one likes to know a few things about it. To whom is the book directed, and who will benefit from reading it? What is the book expected to provide the reader? How is the book organized? All are reasonable questions that are frequently not answered in the early stages of reading. This can easily discourage the reader. We will attempt to answer all these questions here, and thus both inform the reader and add orientation that should make the book's progression more understandable.

First, the book is directed primarily to otolaryngologists, but also to any other physicians considering adding allergy to their practice. Two of the authors are otolaryngologists, and the third is an otolaryngic allergy nurse, so it is inevitable that the material presented will be seen primarily from their viewpoint. However, it will be found equally appropriate for the family physician, the pediatrician, and any other primary care giver. Because a large amount of allergy care is provided hands-on by trained ancillary personnel, and because large numbers of personnel have been requesting a book of this type for a number of years, special attention has been given to the needs of this group: as much of the text as possible has been made easy to understand for anyone with a medical background, and well-marked sections indicate areas of special interest to nurses and ancillary personnel, drawn from the experience of an allergy nurse. (It's also perfectly acceptable for physicians to read these sections, found throughout the text as "Nurse's Notes.")

Second, the book is designed to introduce allergy in everyday practice and to prepare physicians and office personnel to begin such a practice and pursue it as extensively as they wish. There can be no such thing as a "cookbook"-type manual on how to practice allergy if the practice is to be carried out in a competent way. The reasons for each decision must be understood, at least to the degree needed to make such decisions. This can be achieved without delving extensively into advanced and theoretical areas of study, which may be of interest in themselves but are not essential to carrying out a successful clinical practice. For those interested in these more obscure aspects of care, references are provided so that they may be investigated at leisure if so desired.

Third, the book is organized to carry the reader step by step through each stage of allergy diagnosis and care, from understanding the benefits of providing such care, to the steps necessary in providing logistic support to a beginning allergy practice, to the more complex aspects of allergy care that may be added as the practice grows and the need arises. Although many practices can benefit from the addition of an active allergy practice, there is a marked scarcity of material designed to help such a practice get started. This book is designed to aid the aspiring part-time allergist in meeting these needs. It also addresses some of the more specialized areas, including pediatric allergy and the relationship of allergy and sinus disease. Finally, the book provides an insight into anticipated future developments in the practice of allergy.

The book is programmed (we hope) for easy reading. The authors make no apologies for areas of repetition throughout the presentations. It can be quite distracting to be directed repeatedly to another part of a book to find material pertinent to the subject being discussed. When found, the material frequently appears in a totally different context, and trying to apply it to the material presently being read interrupts the concentration of the reader. When referrals to other parts of the book are made, it is because the material is too extensive to be contained in the chapter being read.

With these introductory remarks, we welcome you to an introduction to the office practice of ear, nose, and throat (ENT) allergy.

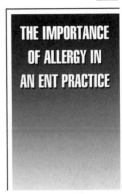

2

THE IMPORTANCE OF ALLERGY IN AN ENT PRACTICE

THE PLACE OF ALLERGY IN CLINICAL MEDICINE

The importance of allergy as a vital element in clinical medicine has become strongly established only in recent years. The burgeoning recognition of allergy has been nothing short of remarkable within the past decade. Not too long ago, much of the medical community and a large segment of the lay public considered allergy a questionable condition at best. The opinion "It's all in their head" was often expressed when the diagnosis of allergy was suggested. Without any real knowledge of the mechanism involved, and faced with the immense diversity of allergy manifestations, the fact that a physician could express such an opinion was not surprising. All this has changed, however. Now, an informed clinician must consider allergy as possibly playing a significant role, either independently or in combination with another medical problem, in the condition of almost any patient presenting for diagnosis. Failure to diagnose and treat the allergic element may easily result in less than optimal results.

Indeed, the pendulum may have swung too far in some regards. The public, once prone to scoff at all but a few manifestations of allergy, has now embraced the condition as a likely cause for almost any undesirable condition. Foods that a patient dislikes are often represented as foods to which the patient is allergic. Unpleasant working conditions may be reported as places harboring substances to which the worker is allergic. Poor performance in school may be blamed on allergies. Whereas formerly clinicians were often reluctant to make a diagnosis of allergy, they may now frequently find it necessary to modify a patient's conviction that some form of allergy is at the root of all present problems.

The lay press, attracted to self-diagnosis, has frequently encouraged this image of allergy. A condition with multiple manifestations, often going unsuspected, makes for good reading. A conscientious physician, aware of the prevalence of allergy, must become at least reasonably knowledgeable as to the true extent of the problem and proper approaches to diagnosis and care.

PREVALENCE OF ALLERGY

To address properly the need for becoming involved in treating allergy, the physician must ask certain critical questions: How important is allergy to a practicing clinician? Is it truly widespread enough and debilitating enough to affect the practice? Becoming active in allergy care might entail a considerable investment in time and equipment. A busy clinician needs to know whether such an investment would be justified, regarding both expense and effect on providing improved patient care.

The exact incidence of allergy is not known, and it may not be accurately known in the foreseeable future. Only one real study on the prevalence of allergy has been performed, in 1987 under the auspices of the National Institute of Allergy and Infectious Diseases (NIAID). The study indicated that about 17% of the population of the United States was suffering from allergy at the time of the survey.[1] The investigators noted that the figure reported was most probably well below the true level, as it considered only patients currently under care, and primarily at large institutions. Most allergy treatment is delivered at the office level, and this body of patients was not included in the study. In addition, many symptoms, such as cough and headache, that in many cases actually represent allergy were not included in the study in the absence of a confirmed diagnosis. Patients previously under allergy care and no longer receiving it were not included, nor could patients with undiagnosed allergies be a part of the total figure. Even without these factors, the study showed that the only condition producing more visits to health care providers' offices than allergy was dental problems.

In addition, the study considered only inhalant allergy patients. Patients hypersensitive to foods may well constitute an even larger group. No estimate of the number of victims of food allergy has ever been made, in part at least because there is as yet no uniformly accepted definition of food "allergy" as opposed to food "hypersensitivity" or simply "adverse reactions to food."[2] This will be the subject of further discussion in Chapter 14. It is evident, however, that inclusion of this body of patients would significantly increase the total percentage of the population affected by allergy.

It is not difficult to see that when all aspects of allergy are considered, this condition may well represent the largest single medical problem seen in the United States today, and probably in the world.

Although generally not life-threatening, from an economic point of view allergy is not a minor problem. Based on figures reported in 1980, allergic rhinitis alone accounted for an expenditure of $224 million annually in physicians' services, and an additional $297 million for relief of symptoms. The same condition produced 2 million days of absence from schools annually, and 3.5 million lost work days, accounting for $154 million annually in lost wages.[3] Evidently, even two decades ago allergy was far from a minor problem. The figures are undoubtedly higher by now, with increased costs and more recognition of allergy as a problem. No primary care physician, or realistically any clinican at any level, can afford to ignore the extent of allergy in the population or the degree to which it can affect the success of a practice.

Current estimates are that allergy in one form or another affects some 30% or more of the general population. Otolaryngologists may expect about 50% of the patients encountered in their practices to have allergy as a major or at least a contributing cause of the presenting problem. Because the ear, nose, and throat area accounts for a large percentage of complaints in a family practice, and an even larger segment of a pediatric practice, an understanding of common findings that are frequently allergy-related should also be of major benefit in these specialties. As a practical matter, any primary care physician should be prepared to identify patients with allergy.

Bearing this in mind, it is reasonable to ask why the presence of allergy is so often overlooked by the clinician. Allergy in many cases may be a rather subtle condition. Its failure to appear in the forefront of diagnostic considerations is not so much a consequence of its absence in the patient (as its prevalence has demonstrated) as of its tendency to appear in forms other than those most widely recognized by the public, and frequently by the unsuspecting physician. Allergy may not be a presenting complaint. Often, unless an allergy has been diagnosed in the past, or the specific presenting complaint is obviously allergic in nature, as with hay fever or violent food allergy, patients may be unaware of an allergic contribution to their condition. In previous generations, allergy was rarely identified unless it was of the classic "hay fever" type, with sneezing, running nose, conjunctivitis, and all the associated problems of itching and irritation. It was not unusual for such euphemisms as "catarrh," "sinus," or simply "postnasal drip" to be reported, and even then, sometimes only in response to specific inquiry. In many cases, because the patient and frequently other family members had had the condition throughout most of life, the symptoms were considered a normal, or at least not an unusual, condition. Unless the clinician carried a high level of suspicion and followed up the physical examination with critical questions, the presence of allergy was easily missed.

To make the diagnosis, the clinician must be alert for allergy. The manifestations are multiple but frequently not obvious unless specifically sought. Allergy has been called "the great masquerader" because of its ability to mimic an immense variety of other conditions.

Some examples of commonly overlooked or missed diagnoses of allergy may illustrate the way in which allergy may produce or contribute to familiar problems. Consider the familiar case of a child with repeated episodes of otitis media from infancy on. If the problem starts before the age of 1 year, in roughly 80% of cases the child will be found to be allergic. (In most cases, when this appears in infancy, the culprit is food. It can be distressing to find that simple dietary control might have saved repeated myringotomies with tubes, and the attendant risks.) The adult who complains of repeated respiratory infections every month or so, especially without fever, merits an allergy evaluation. Many cases of migraine-type headache are actually allergic in origin. A wide variety of gastrointestinal complaints may actually be food hypersensitivities. In short, almost any medical condition may be imitated by allergy. This does not imply that allergy is the underlying or a contributory problem in all such cases, but only that the possibility deserves consideration, especially if the findings are not exactly those expected for the initial presumptive diagnosis, and even more so if the patient has a personal or family history of other forms of allergy.

Although inhalant allergy confines its symptoms for the most part to the respiratory system, even this is not an absolute limitation. As more information becomes available, the presence of concomitant reactions between inhalants and food become more and more evident, blurring the distinction between inhalant and food triggers. In the case of food sensitivity, almost any organ or organ system may become the target of an adverse reaction. Whereas the pathophysiology of hypersensitivity reactions may be quite similar in a wide variety of responses, the signs and symptoms depend on the target organ, and hence may mimic those of an almost unlimited range of complaints. This seriously compounds the difficulty of diagnosis. It is not unreasonable to state that anything from a headache to halitosis to itching feet may be the result of allergy. This does not mean that nearly all medical problems are really allergic in nature, but only that when other diagnostic approaches do not provide the expected results, it may be reasonable at least to consider the possibility of an allergic entity.

REFERENCES

1. NIAID. Task Force Report: Asthma and Other Allergic Diseases. Bethesda, MD: National Institutes of Health; 1979: Publication No. 79-387.
2. King HC. Exploring the maze of adverse reactions to foods. Ear Nose Throat J 1994;73.
3. U.S. Department of Health and Human Services: Asthma and Allergies—An Optimistic Future. Bethesda, MD: National Institutes of Health; 1980: Publication No. 80-388.

3

**BASIC,
"NEED-TO-KNOW"
IMMUNOLOGY**

As with all new additions to a practice, some basic principles underlying the diagnosis and treatment of allergy must be digested and understood if the care provided is to prove effective. A "cookbook" or "owner's manual" approach may produce some early successes, but as soon as the first case arrives that presents some atypical patterns, this type of approach may be expected to fail. Such failure may discourage the patient, and repeated failures may easily discourage the physician and undermine the credibility of the practice.

It is not necessary to understand fully all the underlying mechanisms by which allergy affects the body. (This is fortunate, as science does not as yet fully understand all these mechanisms.) Nor is it necessary to keep at one's fingertips all the principles of each test devised for the diagnosis of allergy. What is necessary is a basic, general knowledge of the immunologic mechanisms governing allergy as far as they are understood at present, and of how these mechanisms apply to allergy testing and treatment. Details, as presented here, should be gone over and understood, but they may then be relegated to the realm of "know where to find when needed."

"NEED-TO-KNOW" IMMUNOLOGY: BASIC IMMUNOLOGIC PRINCIPLES

There are numerous texts on immunology. Most are written by immunologists for immunologists. Most primary care physicians would just as soon spend as little time with immunology as possible. The study of the immune system is extremely complex and appears to change every day, with bits of knowledge being added via research. The immune system appears to have a major place in the body's function, but the specific aspects of how this is achieved seem highly theoretical and often incomprehensible. Many of us would like to pay our respects to the immune system, and then move on to something more understandable and of clinical use.

Unfortunately, allergy cannot be understood or practiced without some knowledge of immune system function. Allergy is a genetic defect in the immune system. The immune system must be, and can be, manipulated to some degree to achieve long-lasting benefits in allergy care. Like all aspects of medicine, practices keep changing as new knowledge appears, and an understanding of immunologic principles involving allergy is necessary to evaluate new procedures properly and integrate them into the practice as needed. It is a familiar situation to find practitioners of allergy still using techniques and procedures established several decades ago and since found to be less than optimal, if not actually ineffective. Every attempt will be made to limit the immunology discussion to what is needed to understand basic aspects of allergy, and to some degree communicate them to the inquiring patient. The first portion of the following discussion is on overall view of the immune system in the normal individual. It is needed as background. The reader should note the ''need-to-know'' caveat at the end of the following section before becoming discouraged.

Function of the Immune System

The immune system provides the means by which the body relates to the environment. The environment provides the body with all its needs for growth and subsistence, so the relationship is obviously a necessary one. Much of the environment is beneficial, such as food and oxygen; much is neutral, neither benefiting the body nor hurting it, and some is distinctly harmful. It is the job of the immune system to sort out the various items encountered in the environment, accept those benefiting the body while eliminating those threatening it. In addition to items from the environment, aging, decaying, or malignant cells appearing within the body must be identified and eliminated if the body is to survive. This also is the job of the immune system. Immunologically speaking, the immune system differentiates between ''self'' and ''nonself,'' but its function goes beyond that, as it must be able to distinguish between beneficial ''nonself'' (nutrients) and harmful ''nonself'' (bacteria and viruses, for example.) Not all the means by which these actions are performed are fully understood, but the basic format is known.

The immune system is made up of a variety of cells present in the circulation and the body tissues, in addition to chemical substances produced by these cells that affect foreign invaders, other cells of the immune system, and at times other cells of the body.

When a foreign substance enters the body, it is picked up by a macrophage and ingested. In the lower animals, the substance may simply be digested and eliminated. In humans, however, the substance is carried through the circulation, undergoing some processing en route, until it can be presented to a specific lymphocyte. In the higher animals, with immune system memory, these foreign substances are known as *antigens*. The lymphocytes are the basic cells of the immune system, and they form the source of the immunologic "memory" differentiating the human system from that of the lower animals. The lymphocytes are all produced in the bone marrow, but after release into the circulation, they differentiate into two distinct types, B lymphocytes and T lymphocytes. The B lymphocytes are further processed in the bone marrow (hence *B* for bone marrow-dependent lymphocytes) and acquire a multitude of antigenic attachment sites able to react to a single type of antigen on their surfaces. These sites are highly specific and genetically determined. They cannot be altered. Each B cell has a specific configuration of its antibody sites. Each B lymphocyte is thus capable of reacting to a specific antigen, should it ever encounter that antigen. This encounter does not always occur. It has been estimated that at least five exposures to even a highly sensitizing antigen are needed to induce sensitization (Walter N. Lewis, *personal communication*). If no such exposure ever occurs, the cell never becomes sensitized.

As a whole, a person's B lymphocytes may display as many as 10 million different attachment configurations for different antigens. In addition, most foreign substances carry a variety of antigens, and antigenic attachment sites may react with structurally similar antigens, expanding the possible range of sensitization. This is one of the factors producing cross-reactivity, and concomitant allergy between foods and inhalants. (The immune system does not recognize the route by which an antigen enters the system, only its presence in the circulation.)

When and if the monocyte carrying the antigen reaches an appropriate lymphocyte, the antigen reacts with the antigenic attachment site and sensitization occurs. The B lymphocyte is now immunologically committed. It will go on to mutate into a host of identical cells, now known as *plasma cells*, each of which produces a substance known as *antibody*, specific to the antigen producing the sensitization.

Antibody has a variety of functions, but the most important is to bind to antigen, aiding the body in removing the offender. In the case presented, however, if no further factors were interposed, antibody would be produced in uncontrolled amounts. This production must be moderated for the body to benefit. Control of the antibody production process is the function of the other type of lymphocyte.

The other type of lymphocyte undergoes processing in the thymus gland to become a T lymphocyte (thymus-dependent). The T lymphocyte also has attachment sites on its surface, but it reacts differently to antigen exposure. It may become a T helper or a T suppressor lymphocyte, increasing or decreasing the antibody production of the B lymphocyte to meet the body's needs. The T lymphocyte is also active in cell-mediated immunity, presented later in this chapter.

Both B lymphocytes and T lymphocytes may become memory cells, storing the identity of the invading allergen and able to recognize the pattern on subsequent appearances and institute appropriate defensive action.

A significant portion of the immune process is affected by protein hormones known as *cytokines*. The cytokines that are involved in the natural immune processes are largely produced by mononuclear phagocytic cells, and may also be known as *monokines*. In an immune response to antigenic stimulation, activated lymphocytes produce cytokines, which are sometimes known as *lymphokines*. A final family of cytokines are the colony-stimulating factors, which enhance the growth and differentiation of stem cells and immature bone marrow cells. Because the principal source of cytokines is the leukocyte, and because their biologic activity is primarily directed at other leukocytes, they are often generically known as *interleukins*. Current terminology numbers these interleukins (abbreviated as IL), so that common designations are IL-1, IL-2, etc.

The generally accepted functions of cytokines are to (1) mediate natural immunity; (2) regulate lymphocyte activation, growth, and differentiation; (3) regulate immune-mediated inflammation; and (4) stimulate cell growth and differentiation. The effects and target cells of cytokines remain under active investigation, and this base of knowledge is constantly expanding. The serious student may consult other sources for more detailed information,[1-3] but for purposes of this discussion, the general concept explained here will suffice.

One further component of the immune system requires mention: the complement system. This is actually a group of enzymes that react in a cascade pattern when stimulated by an antigen, gaining strength and amplifying as the cascade progresses. An exact knowledge of the routes involved is rarely necessary for the clinician. The end result of complement activation is to produce one of three responses: (1) Complement may aid the ingestion of offending cells (invaders or dying or diseased body cells) by the major phagocytes of the body. (2) Complement reacts with various other immunologic components to produce direct cytolosis of invaders. (3) Complement may facilitate immune complex reactions, which are discussed in the following section on the malfunctions of the immune system involved in allergy.

This has been, despite appearances, a very cursory introduction to the basic functions of the immune system. Even so, trying to absorb even this much may seem daunting. How much of the above does one actually "need to know" to understand the position of allergy in the much larger field of immunology, and therefore how allergy can be diagnosed and treated? Certainly, not everything must be committed to memory. Reading it through to establish a familiarity with the terms should provide a reasonable introduction to the aspects of the immune system directly involved in allergy, and therefore of importance as background material to the clinician. One may then go back to review parts of the discussion as needed, if portions of the sections on testing and treatment become confusing.

ALLERGY AND THE IMMUNE SYSTEM

Allergy is a malfunction of the immune system. The normally functioning immune system identifies true environmental threats to the body, as well as internal cellular disorders, and attempts to remove the offenders from the body. The allergic immune system identifies as dangerous environmental invaders that may not actually present any threat to the body, and institutes defensive action. The defensive action may be limited, or it may be greater than that needed to defend against true offenders. This situation is genetically determined. By this is meant that the potential for development of an excessive response to harmless exposures, such as dust, molds, pollens, and certain foods, is predetermined in each individual. If the exposure to the potential allergen does not occur, the individual will never show a response. (In the allergic patient, "antigens" become "allergens," as they are capable of inducing an allergic reaction.) Conversely, if the individual is exposed to a substance to which no antigenic attachments exist in that person's immune system, that person cannot become allergic to the substance. Although it is true that most allergic patients do respond to a variety of offenders, the lay designation of the patient who is "allergic to everything" does not exist. The potential number of allergens to which any one patient may react is large but limited. This fact may be of some importance in preparing a testing program for a patient. Although sensitization may occur at any stage of life, and rarely occurs on limited or early exposures, a patient who has lived for years in the same place with no significant change in activity or occupation will usually have had enough exposure to the potential allergens present to induce a reaction, if one can occur. If the patient has had extensive testing and treatment and has been doing well, and suddenly has a marked increase in allergy symptoms, it is rarely necessary to repeat the previous tests. Instead, a diligent search for a new exposure and sensitization is indicated.

TYPES OF ALLERGIC MECHANISM

Allergy may appear as a malfunction of any part of the immune system, and frequently more than one mechanism is involved. The complexity of the problem led two investigators, Gell and Coombs, to divide allergic reactions into four types. Although not a perfect delineation, as it is quite possible for more than one reaction to occur simultaneously, the designation is of great use in understanding and treating allergy.

Type I Reactions

Type I allergy (Fig. 3–1), also known as *atopy* or *immediate hypersensitivity*, is the best-known form of allergy and is the type usually associated by the public with the diagnosis of allergy. As far as is known, all inhalant allergy is a type I reaction. A small percentage of food allergy represents a type I reaction. Insect sting allergy is also type I, as is penicillin sensitivity. This is the only potentially life-threatening form of allergic reaction commonly seen, and it can proceed to anaphylactic shock and death. Type I reactions are produced by immunoglobulin E (IgE), a substance present in greater than

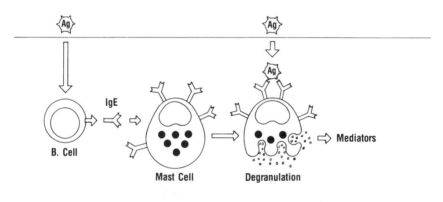

| B. Cell Sensitized IgE Produced | Mast Cell Sensitized IgE Binds to Surface | Antigen Bridges 2 IgE Molecules, Mast Cell Degranulates | Released Mediators Produce Allergic Symptoms |

FIGURE 3–1. Gell and Coombs type I reaction. Type I hypersensitivity. An antigen passing through the respiratory or gastrointestinal mucosa sensitizes a B lymphocyte, which in turn initiates production of IgE. The IgE binds to the surface of mast cells, sensitizing them. A second exposure to the antigen results in bridging of the IgE molecules and triggers degranulation of the mast cell, resulting in the release of mediators that produce hay fever, asthma, utricaria, etc. (Adapted from Roitt et al. Immunology. St. Louis: C.V. Mosby Co.; 1985; and Mygind, N. Essential Allergy. Oxford: Blackwell Scientific Publications; 1986.)

trace amounts in an estimated 20 to 30% of the population. This type of allergy is the only form that can be diagnosed reliably by skin testing and also by in vitro testing, leading a large percentage of the allergy community to consider this condition the only true form of "allergy" and to refer to all other adverse reactions by a different designation. (The controversy about the definition of allergy is discussed in some detail in Chapter 14.)

Type I allergy produces an immediate reaction in most cases, occurring within seconds to minutes. If the target organ is the upper respiratory tract, the classic "hay fever" pattern will be seen, with extensive sneezing, rhinorrhea, often conjunctivitis, and frequently itching. If the target organ is the lower respiratory tract, cough, increased sputum, and wheezing may occur. Systemic type I reactions may include urticaria, angioedema, and, in the extreme case, anaphylactic shock resulting in death.

The mechanism is shown in Figure 3–1. After entering the body, either via the respiratory tract, the gastrointestinal tract, a venomous insect sting, or a hypodermic needle injection (which may apply to any drug, not only an allergenic extract), the allergen is picked up by a macrophage and carried eventually to a lymphocyte containing the appropriate attachment sites; this lymphocyte then becomes sensitized. The lymphocyte next becomes converted into replicating plasma cells (B cells). Up to this point, the reaction is that of a normal immune system. In the allergic patient, however, the plasma cells now begin to produce large amounts of allergen-specific IgE, which binds to mast cells throughout the body. Within the mast cell are multiple granules containing histamine and various other chemical mediators, which the system produce the type I allergic reactions described. When a second contact with the allergen occurs, the allergen is able to bridge two IgE molecules on the mast cell, triggering the mast cell to release its granules.

The chemical mediators released do not stay in the system long, but many of the lymphocytes have now become "memory cells," able to identify the allergen and re-establish the entire sequence rapidly on additional exposures. Once sensitized, most patients with this type of allergy remain so for many years, or a lifetime.

Through the years, there has developed a tendency to identify the eosinophil with allergy. Eosinophils appear in profusion in the presence of allergy, drawn by the chemicals released by the mast cell, but it now appears that their function may not be one of producing the allergy, but rather in shutting down the inflammatory reaction induced by the mast cell. The eosinophil appears in other conditions, and its complete function is as yet not fully understood.

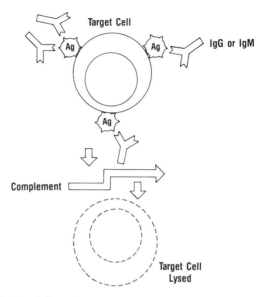

FIGURE 3–2. Gell and Coombs type II reaction. Type II hypersensitivity. Antigen binds directly to the surface of the target cell; a degenerating erythrocyte, an invader, or in allergy a healthy body cell. IgG or IgM antibodies attach to the antigen, and by direct action of complement the cell is lysed. This is a beneficial action in normal homeostasis, a destructive one in allergy. (Adapted from Roitt et al. Immunology. St. Louis: C.V. Mosby Co.; 1985; and Mygind N. Essential Allergy. Oxford: Blackwell Scientific Publications; 1986.)

Type II Reactions

Type II allergy is an abnormal modification of one of the body's standard mechanisms for removing invaders or degenerating body cells. In its normal format, the antigen binds directly to the surface membrane of some tissue or cell of the body. Attached there, it reacts with and binds to specific immunoglobulin G (IgG) or immunoglobulin M (IgM) circulating antibodies. When attached to the antigen, these antibodies activate the complement cascade, which in turn lyses the cell (Fig. 3–2). When the cell in question is an invader or degenerating cell, the reaction is beneficial. When the cell is a normal body cell, incorrectly identified by the immune system as an invader or degenerating cell, the body is harmed. An example of a Gell and Coombs type II reaction is the hemolysis that occurs following a transfusion with incompatible blood.

Type II allergy does not appear to be involved in any form of inhalant allergy. At times it is a component of food allergy, but the prevalence has not as yet been determined, although it does not appear to be a major compo-

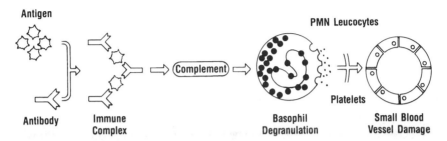

FIGURE 3–3. Gell and Coombs type III reaction. Type III hypersensitivity. Antigen and antibody, usually IgG, combine to form a large immune complex. These complexes attach to small vessel walls and through the action of complement induce basophil degranulation, polymorphonuclear leukocyte attraction and activation, and platelet activity. This results in small vessels vasculitis with retraction of endothelial cells and leakage of fluid into the tissue of the target organ. (Adapted from Roitt et al. Immunology. St. Louis: C.V. Mosby Co.; 1985; and Mygind N. Essential Allergy. Oxford: Blackwell Scientific Publications; 1986.)

nent of food sensitivity. More details about adverse reactions to food are presented in Chapter 14.

Type III Reactions

Type III allergy involves the formation of immune complexes, with subsequent tissue damage. When an allergen molecule enters the body, it reacts with a circulating antibody molecule, forming a large, irregular molecular aggregate known as an *immune complex* (Fig. 3–3). This occurs whenever an allergen enters the body, but under normal circumstances the immune complexes are cleared from the circulation promptly by the reticuloendothelial system. If the patient has become sensitized to the allergen, however, and has a large amount of circulating antibody, the number of immune complexes may be too great to be cleared promptly, and they may produce an allergic reaction.

The circulating immune complexes do not react, but they have an affinity for the small vessels of various target organs and attach themselves to these vessels. Here, they produce an inflammatory reaction by several mechanisms, including activation of complement and attraction of basophils, polymorphonuclear leukocytes, and platelets. These cells in turn release biologically active substances that cause retraction of the endothelial cells lining the small blood vessels of the target organ. This in turn allows the leakage of fluid and inflammatory substances into the tissues of the target organ. It is the presence of this excess fluid in the tissue of the target organ and the action of the inflammatory mediators in the fluid that produces the patient's symptoms. An example of a Gell and Coombs type III reaction is the delayed penicillin reaction, or "arthus phenomenon."

The mechanism of action is essentially the same in all type III reactions; however, the effect on the patient will be widely different depending on the target organ. To give examples, the most common target organ for a type III reaction is usually considered to be the upper respiratory airway, followed by the lower airway and then the gastrointestinal tract. If the target organ is the upper airway, the patient's symptoms will be those of allergic rhinitis. If it is the lower airway, the result will be asthma or allergic bronchitis. Reactions in the gastrointestinal tract may be diarrhea, cramping, or even ulcers or colitis. In the skin, urticaria or angioedema will appear. Thus, although the effect of the attached immune complexes may be essentially identical on the underlying tissues of any target organ, the effect on the patient will depend on the normal function of the organ and how inflammation affects this function. This almost unlimited diversity of symptoms is the factor that has made identification of offenders in type III allergy so difficult.

Type III allergy is presumed to be the most common form of allergy seen in food hypersensitivity. Various types of laboratory tests have been developed for this type of reaction, but none has proved uniformly reliable. More details are presented in Chapter 14, but some examples may be of value at this point in terms of clarification. First, the precursor of the type III reaction is the reacting antibody, which is usually IgG. This may be measured, in the same manner as IgE. However, IgG is normally formed by everyone on eating a food, and at what point the amount of specific IgG produced becomes abnormal has not been established. Second, circulating immune complexes may be assayed, but the cost is prohibitive for an individual, and in any case it is not the circulating complexes that are the offenders, but rather those attached to the small vessels of the target organ. This is the type of problem that has made the development of simple, clinical allergy tests so difficult.

To further confuse the clinician, type III allergy may develop rapidly or may be delayed for hours or, under some circumstances, days. This greatly compounds the difficulty of establishing a cause-and-effect relationship between the allergy exposure and the resulting symptoms. At this point, it is necessary only that the clinician be aware of the problems occurring. The various approaches and their limitations are discussed in the sections on diagnosis.

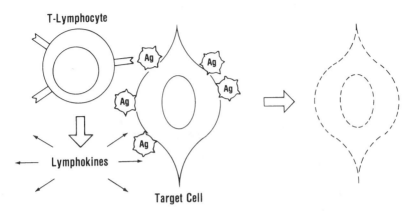

FIGURE 3–4. Gell and Coombs type IV reaction. Type IV hypersensitivity. Sensitized T lymphocytes contain receptor sites on their surfaces. These attach to antigen bound to the surface of target cells. The target cell may be lysed directly without the intervention of complement. The T lymphocytes also produce lymphokines that attract other protective cells, increasing the action. This is delayed hypersensitivity and may not appear for days after the exposure. (Adapted from Roitt et al. Immunology. St. Louis: C.V. Mosby Co.; 1985; and Mygind N. Essential Allergy. Oxford: Blackwell Scientific Publications; 1986.)

Type IV Reactions

Understanding this form of allergy is essential to clinicians, even though their influence on the course of the reaction is greatly limited. Type IV allergy is most frequently seen in such conditions as poison ivy. It has been demonstrated to appear at times in food hypersensitivity, but the degree to which this occurs is not known.

In type IV allergy, the presence of complement is not required. The T lymphocyte has antibody receptors on its surface; these react with specific antigens in the same manner as those of the B lymphocyte (Fig. 3–4). As with the B lymphocyte in type I allergy, previous sensitization is required to establish the necessary condition on the lymphocyte surface. Once the sensitization has been established and activated by a new contact with the antigen, the T lymphocyte releases a variety of substances that mobilize other inflammatory cells, which in turn produce a direct effect on the target organ.

The distinguishing feature of the type IV reaction is its delayed nature. It takes time for the cellular mobilization to occur. Thus, a type IV reaction may occur 24 to 48 hours after contact with the allergen, or even later. A classic example is that given, poison ivy. The reaction does not appear immediately after contact, but a day or so later, and it may continue to proliferate for up to several days thereafter. This delay in appearance is the factor that has led to the lay belief that rupturing the blebs of the skin reaction spreads the rash, whereas actually the extent of the reaction has already been established by the extent of initial skin contact with the ivy allergen. This delay makes establishing a cause-and-effect relationship between exposure and reaction in reactions other than poison ivy all but impossible to establish.

CLINICAL CLASSIFICATIONS OF ALLERGY

Immunologically, there are four Gell and Coombs types of allergy, whereas, clinically, allergy is divided for practical purposes into two types: fixed and cyclic. This division is largely accepted by all physicians practicing allergy, regardless of specialty background. Although the designation is essentially clinical, there is an immunologic application that is usually, although not always, comparable. Most of the considerations of fixed and cyclic allergy relate to food sensitivity, and they are discussed in considerably more detail in Chapter 14. At this point, however, a brief overview may be helpful in avoiding later confusion.

Fixed Allergy

In general, the designation of *fixed* applies to IgE-mediated responses, including all forms of inhalant allergy, as far as is known, insect sting allergy, and most forms of drug allergy. Some forms of food sensitivity fall under this category, but the number is limited. This type of allergy manifests as an immediate reaction, occurring within seconds to at most a few hours after contact with the allergen. It normally occurs every time the patient is exposed to the allergen once the sensitization has occurred. At times, if there has been no contact with the allergen for several years, the reaction may not occur immediately on a single exposure. This is most frequently seen with drug sensitivity. The reaction is not predictable, however, and a single exposure without a serious reaction is not grounds for assuming that the allergy has disappeared. When such a situation does present itself, another exposure or two, even in minimal amounts, will usually fully re-establish the sensitivity in all its severity. Because a single dose of an antibiotic will provide little in the way of benefit, once a fixed reaction has been demonstrated, it is best to consider the sensitivity permanent and avoid the offending allergen indefinitely. This type of allergy may be life-threatening and requires the most scrupulous control.

Cyclic Allergy

All types of allergy other than fixed are designated *cyclic allergy*. For the most part, this designation is applied to food sensitivity. This form of allergy is both dose- and frequency-related, meaning that the patient may encounter a small amount of the allergen without sustaining a reaction unless the contact is repeated. Several doses in rapid succession, however, will usually trigger a reaction even if the doses are small. A single dose may also trigger a reaction if it is large enough. Although the designations of fixed and cyclic allergy are used primarily in connection with food sensitivity, both conditions actually apply to both inhalant and food allergy. An example of incremental effects in inhalant allergy is seen in the "priming effect," in which at the beginning of an allergy season the patient may have little trouble, but as the season progresses the allergy becomes more severe, and less exposure is required to produce symptoms. In addition, the entire immune system becomes progressively more sensitive, so that by the end of the season the patient is found to be sensitive to other minor allergens that did not cause a reaction earlier in the season.

Except for the "priming effect" described above, which is not really a form of true cyclic allergy, a primary consideration in cyclic allergy is that by definition it is not IgE-mediated. IgE-mediated sensitivity is much more severe, and although repeated exposures do increase the reaction, the increase is very rapid and severe. (A good example is penicillin sensitivity, in which the first reaction may be only itching, but the next may well be angioedema, asthma, and anaphylaxis.) Cyclic allergy tends to be occult and difficult to recognize, and there tends to be little evident cause-and-effect relationship between allergy exposure and symptom onset. The patient may even feel temporarily better after some exposure to the allergen, although the overall effect is deleterious. This phenomenon, known as *masking*, is discussed in detail in Chapter 14. It is most pronounced in food allergy.

"NEED-TO-KNOW" IMMUNOLOGY: SUMMARY

The preceding discussion, despite its length, has been a very basic overview of immunology for the practicing clinician. More information on the subject is readily available for those wishing to expand their understanding of the field. The preceding material has been presented as a basic referral source for practical approaches to allergy diagnosis and care that are described later in the book. In other words, if the reader is confused by some test or treatment modality discussed later, a review of the preceding material on basic immunology may help to clear up the confusion. It is not intended or necessary that the clinician carry all the details of the function of the immune system fully in mind at all times. Although they are interesting, this would be a waste of concentration. Certain aspects of the immune system's function, however, do need to be understood and immediately available to evaluate properly a patient's complaints and plan appropriate definitive testing and treatment. This is "need-to-know" immunology, which, then, includes the following items:

1. The immune system is a complex mechanism designed to protect the body against stress, both internal and external. Allergy is a malfunction of the immune system, in which the body attempts to protect itself against substances that really pose little or no threat to its safety. Allergy is essentially an overshooting of the immune mechanism.

2. Immunologically, there are four types of allergic reaction, but clinically only fixed and cyclic reactions need be considered in the majority of cases. Fixed reactions are normally immediate and severe, and they may be life-threatening. They are all caused by IgE, a substance present in significant amounts in only 20 to 30% of the population. This is a genetically determined characteristic of the immune system in this group of people. Others do not form IgE in more than trace amounts. Therefore, not everyone is even somewhat allergic, regardless of the exposure, at least in this type of allergy, which is what most of the public recognizes as allergy.

3. All inhalant allergy and insect sting allergy and most drug allergy is caused by IgE. Only a small proportion of food allergy is a result of IgE reactions, and this type is usually very obvious (e.g., an immediate onset of itching, wheezing, and shortness of breath).

4. IgE-mediated allergy may be diagnosed by skin testing or by laboratory testing on blood: radioallergo sorbent testing (RAST) or enzyme-linked immunoadsorbent assay (ELISA). Other allergies may not be diagnosed by this method with any reliability.

5. Food sensitivity may be either fixed (IgE-mediated, a small percentage of cases and usually obvious, as above) or cyclic, mediated by other branches of the immune system or even mechanisms outside the immune system. There is no reliable laboratory test for this type of sensitivity. The various means of identifying offenders are discussed in Chapter 14.

6. Food sensitivity may affect almost any part of the body, producing an immense range of symptoms. Cyclic food allergy is usually subtle, often delayed, and related to dose and frequency of ingestion. The patient is almost always unable to establish a connection between the consumption of the food and the symptoms produced without very specific help.

With these basic rules of thumb and general information, the clinician should understand enough immunology to progress into consideration of allergy diagnosis and care. For best results, not only the physician but also the ancillary person in charge of administering allergy treatment should be aware of this much immunology, as the patient will be much more cooperative if this person can explain the situation in an understandable manner. Patient confidence in the person providing the actual treatment and taking the ongoing history is a vital component of allergy care.

REFERENCES

1. Fireman P. Immunology of allergic disorders. In: Fireman P, Slavin R, eds. Atlas of Allergies. 2nd ed. London: Mosby-Wolfe; 1996:1–26.
2. Bellanti JA. Immunology. Philadelphia: WB Saunders; 1985.
3. Roitt I, Brostoff J, Male D. Immunology. 4th ed. London: Mosby; 1996.

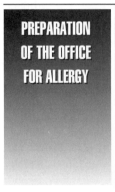

4

PREPARATION OF THE OFFICE FOR ALLERGY

GETTING STARTED: PREPARING THE SETTING

It must be presumed at this point that the physician has decided that adding allergy care to the already existing primary care practice will be of benefit to both the practice and the patients. A large majority of patients resent being shuffled from one physician to another, and wish to have as much of their care as possible handled at one location by a physician who is aware of their problems. Although expanding managed care may have made it necessary for the physician to reduce the time spent at each patient visit, the desire of the patient for a personal relationship with the doctor still exists.

Most patients will readily accept the need for a secondary or tertiary care facility for major surgery or life-threatening problems, but ongoing care of a more or less routine nature is expected to be performed in a familiar setting. Adding this facet of care to a practice can only enhance the success of the practice and increase patient satisfaction. In summary, the project has now received a favorable executive decision and is in the hands of the ways and means committee.

Little if any of this chapter deals with science. The chapter is all logistics. Nothing should be taken as a rigid requirement for a successful practice. All practices are different, and subject to various needs and conveniences. Presented here is the accumulation of several decades of trials, failures, revisions, restructuring, and successes—not only on the part of the authors but also of many of their colleagues nationwide who have introduced allergy into their practices and survived the ensuing struggles. It is to be hoped that it will help the novice to overcome some of the normal problems encountered in starting.

Unlike many of the chapters in this book, this one will be of importance primarily to the physician. This is not an ideal situation. It would be better if the person providing the actual day-to-day care were able to provide input on preparing the area in which allergy care is to be practiced, but more often than not this member of the staff has not yet been employed. This entails some projection of actual needs on the part of the directing physician, often with little experience. On the rare occasion when the member of the staff who will be performing the allergy testing and treatment is already employed in another role, it will be to the directing physician's advantage to discuss the preparation of the area set aside for allergy in advance. Often, this person will be able to identify arrangements that would make the daily procedures cumbersome and require later revisions in the layout. Even if this situation exists, however (i.e., a person already employed is to be given the job of allergy care), no one can anticipate reliably in advance the changing needs of an expanding allergy practice. It is often better to be as flexible as possible until this aspect of the practice is well under way, thereby reducing the need for later major physical revisions in the area in which allergy is to be practice. If the person providing the allergy care has yet to be employed, as is usually the case, the directing physician must prepare the allergy unit with only theoretical information. This is not easy, and it is common either to overestimate or to underestimate the needs in advance. In the following pages, as much help and advice as possible are provided.

Adding allergy entails some expansion of the physical facilities available in the office, but these are smaller and of lesser complexity than many other types of technology used in upgrading a practice. No heavy equipment is needed. If the room chosen already has a sink and an electrical outlet for a refrigerator, no new plumbing or electric wiring will be necessary. Some space is needed, but not an excessive amount and not all positioned close to other parts of the office. An allergy office can be crowded into a small space if necessary (Fig. 1), but if a moderate amount can be allotted, it will make the operation more comfortable. Basic equipment is necessary, but even more important is the acquisition of good personnel. This latter deserves special consideration and is discussed in a special section below. The first consideration, however, is space.

Space

The space needed to perform allergy testing and treatment is not great. A room roughly 8 by 10 ft is more than adequate for testing. (A smaller space is actually adequate but tends to produce a degree of claustrophobia because most such spaces are entirely enclosed.) This testing area need not be an integral part of the rest of the office, although it should not be so far away that the treating physician would have difficulty reaching the allergy testing and treatment area should a problem arise. Actually, there are many benefits in having the allergy section physically separated from the rest of the office. Allergy patients are seen much more frequently than other patients as a general rule. They tend to attach closely to both the physician directing their treatment and the person directly administering it. This is an advantage from

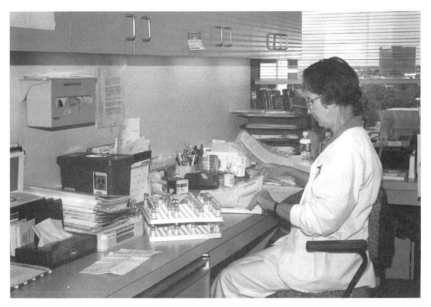

FIGURE 4–1. Finding adequate space may present a problem when allergy is added to an existing practice. However, with ingenuity and careful planning, a small space can be used if necessary.

the point of view of expanding the practice, but it can seriously disaccommodate directing physicians if every patient has the opportunity to intercept them with questions while they are attempting to move efficiently through the office to handle the daily patient load aside from allergy. Separating the allergy testing area from the general office by a door at the very least will normally provide such a division for practical purposes.

It is also advisable to arrange in some way to have allergy patients clearly separated from other patients throughout their visits. This may be accomplished by having a separate receptionist handle and route allergy patients; alternatively, while the allergy portion of the practice is small, the member of the team administering the testing and care may receive the patients in person. (As the practice grows, this will quickly become impractical, but it may work at the start.) Having allergy patients processed through the same receptionist as other patients quickly becomes prohibitively cumbersome. Allergy visits to receive therapy are brief. The patients are in and out of the treatment area in minutes. Testing sessions may be scheduled to occupy predictable time segments. The more the allergy part of the practice can be separated from the rest of the practice, the better and more smoothly it can be run.

There are other reasons to separate the allergy portion of the practice from the general part. These may not seem important initially, but if ignored they tend to produce increasing problems with time. Allergy testing and treatment and the preparation of extracts require careful timing and measurements. Interruptions should be kept to a minimum. There is always the temptation on the part of the physician to call the person involved in allergy treatment away from the procedures being performed when an additional hand would be of value elsewhere in the office. The allergy section may appear quiet at the moment, but if such procedures as skin testing are under way, for example, the person providing the care must time and measure the responses accurately if good treatment results are to be obtained. An unexpected delay in timing may invalidate an entire test series. Even more deleterious is interrupting the person involved in preparing the vials of allergenic extract used in both testing and treatment. Test vials must be remade every 6 weeks if potency is to be maintained. The same procedures used in making testing vials is used in making treatment vials, and a small practice the same vials may be used for both testing and treatment. If these are mismade, as a result of an interruption during the procedure, not only may test results be invalid, but treatment can be compromised. This is comparable with a pharmacist dispensing the wrong drug. Allergenic extracts for treatment, unlike most drugs, are not normally prepared in a central reference laboratory, but in the physician's office. (It is possible to have treatment vials made by a manufacturer of allergy extracts, but this frequently compounds the problem of a difference in the strength of extracts used in testing and treatment. Also, another potential source of error is created by inserting an additional step in the preparation, with another chance for human error.) Careful office preparation of the treatment extracts, free of interruptions, provides the best and standard format for safe and proper treatment of the patient.

Despite the convenience of being able to call in an additional set of hands when it would benefit the other office workers, the directing physician should be aware of the need for concentration in extract preparation. This problem may often best be solved by having the testing and treatment extracts prepared in a location not directly attached to the clinical part of the office, and therefore not readily visible. It is also a good idea to have them prepared by another person, possibly someone more accustomed to laboratory procedure, leaving the person charged with testing and treatment free from these time constraints.

It is quite reasonable at this time to raise the question of whether the extracts might be more conveniently prepared in a central location and shipped to the office. This would reduce the space requirements and bring quality control under a simpler format, as it would basically apply to laboratory conditions. Sometime in the future this may indeed be a practical solution, but that time has not yet arrived. The theoretical benefits still fall short of the practical logistics. Allergy care is an ongoing procedure. Centralization inevitably results in delays, which rapidly undermine the success of treatment. When extracts do not arrive on time, treatment is interrupted, testing schedules are compromised, and results are delayed. Possibly more important, patients are irritated and upset, and the physician's credibility is threatened. This does not bode well for the developing allergy practice.

On a more scientific level, even when basic inhalant testing is performed on an in vitro basis by a reference laboratory, the results must be confirmed by limited skin testing, using extracts prepared in the office. The treatment should be performed with the same extracts. One of the basic tenets of allergy from its inception has been the insistence on treating with the same material used in testing. This has already been violated by the use of in vitro procedures in testing, and one of the surprises associated with the expansion of in vitro testing has been the fact that removing this restriction has not seriously compromised results or produced significant risks. This does not present a carte blanche license to accept laboratory results, however. The closer the treatment material is to the patient, the more careful controls must be. Preparation of extracts in the office by competent and concerned personnel and verification of the results in a controlled manner on the patient who is to receive the treatment is the safest approach yet designed, ensuring that the material tested and that to be administered are identical.

There are many ways in which the time and assigned tasks of the person performing allergy testing and administering treatment can be varied to a successful level. No physician in today's market wishes to employ someone who will be idle a large amount of time, or who may not be put to use elsewhere. The above caveats might seem to preclude dual functions of the allergy personnel, but this need not be the case. Allergy testing and care rarely require urgent responses. After the physician in charge makes the initial determination that allergy testing and treatment are indicated, temporary relief may be provided medically and the patient scheduled for appropriate testing, at which time a more complete history may be taken. If desired, a prepared history form may be sent home with the patient, to be returned at the time of testing. This will not replace a face-to-face history, but it may be of considerable assistance. (More of the details of an allergy history are presented in the sections on history taking in Chapter 5.) This arrangement will allow allergy testing and treatment to be scheduled during predetermined times and performed without interruption. It does not take long for a generally reliable picture to be obtained of the time needed for testing and treatment of a patient, allowing accurate scheduling to take place. Similarly, a time for the preparation of testing and treatment vials without interruption maybe set aside on a regular schedule. The person in charge of allergy may thus be freed to assist in general office needs at other times.

There is a benefit in having the person assigned to allergy be present in the office on a full-time basis. Whereas testing and treatment may be scheduled, questions may not. These will be telephoned in at any hour. Only the person involved in administering the allergy care and in regular contact with the patient will be able to answer these questions accurately and with minimal delay.

A separate section of the physician's office is definitely needed for allergy treatment and testing. A section is also needed for the preparation of the vials of extract used in testing and treatment. This may be a part of the testing and treatment section if space permits, and this is always convenient. It can be separated from the rest of the office simply by closing the door and forbidding interruptions while testing and treatment vials are being prepared. This immediate office space is frequently at a premium, however. It is quite acceptable to have testing and treatment vials prepared elsewhere, where there is more space, although a place in or adjacent to the office is desirable to avoid damage in transferring the vials to the allergy treatment area. Here, a large refrigerator to hold bulk extract and prepared vials and a table for vial preparation are needed. It can easily be seen that there is a benefit in combining this area with the main allergy section; the prepared vials are then immediately at hand, but the alternative is a possibility that has been used successfully in many locations.

The person preparing the vials should ideally be familiar with the patients, as is the regular allergy care giver. The same person may perform both tasks at different times, or another person, possibly a part-time employee, may prepare the vials. This affords the opportunity for another person to become familiar with allergy protocol and the treatment methods in use, avoiding a major hiatus should the regular allergy care giver be ill or absent. This will be discussed again later in the chapter under selection of personnel. It is not, however, practical for both persons to be occupying the main allergy section at the same time. This produces even more confusion than calling on the allergy care giver for other needs.

Furniture

The furniture needed for the allergy section is limited and simple. A standard secretary's desk with a typewriter return is excellent for both testing and

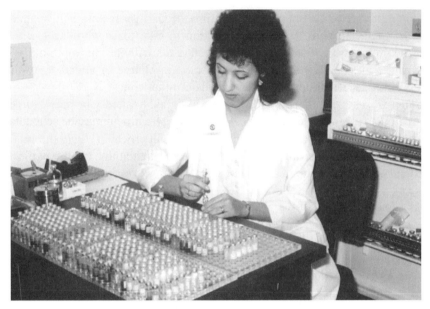

FIGURE 4–2. Sufficient counter space to allow mixing and access to vials is necessary in the plan of an the allergy office.

treatment. A standard secretary's chair, without arms, is ideal for the person testing and treating. It is easier on both patient and allergy provider if the patient is positioned a little above the standard chair level, although this is not absolutely necessary. A bar stool provides a convenient elevation if the patient is to be present for an extended time, as in skin testing. A couple of chairs for family members should be provided. In addition to a sink and refrigerator, plus sufficient counter space for work (Fig. 4–2), the only other item needed is specific allergy material.

The above has been itemized separately, as this may be arranged through general channels; the allergy space can be selected by the physician and the furniture purchased through any civilian source. The rest of the material needed may be obtained through various allergy supply houses.

At this point, it should be mentioned that the description of space and needed furniture applies to the office that does not plan to perform in vitro allergy testing. Under present circumstances, this is the most practical arrangement. In-office laboratories for in vitro testing became very popular in the 1980s, when costs had dropped to a practical level and a certain prestige accrued to performing everything on an on-site basis. Unfortunately, during the early 1990s costs escalated, and third-party payers frequently balked at paying for in vitro testing, although studies confirmed its cost-effectiveness. The final blow for in-office laboratories came in 1988, when they were placed under strict governmental regulation according to the Clinical Laboratory Improvement Act (also known as *CLIA 1988*). As a result of these factors, by the 1990s this type of testing became impractical in the small office. However, times and conditions change. It is quite possible that governmental regulations will be relaxed to a degree, or that increased refinement of technologies may bring back the practicality of the office in vitro laboratory again. For the present, however, it is far more practical to have the patient's blood sent out to a reference laboratory. Results are controlled, and the turnaround time is close to what could be achieved in the private office. The physician needs to understand the principles and mechanism of in vitro testing to assess and apply results, but it is more practical to leave the actual performance to the reference laboratory, which is better equipped to assume the necessary controls. The office must still check the results against the patient, but it need not cope with all the problems.

Allergy Equipment

Although both may be obtained from the same source, for convenience the special equipment needed for allergy testing and treatment and the actual allergenic extracts are discussed separately.

The basic equipment needs are simple: glass vials, racks to hold the vials, syringes, and bottles of diluent to be used in preparing the vials. These are considered one by one, and suggestions are made regarding purchasing. Although other formats are available, skin endpoint titration (SET), which is used by most otolaryngologists as well as many nonotolaryngologists, is the one presented here. It would be impossible to present all possible testing and treatment formats, and SET has a proven safety and convenience record extending over 35 years. An additional reason for selecting this format for discussion is that the group preferring it rarely wishes to convert the entire practice to allergy, and therefore tends to utilize the most reproducible and least subjective method available, producing the fastest results.

Glass Vials

For SET, testing vials are purchased as 5-mL vials with aluminum-protected rubber stoppers containing 4 mL of buffered saline diluent. This saves on-site measuring and time. In the early stages of practice, or if the number of allergy patients is limited, these vials, when properly prepared, may be used for both testing and preparation of individual patient treatment. The details of preparation are presented in the sections dealing with inhalant testing and immunotherapy in Chapters 6 and 9. The number of vials required initially can be computed when the number of allergens that will be on the testing board is known. This is discussed in the section on antigen selection later in this chapter. Six of these vials containing diluent are needed for each antigen. These have to be remade every 6 weeks. Simple multiplication and a cost evaluation based on quantity purchase should provide the necessary information. These vials provide the initial testing board, and can be used to make the patient treatment vials in the initial stages of practice. The preparation of a separate treatment board can be considered when the practice outstrips this format.

Empty glass vials are needed for the preparation of extracts for patient treatment. Most of these vials will also be of the 5-mL size, but when a large number of antigens are needed, a few situations may require a 10-mL vial. A few of these should be on hand. In the early stages of treatment, during build-up immunotherapy, the patient should receive all injections in the office whenever possible, as is discussed in more detail in Chapter 9. In the early phases of treatment, this approach allows for better safety and a better picture of the patient's progress. Later on, when maintenance dose levels are reached (and under special circumstances), the patient will probably take injections at home, or in another physician's office. When this time arrives, it is advisable to make unit doses for the patient using 1-mL vials and at least partly filling them with diluent. At that time, 1-mL vials will obviously be needed, but from the start of allergy practice to this point will usually be a matter of several weeks or a few months. It may be advisable to purchase some 1-mL vials immediately, but the quantity need not be large.

Racks for Vials

Containers for the vials containing the diluted antigens are an immediate necessity. With an SET format, vial racks will contain six progressive dilutions, so that the racks must be at least six rows deep and have sufficient numbers of rows to accommodate each antigen to be tested (and extras for future use). Five-milliliter vials are supplied in most cases in a thin plastic rack, which may be used in an emergency but will not prove adequate during any long-term use for the testing board. They may, however, be used to store treatment vials (Fig. 4–3).

Many physicians have Formica racks made for the office when the allergy section is designed. This arrangement is very attractive, and blends in with the space. The disadvantage is that these racks cannot reasonably be refrigerated,

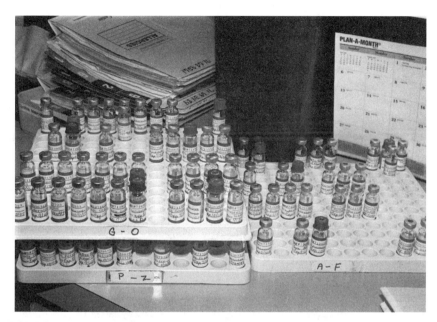

FIGURE 4–3. The plastic trays used to ship empty or diluent-filled vials can also be used to store patient treatment vials if necessary. However, they are not sturdy enough to hold stock antigen dilutions for testing and for making treatment sets.

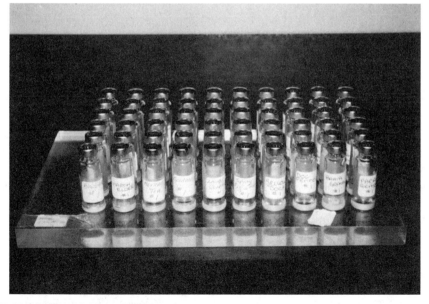

FIGURE 4–4. An acrylic rack serves well to hold the various dilutions of the antigens needed for skin testing and for making treatment sets.

which limits the duration of potency. Refrigeration may almost double the life of vials that are in constant use. However, this time extension is not recommended, as the degree of potency lost is not uniform. Nevertheless, in the early stages, when few patients are involved, refrigerating everything is of appreciable value. Probably the best vial racks are made of acrylic, 10 holes wide and at least six holes deep (Fig. 4–4). These may easily be refrigerated, and when the practice volume increases, they may be used to hold patient treatment vials, which always require refrigeration. Most allergy supply houses are able to provide such racks or direct the physician to a reputable source. Whenever injections are not being given or vials prepared, all vials and antigenic material should be refrigerated.

NURSE'S NOTE

Only the dilutions #1 through #6 of each antigen should be on the testing board. Concentrates are generally purchased in vials larger than can be accommodated on the board. However, even if small bottles of concentrate are being used, to avoid inadvertent administration of an injection or test from a bottle of concentrate, these are never kept on the board.

Only the material being used should be removed from the refrigerator. If testing is being done, only the testing board is removed. If injections are being given, only the patient vials are removed. This not only prevents inadvertently picking up the wrong vial, but preserves the potency of the antigenic material. When made without added glycerine, antigen mixes and dilutions lose significant potency after 6 weeks, and earlier if they are not kept refrigerated when not in use.

Syringes

Two types of syringe with attached needles (labeled *allergy syringes*) are available for use in the allergy office: testing syringes and injecting syringes. Both are available in 0.5-mL and 1.0-mL sizes. Although the two are interchangeable in practice, there are differences, and the person ordering the syringes will be faced with the decision of which, and how many of each, to order. The difference is in the bevel of the needle. A testing syringe has a shallow bevel, allowing the test injection to be made easily in the upper layers of the skin with minimal insertion. The injection syringe has a long bevel, which causes less pain during injection. Each has its benefits, but either may be used for the other purpose when necessary. A good compromise in the early stages is to order an equal number of each (by the case) and, when supplies run low, to use whichever is left in greater quantity until new supplies arrive. After the first few orders, a reasonable proportion should be evident.

Do not try to substitute tuberculin syringes for allergy syringes unless absolutely necessary! These syringes do not have needles as an integral part, and as a result roughly 0.05 mL of the injection material is left in the hub and barrel of the syringe. This makes testing difficult and treatment wasteful. (See Chapter 9.)

Diluents

Through the years, a variety of diluents for allergenic extracts have been utilized, but the current standard is buffered saline solution. Largely for informational purposes, a brief mention will be made of other diluents. Some are still in use, and the novice allergist should be able to compare them with the present standard and validate the position taken.

Normal Saline Solution

This is a diluent of the same consistency as normal body fluid. It is safe and predictable. It lacks any preservative, limiting its potency span. Extracts made with normal saline diluent should be used completely or replaced every 6 weeks. Because it does not contain a bacteriostatic agent, normal saline solution has been largely replaced by phenolated, buffered saline solution (described below).

Human Serum Albumin

For a time, there was much concern over the significance of "walling" of antigen when serial dilutions were mixed. This condition occurs when normal buffered saline solution is used as a diluent. Antigen tends to adhere to the glass of the vials, making successive dilutions less potent. In actuality, it was found in subsequent studies that the degree of walling was minimal, and that concerns about its effect were truly unfounded. In addition, the public became seriously concerned about the possibility of transmitting AIDS or the hepatitis B virus through the use of human serum. Again, in actuality the concern was unfounded; both viruses are highly heat-sensitive, and all human serum albumin products were heated far above virus survival level before being placed on the market. The product was more expensive than buffered saline solution, however, and this coupled with public concerns have limited its use.

Buffered Saline Solution

After years of experimentation, this product is again the standard. Buffered saline solution is normal saline solution to which two important additions have been made. Phenol, in a concentration of 0.04%, is bactericidal and viracidal. Sodium bicarbonate or a similar compound is added for pH adjustment. Buffered, phenolated saline solution is inexpensive and practical. It may be bought in bulk and kept for a long period, as designated by the expiration date on the bottles supplied.

Glycerine

Glycerine is not a diluent per se, but it is a preservative. A moderate supply, a few hundred milliliters of 50% glycerine, should be purchased. This is used in the preparation of treatment vials in the format described in Chapter 9.

In addition to the materials mentioned, the allergy office will require a large supply of cotton balls, alcohol, and/or alcohol wipes. An occasional patient will require a spot bandage to prevent bleeding from an injection site from staining clothing. With these supplies, and antigens selected and purchased appropriately, the physician has made the necessary physical preparations to begin adding allergy to the practice.

SELECTION OF PERSONNEL

Clinicians vary in their approach to allergy testing and care. Most otolaryngologists, most family physicians, and many pediatricians delegate much of the actual testing and treatment of allergy to ancillary personnel. This is a perfectly acceptable approach if the person involved in the testing and treatment is well trained and concerned. Decisions regarding rapid dose escalation and terminating therapy remain, of course, in the province of the clinician directing the treatment. However, day-to-day changes in therapy, answering questions, and communicating expected responses may often be better handled by the person scheduling the testing and actively administering the treatment. This person is in closer contact with the patient, observes the patient's attitude, hears the patient's comments, which often are not voiced to the doctor, and provides an invaluable liaison for adjusting therapy to achieve better results. Despite the changes in the public's view of medicine, in most cases the doctor still is viewed with a certain degree of awe, and the patient adjusts the history to whatever will provide the best personal image. This image may not be totally accurate, a situation that may impact on effective diagnosis and treatment. The allergy nurse or assistant, who performs testing and provides regular treatment, comes much more in personal contact with the patient, and is usually viewed more as a confidant than a provider. Such an attitude on the part of the patient allows this key team member to obtain an ongoing history, identify weaknesses in the treatment program, detect new exposures, and provide the treating physician with the material necessary to direct the treatment program accurately. It should go without saying that selection of this person or persons may be the most important single decision in preparing to provide good clinical allergy care.

Personality Type

Not every person with a medical background is ideal for the position of allergy care provider. Although nurses may make excellent members of the allergy team, some are not temperamentally suited for this type of practice, and conversely, a nursing background is not necessarily a prerequisite for becoming an excellent allergy assistant. Regardless of background and experience, such persons must have certain traits and interests if they are to provide good care and if they, the patient, and the treating physician are all to be pleased with the result. First, the person must desire ongoing patient contact. Not everyone has this wish. Many prefer to do a good job during their assigned time, and then go home and not be concerned with the job until the following day. These people are much better fitted to hospital environments, where ongoing patient care is not particularly expected. They may do an expert job, but on the following day the shift, patient load, and area may be entirely different. Good allergy care givers are frustrated by not knowing the outcome of the treatment given to each patient, and want to follow the case. They will have ample opportunity.

Second, the ideal person for this job wants a definite degree of autonomy. This is not to say that such a person should be expected to make overall treatment decisions. These fall under the treating physician's jurisdiction, and the allergy care provider should always be able to turn to the treating physician for advice and instruction. It is to be decried that even today, some physicians practicing allergy send their care providers to educational courses, and then rely on them for critical decisions. The physician directing treatment should always be better educated than the ancillary personnel, as the physician must be held responsible for errors in treatment direction. The person providing the day-to-day care, however, should be prepared to plan testing, adjust treatment, and work with the patient on a plan to achieve the best results. This provider should take pride in making strides in improving the patient's condition; in return, the majority of patients will credit their improvement primarily to the provider. If the directing physician is both secure and competent, the work of the care provider will be both acknowledged and appreciated. The treating physician will always be available for consultation and help and will check the patient at regular intervals so as not to lose control at any point, but will credit the provider with results obtained. This mutual recognition and respect provide optimal patient care.

The best allergy care provider is endlessly curious. This interest impacts the provider at two levels. First of all, the provider is the ongoing source of the individual patient history. The uncommunicative allergy provider will miss most, if not all, of the patient's changing problems. Chatting with the patient while giving therapy and observing the result, as well as discussing additional testing, provides an opportunity to identify new allergenic exposures and to perceive unrelated conditions easily confused with allergy. Once the patient is receiving allergy care, there is a strong tendency to identify any new problems as directly allergy-related. The physician does not see the patient on every visit, and may not be as well able to spot an unrelated situation as is the regular provider. Secondly, allergy is a regular feature in both the paramedical and lay press. The curious provider will spot frequent references in both of these, and bring them to the attention of the treating physician for discussion. Many of these references from the lay press will be of no importance, but some will stimulate the physician to further investigation, and it is not unusual to have such information provide a breakthrough in a difficult situation. In addition, this provision of advance warning will prepare physicians to field questions that may be directed to them by allergy patients on subsequent visits.

Training

The allergy care provider should be well trained and knowledgeable in the field of practical clinical allergy care. A significant degree of autonomy in daily performance requires this knowledge. Because the allergy care provider is an employee, it is not reasonable to expect this training and knowledge to be a prerequisite to employment. This is the ultimate indication for on-the-job training. There are situations in which previous experience with allergy care may be a benefit, but unfortunately they are few and far between. The range of specialties involved in treating allergy, and the years during which allergy has been treated with a limited knowledge of the underlying mechanisms involved, have led to a diversity of approaches to the field. Although today there is little disagreement regarding the principles involved, ancillary personnel trained in one approach or another without an extensive immunologic background may often have difficulty adjusting from one approach to another. It is usually to the benefit of the primary physician to arrange to have the allergy provider educated in the specific approach to testing and therapy that is to be employed in this particular practice. The treating physician has the ultimate responsibility in directing care, and therefore should be even more familiar with current knowledge and approaches to practical allergy care than the employee. Fortunately, this familiarity is not difficult to acquire. A variety of courses in basic approaches to allergy care are offered by nationally accredited organizations, most notably the American Academy of Otolaryngic Allergy (AAOA; see below). These courses should be attended by both the treating physician and the employed allergy care provider. Ideally, both should attend together, so that the primary care physician has the opportunity to clarify any material presented that may be too technical for the allergy care provider to understand. This interchange between employer and employee can prove of inestimable value in future treatment considerations. The approach described has been proved effective repeatedly by the authors during decades of practice. Not only does it provide an opportunity for cooperation between employer and employee, but it also affords a familiarity with the same material, allowing appropriate evaluation and application of such material by both members of the team.

The AAOA is the national organization most directly involved with introducing otolaryngologists to the clinical practice of allergy. This is the oldest allergy organization in the country. The AAOA is separate from, but works in close cooperation with, the American Academy of Otolaryngology-Head and Neck Surgery (AAO-HNS) and other related specialty societies. The AAOA presents regular courses, both basic and advanced, and advertises them through mailings to all otolaryngologists, as well as to other physicians who have expressed an interest. The AAOA also has available other teaching aids to supplement the scheduled courses. Full details may be obtained through the AAOA headquarters at 8455 Colesville Rd, Suite 745, Silver Spring, MD 20910-9998. The American Society of Otolaryngic Allergy Technicians (ASOAT), an arm of the AAOA, works to foster continued education and elevation of standards among ancillary personnel involved in delivering otolaryngic allergy care. In recent years, a survey of ASOAT membership showed it to be composed of 34% professional nurses, 24% certified medical assistants, 14% persons with a college degree, and 28% with ''practical experience.'' More than half those surveyed had been in the field of otolaryngic allergy for 2 to 5 years, and 10% for more than 10 years.

Several universities also present teaching programs in allergy for otolaryngologists at varying intervals. These are usually advertised through direct mailings, and most are accredited for continuing medical education (CME). Further information on these courses is available from the sponsoring institutions. Most if not all such teaching programs are open not only to otolaryngologists but also to ancillary care personnel, as well as physicians in other medical fields. Family physicians especially are in frequent attendance.

Reference books, monographs, and comprehensive articles are unfortunately in somewhat short supply for the beginning clinical allergist. Indeed, this was the impetus for the present text. Books and monographs may serve as excellent supplementary sources of information, but they cannot be expected to substitute for experience. This should be supplemented by individualized teaching, such as at an approved course or at the hands of a mentor. The field of allergy is far too large to lend itself to ''cookbook'' approaches. The size of the field should not overwhelm the novice, however, or frighten the new allergy care provider. It is quite possible to diagnose allergy safely and effectively and care for a large percentage of allergic patients, so long as practitioners recognize and respect the limits of their capabilities. As in any field of medicine, more extensive knowledge comes with time, and some early failures may later be converted to successes. And, as in all of medicine, care and caution are necessary, especially in the early stages of the allergy practice. Experimental and unproven approaches are to be avoided, even though many of these have eventually proved effective through the years. When both physician and allergy care provider are well established and secure with basic material, consideration may be given to undertaking more advanced aspects of care.

Once the basic training has been completed through courses and reading material, a final step will greatly benefit the addition of allergy to the practice. Both the allergy care provider and (preferably) the physician should communicate with a practitioner who has been in practice for some time and arrange to visit the office. Most such practitioners, and especially those involved repeatedly with teaching courses, are quite amenable to having visitors. This visit gives the physician and care provider the opportunity to see allergy care in action. Office patients will usually range from new patients' just referred for care after an initial evaluation, to patients in later stages of care and those being evaluated for discontinuation of care. This spectrum cannot be adequately presented at a teaching course, as the necessary didactic material simply takes up too much of the course time. Most good courses, whether in allergy or any other facet of medicine new to the persons attending (and most courses will contain much material new to the persons attending, otherwise there would be no need to attend), strive to compress weeks or months of learning into a few days. Many people leave a course at its conclusion feeling that they have been overwhelmed by the volume of material presented. If they immediately begin to apply the very basics of the material they have been exposed to, however, they begin to remember other items temporarily forgotten but recalled as the need arises. Visiting a working allergy practice greatly facilitates this recollection process and allows the neophyte practitioner to put much of the material previously learned only didactically into practice.

An additional benefit of an office visit is the opportunity of seeing how a successful practitioner and allergy care provider have selected material appropriate to their individual practice from the extensive material presented at a course and adapted it to individual use. Every practice is different. The type of patient entering the allergy care program will be determined by the type of population living in the area. A large geriatric population will not have the same needs as a large pediatric population. Climate, local occupations, industry in the area, an urban versus an agricultural setting—all influence allergy care equipment and procedure needs in the same way that they influence the overall medical practice from which the allergy patients will be drawn. Courses and reference books of necessity must attempt to include information appropriate to all practitioners in all areas. Only a fraction of this will be pertinent to one specific practice. Analyzing specific needs in advance will provide a major saving in equipment and supply costs, and usually will make both physician and care provider more comfortable with starting the new aspect of the practice.

Job Description

The need for the allergy care provider to concentrate on one job only may present a problem in the early stages of the allergy practice, when there is not enough allergy business to keep the care provider fully occupied. This can be circumvented by limiting the time set aside for both allergy care and vial preparation. Rarely is allergy testing or care, at least in office practice, of an emergency nature. It can be made clear to patients through an office informational handout or by a sign in the office at what times allergy testing and treatment will be provided. This serves the dual purpose of controlling the allergy schedule and advertising to the patient population that allergy care is available. Once the allergy schedule is established and strictly adhered to, the allergy care provider may be free at other times to share in the general duties of the rest of the staff.

Once the allergy portion of the practice becomes active, another consideration will be necessary. As noted, providing allergy care is a specialized job, requiring advance training and on-the-job experience. It is to be hoped that the physician in charge will be significantly more knowledgeable about the field than the specific care provider, but the physician already has major time requirements in place. If the allergy care provider becomes ill, goes on vacation, or leaves the practice, the physician will be faced with a serious problem. A scheduled absence of a couple of weeks can be arranged, with injections prepared in advance, but an unexpected or prolonged loss of this specially trained person may seriously impact the practice.

There is really only one solution to this problem: Fully train a second allergy care provider. This may be another full-time member of the staff, or consideration may be given to a part-time employee. The expense of formal training must be borne, of course, by the physician, but the on-the-job portion may be provided by the already active allergy care provider. In most practices, it will not be long before this second person is active a good deal of the time, the primary person in vial making and giving treatment injections and filling in during absences. Of course, it is possible for both such care providers to be part-time employees, but having someone in the office full-time, answering questions on the phone and providing the continuity of care the allergy patient in particular has come to expect, is highly desirable. One of the benefits of an allergy practice is continuity of patient flow, as opposed to the fluctuations of the primarily surgically based practice. This benefit should be protected.

PAPER GOODS

Informational Literature

Time is an essential ingredient of allergy care. The condition is an ongoing one, and if good results are to be obtained, the patient must interact with both the directing physician and the specific allergy care giver. Questions come up repeatedly and must be answered. To accomplish this in a manner consistent with the demands of an otherwise busy practice, as much use as possible must be made of informational material that the patient may study at leisure. Several pamphlets are available through the offices of the AAO-HNS and the AAOA. These are inexpensive and provide the patient with something to take home, which is also a good advertisement for the practice. In addition, informational pamphlets are available through the U.S. Department of Health and Human Services, National Institutes of Health, Bethesda, MD 20205. These may be ordered through the Superintendent of Documents,

Government Printing Office, Washington, DC 20402. These provide good, noncontroversial information from a well-established source. Many books and monographs on allergy are available to the lay public. Most are good sources of information. A caveat must be expressed here, however. There are today a variety of approaches to allergy care, all of which are effective to varying degrees. Despite efforts to maintain an objective approach to the different formats, many publications tend to denigrate any approach except that practiced by the originator of the publication. This often results in a patient suddenly becoming upset and questioning the expertise of the practitioner. Many patients do not realize that this same diversity of opinion exists in many overlapping medical specialties, often resulting in a turf battle of greater or lesser severity. If a patient asks about a specific publication, it is a wise precaution for the practitioner to check the publication personally and to be prepared to counteract any adverse comments therein. Of course, this requires that the practitioner be knowledgeable and practicing well within reasonable, self-imposed limitations. It is regrettable, however, that the field of medicine should ever become involved in the type of vindictive attack frequently seen in print.

One additional printed source of information should be made available to the patient. This will save the largest number or questions and lost time. Any office practicing allergy will be wise to design a booklet describing exactly how allergy care is delivered in that specific office, what the patient may expect in the way of tests and treatment, and how payment is to be handled, and answering all the other questions almost every patient will ask about the logistics of care sooner or later. Part of this can be prepared in advance, and as the patient load increases, additions can be made. This material will prove invaluable as a teaching tool, a time saver, and a reference when patients fail to remember what they have been told. It is helpful to deliver the initial printed information within a folder that has pockets into which future material may be placed, so that the patient can easily find and refer to it.

Allergy Records

As in all areas of medicine, in allergy detailed record keeping is necessary. Allergy care is a specialty involving multiple brief visits, both for testing and for treatment. This, of course, means that multiple notations must be made on the patient's record. Fortunately, most of these will be brief. Because allergy care is an ongoing situation, involving a period of years if immunotherapy is elected, there is always a good chance that the patient will move out of the area, or for one reason or another will change allergists. (This will probably become more common if managed care continues to expand.) It is important, therefore, that allergy records be easily understood by any trained physician providing care. It has been an unfortunate experience that many such records prove completely incomprehensible to a different physician. Abbreviations well understood in the office may be meaningless to an outsider. This situation may easily impact the office itself if the usual allergy care provider is on vacation or ill, or leaves the practice.

With ever-increasing risks of litigation associated with medical care, it has been impressed repeatedly on physicians that all records should be easily comprehensible to anyone in need of reviewing them. This holds equally true for allergy records. Here, however, some specific problems may arise.

It has long been recognized that there are several schools of allergy with basically different attitudes. The groups particularly involved are the general allergists, with training based on the format of the American Board of Allergy, Asthma and Immunology, a conjoint board of internal medicine and pediatrics, and the otolaryngic allergists, with training based on the format of the AAOA. The latter organization is a subspecialty group recognized by the American Medical Association, with representation in its House of Delegates, and has long been the driving force in otolaryngic allergy activities. Actually, there is no real difference in beliefs between the two schools, only in the logistics of the therapeutic approach. The actual format is discussed in more detail in the chapters on testing for inhalant allergies and on immunotherapy (Chapters 6 and 9). It is necessary at this point, however, to recognize that the approaches differ and that therefore the documentation of testing and of treatment will differ depending on which format is being followed.

Because the authors of this book include two otolaryngic allergists and an otolaryngic allergy nurse, the approaches described here will of necessity be primarily those of the otolaryngologist. This specialty has dedicated itself to providing the training and material necessary for physicians of any background planning a limited allergy practice to perform this service in a competent manner. The concept of the regional specialist has long been dear to the heart of otolaryngology, and the inclusion of allergy care in the physician's armamentarium is no exception. The American Board of Otolaryngology requires that allergy be a part of the training program for residents in the specialty. Although "turf battles" between the two groups continue, unless radical restrictions are placed on allergy care by managed care programs, there will continue to be an ample number of patients to keep competent practitioners well occupied.

Allergy records, both for testing and treatment, should be easily understood by any other practitioner using the same format. Fortunately, basic skin testing forms and treatment record forms are usually available from allergy supply houses. The AAOA has spent well over a decade attempting to encourage all those receiving training under their auspices to use the same forms to facilitate this benefit. Appendix 3 includes an example of a typical allergy history and a skin endpoint titration (SET) form should the new practitioner find commercial forms unavailable or desire to modify such forms for individual use. These basic forms may be individualized on the computer to meet office needs. It is, of course, necessary to insert the individual allergens to be tested in the appropriate locations. Each region of the country will have different allergens.

It is especially important to document the exact contents of each treatment vial. This documentation may determine whether another physician taking over the care of an established patient will be willing to accept the stage of treatment the patient has reached and continue previously successful therapy, or will demand a complete retest and new escalation of treatment. If the physician insists on this second approach, there will be a considerable delay in bringing the patient to maintenance levels. Of course, if the patient is not doing well, new testing may be indicated in any case, regardless of who is providing the care.

Most testing forms include a section indicating the makeup of the initial treatment vial. As the dose is escalated to progressively stronger treatment vials, the contents of each must be fully documented. The source of the antigen (i.e., the laboratory supplying the extract) should also be documented; this is extremely important when records are transferred. The expiration date of the treatment vial should always be recorded. Keeping all this information as a part of the ongoing practice may save the patient extensive repetitions of previously successful immunotherapy, with no guarantee of an equally good result.

It would seem that if an initial immunotherapy course had been successful, a second would certainly be equally so, but this is not always the case. There is still much to be learned about the function of the immune system. When a patient is doing well, it is wise to make as few changes in therapy as possible. This is considered in more detail in Chapter 9, along with appropriate sources of antigen for a patient who is transferred and appropriate safety checks and controls.

SELECTION OF ANTIGEN FOR THERAPY

Once the physical necessities for providing allergy care and the personnel who will be utilizing them have been acquired, it is necessary to consider the specific antigens needed for treatment. Today, the number of antigens available from reputable supply houses is almost unlimited. The physician looking at a catalogue of antigens and supplies for the first time may experience a moment of panic: How is it possible to select appropriate antigens for the practice from so large a list? How many will actually be needed? This can be a daunting experience.

As an aside, it is precisely the great number of available antigens that resulted in the reluctance of third-party payers to provide coverage for allergy care for a large number of patients, especially in the early days of in vitro testing. In the past, some programs were developed in which any physician, regardless of training, could send blood to a reference laboratory for specific testing, and have an antigenic vaccine returned with instructions for administering immunotherapy. This approach is discussed in Chapter 6. There was a strong tendency for the laboratory to perform tests for an immense number of allergens, many not indicated, thus running up a huge bill that third-party payers would in turn reject. The package produced a generation of untrained physicians dubbed "venipuncture allergists," a group not accepted by any school of physicians dedicated to providing good allergy diagnosis and care. This approach seriously damaged the acceptance of in vitro testing as a cost-effective approach to allergy diagnosis, and left a damaged image for the basic procedure that still exists today to some degree, despite evidence that in vitro testing, properly performed, is in fact quite cost-effective.[1]

The "venipuncture allergists" received the greatest publicity in allergy care abuse, and because of this they have largely disappeared. However, it has not been uncommon for other allergists employing skin testing of some variety to augment deliberately the number of tests actually indicated for allergens needing to be investigated. The mere availability of an immense number of allergens does not indicate that such a number should be in the armamentarium of the clinician. All, or even a large percentage, are not needed to provide good diagnosis and care. A geographic, seasonal, and personal analysis by history will provide a good list of allergens that should be available to the practitioner, and determine how many should be used in the initial testing of any one patient.

Regional Allergens

Not all allergens are present in all locations in the country. It is actually rather rare to have more than 30 to 40 inhalant allergens of any significance in any one locality. The new practitioner may not find it necessary to have even this large a number immediately available, as more can easily be added when necessary. What is needed is a determination of the major allergens so that initial testing can be performed, allowing the physician to be prepared to offer treatment for the significant offenders in a timely manner. Acquiring this information requires a critical look at the area, specific exposures, and the individual patient.

For practical purposes in selecting appropriate allergens and evaluating the patient's history, allergens are divided into seasonal and perennial groups. Both need to be considered in selecting a supply of allergens for care, and in deciding which to test for in any one patient.

Seasonal Allergens

Seasonal allergens are those that produce the symptoms usually recognized by the lay public as allergy. These are represented primarily by pollens. Actually, pollens often do not constitute as serious a problem as other allergens, not because of any lack of severity of symptoms but because of the short duration of their presence in the air. The patient sensitive to only a specific group of pollens present during a single season may often be treated with a less definitive approach than immunotherapy with good results, if the patient so desires. The tendency of allergy, however, is to become worse when untreated. The usual pattern seen in a patient becoming allergic is an initial complaint of symptoms during a specific season, such as fall, and an expansion of symptoms as the years progress to occur also in the spring, then the summer, and finally all year round. Thus, seasonal symptoms deserve investigation if the patient is interested in a definitive approach to care.

Although it might seem more likely that a patient would elect a simple medical approach to allergic symptoms when time is limited, the fact is that most patients presenting in the physician's office for care are interested in immunotherapy. With the wide range of antiallergic drugs available over the counter today, most allergy sufferers have already availed themselves of the opportunity to try a number of these; they have either been satisfied, in which case they will not have made a doctor's appointment, or have been dissatisfied, in which case they are interested in a more definitive approach, specifically immunotherapy. The treating physician must therefore become acquainted with the pollen allergens in the area and the degree of importance of each. This is really not as daunting as it sounds.

Some allergy supply houses have available regional maps indicating the major allergenic offenders in each specific area of the country. These are of great value and should be available to the novice allergist from the start. Such maps have been developed from pollen counts in each specific area, either provided by a botanist employed by the allergy supply house or obtained from studies performed by local botanical gardens, universities, the Department of Agriculture, or private organizations. The best are those that deal with a small local area, as the overall region covered by some guides may be excessively large and subject to more variation. In the past, it has been possible at times to obtain pollen counts based on postal zip codes, the information being provided by allergy supply houses. The current availability of such information is limited. A local listing of pertinent aeroallergens may be obtained on request from Windsor Park Laboratories Inc, 190 West Englewood Ave, Teaneck, NJ 07666-3512. Other laboratories may supply a similar service from time to time, and it may be worth asking the supply house.

The American Academy of Allergy, Asthma and Immunology (AAAAI) makes available an annual pollen and spore report, showing pollen and mold spore data from their 80 counting stations. This is summarized in a series of graphs that show peak periods and highest total counts for each station for 10 pollens and 10 fungal spore types. For further information, the AAAAI may be reached at 414-272-6071.

The veritable "bible" of regional allergens is a text by Walter Lewis, which should be consulted by those interested in the most detailed picture of each region.[2] This is a valuable addition to the allergist's library. However, some of the allergenic pollens Dr. Lewis records are not available commercially, and therefore cannot be used in treatment. It is for this reason that the allergy supply houses' regional lists are a more practical source.

The best lists of regional allergens include a category noted as index allergens. These are the allergens whose extracts are in greatest demand, indicating a high degree of allergenic significance in the area. A list of such regional allergens appears in Appendix 2. The physician just starting an allergy practice might do well to begin by simply including the index pollen extracts in the treatment supply set, adding others as the need appears. If the index allergens are supplemented by allergens appearing repeatedly in local pollen counts, a good treatment base for pollens will have been established.

Blooming Seasons

No matter where one practices in the continental United States, certain categories of plant bloom at certain seasons. The actual start and termination of the season may be affected by the latitude, prevailing winds, rainfall, and a variety of other factors of local significance, but the overall sequence of pollination remains very similar in all locations. This sequence of blooming, both over the entire country and in the local area, represents one of the things the person taking both the initial and ongoing history from the patient must keep constantly in mind, as opposed to other factors that may be researched when needed. The patient's response to the blooming seasons of various categories of plant indicates whether the problem is a seasonal or a perennial one, which will affect both the testing to be performed and the treatment plan; if the problem appears to be seasonal, the response also indicates which category of plant should be tested. Nothing other than confusion is likely to be the result of testing plants that bloom in a season in which the patient is symptom-free. (In addition, such testing tends to indicate to any knowledgeable third-party payer that the testing physician is poorly informed, and payment for services may subject to question.)

The overall pattern of the blooming season in the continental United States is simple and clear. Trees bloom in the spring. The starting date may be affected by the local environmental factors mentioned above, but spring is the season for trees. Elms may actually start to pollinate in appropriate areas while snow is still on the ground, and they may pollinate again in the fall. The blooming season for trees may last from 6 to 12 weeks, depending on the area of the country. Rarely to trees continue to bloom into the summer months. However, exceptions to this rule exist (e.g., mountain cedar, which pollinates during the winter), and the allergy team must be aware of this possibility as it applies in their specific area.

Grass is the summer offender. As with trees, the actual start of the blooming season varies, and in some subtropical areas grass blooms all year, but even there the blooming season is concentrated in the summer. Grass is an offender of major importance, as it is a highly potent allergen easily capable of inducing anaphylaxis. Our knowledge of grass pollen as an allergen goes back to the earliest investigations into the nature of allergy. Charles Blackley in 1873[3] used grass pollen to demonstrate the parallel between skin reactivity and ''hay fever'' symptoms, and Leonard Noon in 1911[4] used grass pollen, an extract of timothy (known at the time as *Phleum*), to establish the original Noon unit of allergy, the first quantification procedure for allergic sensitivity.

The grass-blooming season, like the tree-blooming season, usually lasts about 6 to 12 weeks in most temperate regions. The later stages of blooming may well overlap the start of the weed season.

The fall is the weed-blooming season. This may start as early as July in some warm areas of the country, but usually occurs from mid-August to the first frost. Weeds are widely known for their allergenic effects. In much of the country, especially the northeast, ragweed is the key offender, so much so that ragweed is used as the index plant in the majority of allergy studies. Ragweed is far from the only offender, however. The range of weeds of allergenic significance is discussed below in more detail, and still more information can be obtained from examining regional and seasonal charts as presented in the appendix and provided by allergy supply houses.

Winter in most of the country shows little in bloom. Most people spend most of their time indoors, with the heat on. The primary winter offender, therefore, is likely to be dust. Dust is a mixture of many items, and cannot realistically be considered a seasonal allergen. Details of perennial allergens, including dust, are discussed in the section on perennial allergens later in this chapter.

Seasonal allergens are members of the group that has been the subject of the most extensive study. Pollens lend themselves to more objective examination than many other allergens. All inhalant allergy appears to be IgE-mediated, and as such the specific allergens in each pollen extract may be identified. The details of this procedure are not relevant to a clinical discussion, however. The clinician faces a large enough problem in selecting allergenic extracts pertinent to the practice. A brief presentation of the method used to determine IgE-mediated cross-reactivity appears at the end of the section on cross-reactivity, but this is for information only and is not essential to the clinical part of a practice.

Thommen's Postulates

Not all pollens present a significant allergenic problem. Actually, it is probable that the majority of pollens are not significantly allergenic. Aware of the difficulty in evaluating all pollens as possible offenders, Thommen, in conjunction with Coca and Walzer, in 1931 described a group of requirements to be satisfied for a pollen to be considered an allergenic offender. These requirements are known as *Thommen's postulates*:

1. The pollen must be wind-borne.
2. The pollen must be produced in large quantities.
3. The pollen must be buoyant enough to be carried by the wind for considerable distances, with a diameter between 15 and 58 μm.
4. The plant must be abundantly distributed, or habitually grown close to human habitation.
5. The pollen must be allergenic.

Patients tend to associate allergic symptoms with flowering plants that are easily recognized. Actually, most such plants produce pollen that is carried by insects, which is the reason for the visible flowers. Some pollens are quite visible, such as pine pollen, which coats driveways and cars during the pollination season. Such pollens are primarily carried by water, small animals, and birds. Rarely are they airborne. Patients usually need to be advised of the fact that the most visible sources of pollen are frequently the least allergenic.

Today, it is known that Thommen's postulates are not always accurate. In areas of high humidity where pollens cannot easily become airborne, plants producing copious amounts of pollen still may present a problem. The exact mechanism is not clear; the pollen may become attached to foodstuff and ingested, or be carried by birds and animals, but sensitivity on the part of the patient can be demonstrated. In addition, some flowering plants have developed an airborne contingent. Overall, however, Thommen's postulates are generally accurate for most of the country and provide a useful guide for developing a suspicion of offenders.

Cross-reactivity

A factor of significant importance may save the clinician even more time and supplies. It has already been mentioned that pollens, as well as all other allergenic entities, contain more than one allergen. Many plants causing inhalant allergenic activity contain a variety of allergens that are identical or very similar to those of other plants in the same family. Because sensitivity is based on the response to the specific allergen, it is not necessary or desirable to treat for a variety of pollens all containing the same allergen. This would result in overtreatment, and large local reactions. Treating adequately with the pollen extract containing the largest number of allergens to which the patient is sensitive should adequately control the problem in the great majority of cases.

Not all cross-reactivity is fully documented. Appendix 1 contains a fairly complete listing of major allergenic plants, including their approximate degree of cross-reactivity. The tables also contain a listing of foods derived from or related to these plants, which may be expected to cross-react with the plants themselves. When the plants are pollinating, ingestion of these foods may produce an enhanced reaction, often referred to as a ''concomitant food reaction.''

A simple means, usually reasonably reliable, for determining cross-reactivity between allergenic plants is to check the scientific name of the plant. If the first term in the name is the same in both plants (i.e., *Quercus*, or oak), the probability of fairly extensive cross-reactivity exists. This is not completely reliable, especially for trees. It is best to choose the most prevalent member of the family in the area and start with that allergen, adding others if the result does not appear satisfactory after a season of trial.

Grasses

Among plants, the most extensive degree of cross-reactivity is seen in grasses. This is of special importance because grass has a reputation of frequently causing anaphylactic attacks.

All grasses belong to the same overall family: Gramineae. From this family, subfamilies of importance are identified. From a practical allergenic viewpoint, there are three common allergenic subfamilies of grasses: Pooideae, Chloridoideae, and Panicoideae. Cross-reactivity within each subfamily is extensive enough to justify treatment with only a single grass in any family.

The Pooideae subfamily of grasses contains most of the common wild and cultivated grasses: brome, june, perennial rye, fescue, sweet vernal, orchard, and timothy. The grass containing the most allergens in the Pooideae subfamily is timothy. In an area in which this family of grasses is widely distributed, it would be appropriate to test and treat only with timothy, or alternatively with whatever grass in the same family is most widely distributed in the area. Treating with two grasses in the same family would not only be unnecessary, but might well be a major mistake, as it could easily result in overtreatment with the same shared allergens, increasing the possibility of an adverse reaction. This is an error that the authors have commonly encountered in reviewing problems in the practices of novice practitioners of allergy.

NURSE'S NOTE

Grass is the most potent antigen which the allergist will utilize, and grass overdose is the most common error of the novice. Not only should cross-reacting grasses not be included in the treatment mix, but it is necessary to realize that cereal grains (e.g., wheat) cross-react with grasses, as they are members of the Pooideae. Thus, the grass-allergic patient who repeatedly consumes cereal grains is ingesting what is called a "concomitant food," and this may lead to larger than expected reactions to injections containing grass.

The subfamily Chloridoideae is more prevalent in the subtropics. It includes Bermuda and grama grasses. Bermuda is the more representative, containing most of the significant allergens. There is strong cross-reactivity within the subfamily, but little cross-reactivity between the Pooideae and Chloridoideae subfamilies.

The Panicoideae subfamily includes Bahia grass, crabgrass, Johnson grass, and various others. Bahia is the only member of the family uniquely allergenic, and therefore requiring treatment without regard to cross-reactivity.

A practical use of grass cross-reactivity has been described for the Pooideae subfamily: treat with the grass in the subfamily containing the largest number of allergens, or if that grass is not prevalent in the area, the member of the subfamily most prevalent. The same consideration applies to the other grass families: select the member of the subfamily most prevalent in the area and test and treat with it only. This provides adequate coverage for the allergen without risking overdose treatment.

Weeds

Weeds are more of a problem. Here, the degree of cross-reactivity within a family is less. There are four important families of allergenic weeds: Compositeae, Chenopodiaceae, Amaranthaceae, and Plantaginaceae. Even within any family, cross-reactivity is often limited.

The Compositeae family contains a variety of tribes, several of which are allergenic.

The first tribe is Astereae, of which groundsel is the most significant member.

The second tribe is Heliantheae. Ragweed is the most significant member of the group, with some 10 or 12 different types. Fortunately, all cross-react well, and selecting the type most prevalent in the area and using it for treatment is normally quite adequate. There is some cross-reactivity between ragweed and other members of the tribe, such as elder, poverty weed, and cocklebur, but testing for these independently is wise.

The third tribe is Helenieae, which contains no significant allergens.

The fourth tribe is Anthemideae, containing dog fennel, wormwood, sage, and mugwort. The various wormwoods, sages, and mugworts will probably cross-react, but the degree to which this occurs has not been determined, and beyond this, cross-reactivity is limited. Those weeds prevalent in the area should be tested and treated individually.

The Chenopodiaceae family contains multiple members of the atriplex group, such as the various scales and saltbush, which will cross-react fairly well. The family also contains lamb's quarters, Mexican tea, Jerusalem oak, and Russian thistle, which will require independent testing and treatment when prevalent in the area.

The family Amaranthaceae contains a variety of allergenic plants, including water hemp, careless weed, and pigweed. These show limited cross-reactivity and should be treated separately when indicated.

The Plantaginaceae family includes plantain, as well as buckwheat, sorrel, dock, and other weeds.

The above information is presented a guide. It need not be memorized, and it would not be productive to do so. By using the pollen guides as a starting point, the major weeds in an area may be determined, and then the cross-reactivity described may be applied, reducing the total number under consideration. After this, a list of those antigens actually needed for treating the major weeds present may be determined. Remember, the information given is designed generically for the entire country. No one area will contain a prohibitive number of weeds that do not cross-react.

Trees

If cross-reactivity between various types of weeds appears limited, cross-reactivity between trees is truly minimal. This does not indicate that no cross-reactivity exists, but it is usually significant only within closely related subfamilies. In general, one type of oak will usually cross-react with other oaks, although even here the reaction is not complete. On the same basis, elms will all largely cross-react, as will birches and other closely related subfamilies. Beyond this, however, the cross-reactivity potential is problematic. With trees, taking the species name (i.e., *Quercus* for oak, *Juniperus* for juniper) and selecting the most prevalent member of the group present in the area is probably the most realistic approach. The testing and treatment board may be expanded later if indicated, without compromising the treatment already under way.

Seasonal Allergen Selection

Seasonal allergens for testing and treatment, then, are selected by reviewing the regional maps, checking the index allergens for the area, and ideally making some attempt to become familiar with the common allergenic plants present to which the patient is likely to be exposed. Even if the clinician has a very limited knowledge of botany, this need not be an obstacle. Nearly every town has some botanists. Most of them are only too glad to introduce the novice to the significant flora of the area. Armed with a list of potential offenders, the clinician can call a local college, junior college, department of agriculture, or other organization in the area and usually be provided with any additional information needed. Usually, the botanist will be able to inform the clinician in advance as to which plants are in the area in significant quantity and which are limited or absent. This will help reduce the total number of extracts needed for testing and treatment. Those present in significant quantities may then be identified. Bearing in mind the different blooming seasons, the clinician should be prepared to make three field trips (in the spring, summer, and fall) to observe firsthand which plants are common in the area. The clinician will need to know which regional plants have allergenic propensities, as most botanists do not possess this knowledge. Once familiar with the appearance and distribution of the allergenic plants in the area, the clinician will easily note major increases in their quantity and prepare for increased problems. In addition, a familiarity with the appearance of allergenic offenders greatly enhances the physician's credibility. When this preparation is followed, most testing and treatment boards will contain, initially at least, not more than 20 seasonal allergenic extracts. This will be adequate for a good start, and will provide appropriate treatment for probably 80% of patients.

Perennial Allergens

More patients are sensitive to perennial allergens than to seasonal allergens alone. This is not surprising, in view of the fact that the patient is exposed to these allergens during an extended period throughout the year. The perennial allergens of major importance are dust, the various molds, and epidermal allergens emanating from pets. Although these offenders are present throughout the year, they become concentrated during the months in which most people spend most of their time indoors. A generation ago, this produced a definite dust season during the winter months throughout most of the continental United States. This is no longer a dependable pattern. Air conditioning and indoor environmental control have become so much the standard over much of the country that the perennial allergens formerly seen at high levels during only one season may now be present at high levels throughout the year. In the warmer areas of the country, the dust season may actually be reversed, being strongest in the hot summer months, when air conditioning is in constant use and homes receive little, if any, outside ventilation.

Housedust

Because housedust is not only the major allergen producing perennial allergic rhinitis but is generally considered the "universal allergen" by the allergy community, it deserves special mention. By the "universal allergen" is meant that housedust is the most significant allergen to which the usual allergy sufferer is exposed. If the majority of allergists in the country were told that they would be allowed to test and treat with only one allergen, the majority would elect to use housedust. Despite this recognition of importance, the Food and Drug Administration has designated housedust as an inappropriate allergen, and has ordered it to be removed from the market. This is the result of an attempt on the part of the government to produce standardization in all allergenic extracts. All extracts approved for use should now have an identifiable allergenic makeup, which may be standardized in the future when extract standardization is the overall pattern. Unfortunately, housedust is an anachronism. It is not made up of a single allergen, but is composed of some 28 allergenic components, either confirmed or suspected, as reported by the National Institutes of Health.[5] For those interested in such an anomaly, it appears that the actual major allergenic component of housedust is a collection of lysine residues in the process of degradation, which for some reason act as a single antigen. This entity does not meet the criteria of an appropriate allergen extract as established by the FDA, and it therefore is scheduled for removal from the allergist's armamentarium. To date, this scheduled removal has not been activated, probably because of the universal protests emanating from all physicians who practice allergy in any form.

The ingredient of housedust that is most closely comparable with the overall extract is dust mite. The immunologic pattern of dust mite is very similar to that of housedust itself, but the potency is much less. This is not surprising, considering the fact that such common allergens as cotton linter; mold residues, scattered pollens, some almost universal epidermals, and a multitude of other common allergens making up the reported total of 28 have been removed from the overall allergenic source. The background of housedust allergy is an interesting study in itself, but not pertinent to this presentation unless the current regulations change. For the present, it is a reasonable recommendation that housedust vaccine be kept as a part of the allergy treatment package until and unless it is actually removed from the market. Unlike what occurs with some of the pollens, the use of housedust vaccine in conjunction with extracts of the approved ingredients of housedust does not appear to present a problem in the form of possible overdosage. This may be because the significance of each ingredient has never been determined, and therefore the amount of each present in an individual dose is not known. For whatever reason, treating with both an available extract of housedust per se and additional extracts of available known ingredients provides a better result than attempting to test and treat with the individual ingredients available independently.

Dust mite, the most significant single ingredient of housedust, also deserves individual consideration, especially as it appears to be the allergen due to replace housedust extract per se at some time in the future. Dust mite is not a single allergen. There are several species of dust mite, antigens for two of which (Dermataphagoides farinae and D. pteronyssinus) are easily available in the United States at present; antigens for additional types of dust mite will be available in the near future. Some allergens are shared among all varieties of mite, whereas others are not. If dust mite is to replace housedust as the "universal allergen," it will be advisable to test and treat with all mite extracts available. This will still not cover all the ingredients of housedust, but will provide the best substitute possible. If only one dust mite is to be utilized, D. farinae is probably the most appropriate choice.

Epidermals

The allergenic residue of household pets constitutes a major part of both housedust and other individually identified perennial allergens. When taking an allergenic history, the physician is strongly tempted to exclude epidermal allergens from testing when the family reports having no pets. When pressure to limit testing is applied by third-party payers, this exclusion may be necessary, but it is not desirable. With the widespread appreciation of pets, there are very few people who are not exposed to pet allergens. The fact that the patient as an individual does not own a pet does not eliminate the possibility of significant pet allergen exposure. The person with a cat or dog in the household carries the allergen on clothing and hair throughout the day. A sensitive patient in contact with the pet owner will contact the pet allergen in amounts sufficient to produce a reaction. The reports are legion of children sensitive to cat and seated next to a cat owner in school, spending much of the day fighting asthma. Visits to the home of a friend or relative frequently precipitate attacks, and the reason is not usually apparent until inquiry is made about the presence of a cat in the house.

Dog allergen is equally or more sensitizing than is cat. Dog antigen, however, is heavy and quickly sinks to the floor. In addition, dogs do not routinely climb over all the household furniture and draperies, being poorly physically equipped to do so. Dog allergen is therefore primarily a problem for the patient who owns a dog, or who plays on the floor in the home of a dog owner. Under these circumstances, the potency of the dog allergen becomes manifest. Whereas the cause of the reaction to unrecognized exposure to cat antigen in a person who does not own a cat may be somewhat obscure because of the remoteness of the contact, the reaction to dog antigen is usually quite apparent. As with most epidermals, once the source is recognized, avoidance is the best approach to therapy.

Cat and dog allergens are so universally contacted that eliminating testing for them after a negative history of exposure is obtained, or advising patients to avoid such contact, is almost an impossibility. Testing for cat and dog allergy in the patient with multiple sensitivities should be almost axiomatic. These allergens are potent, and when recognized should be viewed as major offenders. Avoidance is indicated to whatever degree is practical, but at the same time it should be recognized that complete avoidance is essentially impossible. A reasonable approach, therefore, may constitute immunotherapy for the offenders, avoidance when possible, and supplemental pharmacotherapy when needed.

Other epidermal offenders may be present on an individual basis. On the farm or ranch, horses, cattle, goats, and other animals may produce a specific problem. When exposure cannot be avoided, or treatment is on an intermittent basis with medications, immunotherapy will usually offer a significant degree of help. Many such problems localized to the farm or ranch, however, are the result of molds present in stalls, animal excrement, or feed. A mixed formulation called ''barn dust'' is no longer available, but discussion with the representative of an allergy supply house may result in the provision of an extract or extracts containing most of the significant allergens of this type, which should be an aid in therapy in selected circumstances.

It should be noted here that epidermals are highly potent allergens. Immunotherapy will usually provide a significant degree of help with the problem, but in many cases some degree of supplementation with medications will be necessary. This should not negate the benefits of immunotherapy, but rather serve to indicate that a single approach may not be adequate when the offender level of exposure is excessive.

NURSE'S NOTE

If a pet is already a member of the household, the family is more likely to get rid of the allergist than the pet. In this situation, it is best simply to work with the family to teach appropriate environmental control. However, there is often an opportunity to give advice on the acquisition of a new pet for an allergic child or adult.

The question of pets for allergic children is a common one. The answer may depend in part on demonstrated sensitivities, but even if no allergy currently exists, continued exposure to a potent antigen such as cat dander in a child with a genetic predisposition for atopy is not a desirable situation. In addition to the obvious avoidance of cats and dogs, the allergic individual would do well not to consider a pet mouse, rat, or gerbil. Pet birds may also be problematic. This is truly a difficult area, and a tank of fish to substitute for another type of pet is sometimes the best solution.

Mold

Based on today's knowledge, mold may be the major offender in the inhalant allergy group. Mold spores are present in the air year round, circulate from ground level to 7 miles up, and unlike allergenic pollen grains, which, as noted, usually range from 15 to 50 μm in diameter, may range from 2 to 200 μm. Many mold spores, being extremely light, travel on wind currents for many miles.

Selecting molds for the allergy testing and treatment supply presents some problems. Distribution maps are available from many antigen suppliers, but the regional prevalence of molds may fluctuate from time to time. A local mold survey, if one can be obtained, is the best guide to the prevalence and distribution of specific molds.

The allergenicity and cross-reactivity of molds is still questionable. The active allergen in molds is the sporehead, and molds do not sporulate well in culture. Allergenic extracts, therefore, must be made from the mold hyphae, in the hope that the same allergens are present in the hyphae as in the sporehead. Molds grow at very different rates at different times in culture, raising the question of the development of variations in the mold type. Most mold allergens are complex carbohydrates rather than the proteins usually seen in other inhalant allergens. These allergens react poorly on skin testing and often on in vitro testing, making reliable quantification difficult. In addition, mycologists have been inconsistent about mold nomenclature, sometimes changing the classification of a mold as new material is discovered. For the clinician, this means that attempting to select molds for testing on the basis of possible cross-reactivity is essentially impossible. In short, cross-reactivity among molds is not known at the present time. How, then, can the clinician select molds for testing and treatment, knowing that molds may represent the largest group of potential offenders year round?

First, the clinician must start with a strong suspicion of mold sensitivity. Perennial symptoms, aggravated in damp, cool weather and in low places, as discussed previously, indicate a probable mold sensitivity. Some molds are present nearly everywhere, and are known as "universal dominants." Among these are *Alternaria, Cladosporium, Helminthosporium, Aspergillus, Penicillium*, and *Pullularia*. Most allergy supply houses have available lists of molds indicating their predominance by region. It will be wise for the clinician to include several major molds, including these important ones and others as identified by the best available regional data, in the testing format. Most molds today may be tested by in vitro studies by reference laboratories. A caveat here is that mold is sometimes said to react less strongly on testing than do other antigens, and therefore if the symptoms indicate mold sensitivity, the clinician should consider treating with molds based on a level of sensitivity by either skin tests or in vitro studies that might be considered insignificant in pollens.

In an area not especially prone to mold growth, eight to 10 molds will usually be sufficient as a start. More molds may be added to the testing and treatment battery if it becomes evident that they are of local significance.

Adding Antigens to the Testing and Treatment Battery

The foregoing information may seem cumbersome at first, and if it were necessary to continue to use so much material, creating and maintaining a battery of allergens would become an impossible task. Fortunately, this is not necessary. To start, the major local pollens are identified by regional maps and pollen counts if available, and if a friendly colleague who has been practicing allergy for a time resides in the area, some further information should be available. A starting list of pollens may number anywhere from a dozen to possibly 20. More may be added later if necessary, but this will provide a good start. The number of perennial allergens initially required is limited. They should include housedust if available, dust mites, cat and dog, and the molds as noted above. These antigens should be adequate for basic allergy testing and treatment, although initial screening with a more limited number of antigens is generally the initial step in testing (as discussed in Chapter 6).

Adding new allergens will become necessary from time to time. Some considerations in determining these have already been discussed. Even with the original battery and necessary additions, the overall selection will not be unmanageable. Additional antigens may be identified in a variety of ways, none of which should involve unnecessary expenses or unusual effort on the part of the novice in allergy. One easy means of identifying needed allergens depends on the concerns of the patient. As has already been noted, most allergenic plants do not have easily visible pollen sources (i.e., no bright flowers or heavy pollens coating cars and driveways). This is not always the case, however. There are instances when such pollens are truly significant offenders. Whether this is the case or not, many patients will insist that they are well aware of the seasonal pollen offenders, based on their personal observation. In most cases, they will be wrong, but occasionally they will be correct. In either case, it is to the advantage of the treating physician to pay attention to the patient's concerns. If the patient is wrong, testing will confirm the physician's initial impression. If the patient is right, a new allergen will be added to the testing and treating battery, and a grateful patient will be the result.

A simple and safe approach, cost-effective for the physician, is to discuss with the patient the offenders that the patient considers important. If the patient is fairly well convinced of the importance of certain offenders, the physician should purchase the minimum amount of allergen extract available for the specific antigen and use it in testing the patient. The testing will usually cover the cost of the small amount of antigen purchased. If the test response is positive, the antigen should be included in the battery, at least for a time. The implication of positive responses would be that at least some patients in the area are sensitive to the allergen indicated. This allergen may then be added to the basic test battery. If, as is often the case, the testing board and treatment board are represented as a single board in the early stages of allergy care, an additional shortcut is practical. Every allergen is delivered with an expiration date. If the expiration date arrives before the dilutions of a questionable allergen on the testing and treatment board are used up, this antigen is probably not a major factor in the area, and more antigen extract should not be purchased (or if the physician feels it is necessary, it should be purchased in the smallest quantity possible). If the supply runs out before the expiration date, the indication is that the allergen being evaluated is in fact significant in the area and should be included in the basic testing and treatment battery. The cost of the purchased allergen has already essentially been absorbed by the initial testing, indicating no unwarranted cost to the physician. This is the most practical means of determining the necessity of adding new allergens to the basic battery, while supporting patients who have reasonable concerns about items that appear to them to be symptom triggers.

Quantity and Type of Antigen Extract Needed

After selection of the appropriate antigen extracts to be included in a basic testing and treatment set, it is time to select appropriate amounts and type of each for an initial purchase. There is no completely reliable guide to this, as various practitioners differ in their approach. The largest concern is that eventually more extract of the same antigen will be needed, and all batches are not identical, even when purchased from the same supplier. Thus, if possible, it is recommended that about a year's supply of antigen be ordered at a time.

Concentrates: Weight/Volume versus Standardized

There has been a gradual movement toward standardization of extracts as mandated by the government, but even when these extracts become available for all allergens, uniformity will be far from complete. Under the still prevailing weight/volume format, properly prepared extracts have been found to vary in antigenic activity by more than 2000%. This will be improved by standardization, but even standardized extracts may vary by as much as 400%. To date, only a very limited number of extracts are available in standardized form; these standardized extracts are replacing the older weight/volume extracts as they become available, resulting in weight/volume extracts gradually unavailable.

Although standardization is a commendable ideal, the way in which it has been pursued has caused more difficulty than improvement. There is no reliable conversion factor between antigens prepared by the traditional weight/volume measurements and antigens prepared by the new, standardized measurements. Therefore, patients under therapy with traditional weight/volume extracts who are undergoing antigen escalation or who have reached maintenance will find it necessary to either face an attempt at conversion of some sort, be retested, or possibly even begin treatment all over. None of these options is an ideal solution. This problem is discussed further in the section on immunotherapy, but it needs to be addressed briefly here because of the dilemma facing the novice allergist in purchasing antigen extracts.

No good answer exists. As new, standardized extracts become available, the older weight/volume extracts are being eliminated, so there will not be a choice. Whatever is available must be selected. Many established allergists have stockpiled weight/volume extracts for the benefit of patients already under care, but this will not be an option for the new allergist. The best recommendation that can be made at present is to purchase antigens in whatever form is available. Conversion figures, as accurate as possible, and other suggested methods of switching from weight/volume to standardized antigens are presented in the section on immunotherapy. When these are used in preparing a treatment vial, it will be necessary to perform an additional vial test, but it may be possible to avoid complete retesting and new build-up immunotherapy.

Concentrate Preservative

Essentially all otolaryngic allergists and many general allergists purchase all their allergenic concentrates in 50% glycerine. Glycerine is a preserver of potency, and extracts provided in this form will remain stable for years. The mandated expiration date is provided on each extract purchased and should be considered reliable, although actual studies have frequently confirmed full potency well beyond the reported expiration date. It is therefore certainly safe to assume that the concentrate provided in 50% glycerine is fully potent during the time described. It is possible to purchase extracts in saline solution alone, without the glycerine preservative. This has been recommended by some practitioners for patients sensitive to beef, and therefore presumably to glycerine. These patients are limited in number, and their degree of sensitivity will probably place them beyond the range of the neophyte allergist. If such patients seek care, referring them to a physician specializing in this sort of problem will be beneficial. Rarely is it possible for a physician incorporating allergy as a part of a more general practice to devote the time necessary to cope with the problems of these exceptionally sensitive patients.

Quantity of Extract Needed

This is the point at which various practitioners have established individual formats. Each approach has its good and bad aspects, and each approach has its adherents. All are based on the consideration that the ideal of allergy care is to treat the patient with exactly the extract that has been used in testing. Because allergy care is an ongoing procedure, such an approach is manifestly impossible. New batches of antigen must be obtained as the old are used up, and the new material must be used in therapy. How this transition from the earlier batch is to be integrated with the new batch affects the quantity of each extract purchased initially.

Practitioners are generally advised to purchase initially the amount of each allergen concentrate that they estimate will be used in the first year. This in itself is difficult when starting a practice. No one knows how well the addition of allergy to the practice will be received initially, and therefore how many patients will seek care and continue with immunotherapy. In addition, if all extracts expire at approximately the same time, it is theoretically advisable to recheck all endpoints when this occurs. This is further complicated by the fact that patients undergoing escalation therapy will be expected to have endpoint changes as escalation proceeds, although these should not affect the course of therapy. These changes will be discussed in more detail in the section or immunotherapy.

Other practitioners gradually introduce new antigen into the testing and treatment supply, replacing about a quarter of the supply every 3 months. This change is rarely abrupt enough to produce an adverse reaction unless the supplier or manufacturing procedure is changed. Any local reaction occurring at any time should initiate a controlled skin test. This will also be discussed at greater length in the section on immunotherapy. As a practical matter, after the allergy practice is well established, stock vials will be used up at varying rates, and new ones will constantly be purchased.

Most allergenic extracts are available in vials of 5, 10, 30, and 50 mL. The most common vial is the 30-mL size, which should last for most of the first year at least, although the expiration date will probably be about 2 years after the date of purchase. Amounts smaller than 30 mL may be purchased but usually will be used up in a short period, necessitating earlier blending of new and old extracts with an additional loss of time and labor. The expiration date of glycerinated extracts is a matter of about 3 years, leaving a reserve if the use is less than anticipated. After the first year, a much better picture of the amount of extract needed on an ongoing basis can be seen.

One unanticipated benefit of the allergy care format was produced by the ever increasing use of in vitro testing. The in vitro method basically violated the requirement that the antigens used in testing be identical to those used in treatment. With in vitro testing, this was impossible. Despite initial concerns about possible severe reactions when treating with an antigen produced elsewhere, it was soon found that when such safety procedures as vial tests were regularly performed, adverse reactions did not present a significant problem. In like fashion, blending new and old extracts has proved practical, as long as care is used in progression. This a subject, which frequently produces a large amount of misunderstanding, requires a detailed discussion, found in Chapter 9.

NURSE'S NOTE

For the beginner, it is extremely helpful if as many as possible of the allergenic concentrates being used are at the same strength. This is generally a 1:20 weight/volume concentration, or 30,000 allergy units or biologic allergy units per milliliter for standardized extracts. Although some antigens are sold at 1:10 or even 1:33 weight/volume concentrations, and it is possible to carry out dilutions so that the #1 dilution is always a 1:100 weight/volume concentration, to do so introduces an additional source of error and confusion for the neophyte allergist.

It is best to start with as many antigens as possible at the same dilution. If in the future it is desired to purchase antigens at other concentrations, it must be realized that diluting them will result in a variance from the general rule that concentrate contains 50% glycerine, and this will affect the stability of the board prepared from these sources.

For the initial purchaser, buying the strongest concentration available for each antigen, be it weight/volume or standardized extract, is often advised as a cost-saving measure. However, as noted above, this is not without drawbacks. A 30-mL vial of each antigen is a good initial investment. If the physician wishes to proceed with caution, a smaller vial of concentrate may be adequate, but if the practice enlarges rapidly, a new supply will soon be necessary. All should be purchased in 50% glycerine.

When this battery of allergenic extracts has been purchased and added to the equipment and personnel already discussed, the physician and members of the allergy team are prepared to embark on their sojourn into the delivery of allergy care.

REFERENCES

1. Nalebuff DJ, Fadal RG, Ali M. Determination of initial immunotherapy dose for ragweed hypersensitivity with the modified RAST test. Otolaryngol Head Neck Surg 1981;89: 271–274.
2. Lewis WH, Vinay P, Zenger VE. Airborne and Allergenic Pollens of North America. Baltimore, MD: Johns Hopkins University Press; 1983.
3. Blackley CH. Hay fever: its causes, treatment and effective prevention. Experimental Research. (2nd ed). London: Baillière, Tindall; 1880.
4. Noon L. Prophylactic inoculation against hay fever. Lancet 1911;1:1572–1573.
5. NIAID. Dust Allergy. Bethesda, MD: National Institutes of Health; Publication No. 83-490 (revised Nov. 1982).

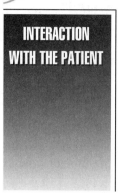

5

INTERACTION WITH THE PATIENT

INITIAL ENCOUNTER

The office is now prepared to receive allergy patients. (Of course, it has always received allergy patients, but definitive approaches to diagnosis and care have not previously been undertaken.) The allergy portion of the office has been completed, and the person who will be in charge of administering allergy tests and treatment, as well as rapidly becoming the allergy patient's sounding board, has been hired.

Certain changes in the office layout, subtle or otherwise, have been made to inform the patient that allergy care is now a part of the available treatment menu. It is certainly to be expected that both the directing physician and the allergy care giver have received appropriate training in allergy diagnosis and care. The patient now entering the office encounters a new aspect of care not previously known to be available here. A new algorithm is established.

Some offices, reacting to the needs of increased efficiency in today's medical market, have established a sort of limited triage format in screening new patients. When a practice offers multiple aspects of care, this approach may provide a saving in time and an avoidance of delay for both patient and physician. When the office uses this approach, the patient is initially seen by a physician's assistant, a nurse, or some other paramedical person, who makes an initial evaluation of the nature of the problem and channels the patient along appropriate lines. This is especially effective when a group practice is involved in which not all members of the group are equally qualified and interested in all aspects of the field. This approach may escalate in the future, but at present a majority of practitioners feel that the physician is the best-qualified member of the group to make an initial decision regarding both the nature of the patient's condition and the best approach to care, and therefore should serve as the first professional contact with the patient other than the office receptionist or the physician's personal assistant. The directing physician, then, should be aware of the signs of allergy, and be prepared to factor this knowledge into diagnostic considerations and eventually plans for therapy. It is even more beneficial, to both the practice and the patients, if other members of the office staff are also alert to the indications of allergy. Some signs and symptoms of allergy may be observed even before the physician sees the patient.

Because many patients with allergy will not arrive at the office with this as their primary complaint, it is advantageous for most or all of the office staff to have some ability to recognize the allergic patient when first seen, even before a formal visit has been established. Because all the office personnel will eventually encounter and be forced to deal with the allergy patient, it should be beneficial for all to recognize allergy, as this will aid them in understanding the various complaints that will appear over time. The allergy patient may be expected to have ongoing problems, and will usually be a frequent visitor. Identifying the allergic patient on first encounter, and frequently on first observation, adds to the staff's recognition of the prevalence of allergy and often provides a feeling of personal knowledge and unique ability. In short, most staff members enjoy this silent exercise in diagnosis. Once the presence of allergy has been recognized, and the decision regarding how the condition is to be treated made, the patient will usually be turned over to a special member of the staff with specific instructions on how to proceed.

RECOGNIZING THE ALLERGIC PATIENT

An overall look at findings that strongly suggest allergy should help alert the person making initial contact with the patient, the member of the medical or paramedical staff observing the patient for the first time, and the person taking the initial history and performing the basic physical examination that there is a strong possibility of an allergic element being present. Because the ears, nose, and throat are the portals of entry for all allergens, and because four of the five senses are based predominantly in the ear, nose, and throat area, a major relationship would be expected and does in fact exist. Conditions that offend the senses drive the patient to the physician, often more rapidly than more dangerous conditions. This probably contributes to the frequency of physician visits for conditions caused by allergy.

PHYSICAL SIGNS OF ALLERGY

When the patient with allergy is first observed, certain physical signs are usually evident. This holds true especially for inhalant allergy, but also for food hypersensitivity. As noted, there is a considerable overlap between the two, and patients with inhalant allergy are more prone to food allergy than are basically nonallergic patients. At this point, it is not important that the cause of the allergy even be considered. The fact that the patient is allergic

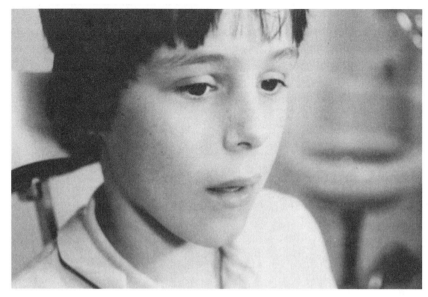

FIGURE 5–1. "Adenoid" facies: short chin, low malar peaks, open mouth, sad expression. (From King HC. An Otolaryngologist's Guide to Allergy. New York: Thieme Medical Publishers; 1990:61.)

should be recognized, and in many cases this can even be seen or suspected when the patient is in the waiting room. The staff member first seeing the patient, and those involved in performing the initial clinical evaluation should observe the patient for the following indications of allergy:

Facial Configuration

The look long known as *adenoid facies* may be equally as indicative of allergy (Fig. 5–1). The cheekbones tend to be less prominent, the nasal bridge is somewhat low, and the mouth tends to be slightly open. The mandible is frequently underdeveloped and the chin recessive. This is a developmental result of any condition that produces chronic nasal congestion and is not diagnostic of allergy, but it should raise an element of suspicion, especially if combined with other, more specific findings. This facial appearance alone is rather subtle and prone to be modified by genetic differences, but the person with this facial format, and a somewhat sad expression, may well be allergic.

Activity

The allergy patient is restless. In most cases, allergy of any type produces a constant annoyance. The allergic patient itches. In a child, the condition may be quite obvious, with the child squirming, twisting in the chair, and often moving about the room. This heightened activity is at odds with the rather sorrowful facial expression. In the adult, the condition may be less marked but will usually be present in some form if watched for. This heightened activity is less obvious than the typical gestures of the allergic patient, but it may supplement other findings.

Gestures

Certain gestures are almost diagnostic of allergy. The most classic is the "allergic salute" (Fig. 5–2). This is most obvious in children. The allergic nose itches and is also congested. Placing the palm flat on the face and pushing upward lifts the flexible nasal tip off the congested turbinates, allowing a brief breath of air to enter the nasal cavity. At the same time, the itch is scratched to some degree. This gesture may be repeated several times in a period of a few minutes. If the allergic salute is kept up for 2 years or more, the supratip crease in the nose, a typical sign of allergy, will develop. These findings are described below in the section on facial stigmata, and when well established may be present throughout life.

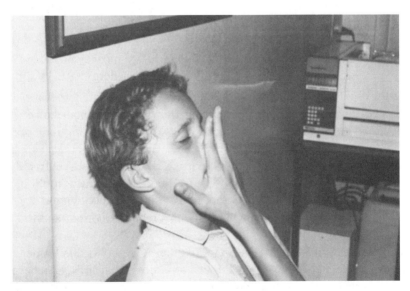

FIGURE 5–2. Allergic salute: the gesture both rubs the itching nose and lifts the nasal tip enough to allow a momentary breath of air to pass above the congested turbinates. (From King HC. An Otolaryngologist's Guide to Allergy. New York: Thieme Medical Publishers; 1990:58.)

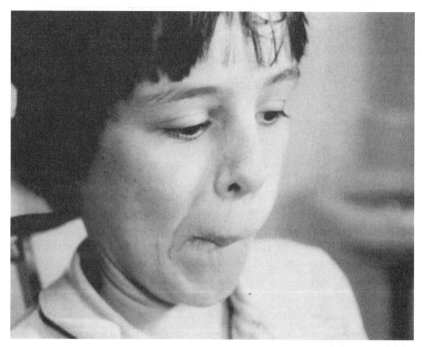

FIGURE 5–3. Allergic grimace: twisting the face replaces the allergic salute. (From King HC. An Otolaryngologist's Guide to Allergy. New York: Thieme Medical Publishers; 1990:60.)

As the child ages, social pressures make the allergic salute less than acceptable. The physical sensations producing the salute continue, however. In most cases, the salute will be replaced by grimacing; twisting the upper lip and midface to move the nasal tip (Fig. 5–3). This may also be unacceptable, inspiring the impression that the patient is "making faces," but is almost unavoidable. It is interesting to observe patients in a waiting room quietly and note the number of adults surreptitiously grimacing to wiggle the nasal tip. This has been referred to as the "bunny rabbit" motion, and the term is singularly appropriate.

One final activity that may need more quiet to be noticed is "clucking." Even in a moderately noisy room, this can sometimes be heard, and it becomes quite obvious in quite surroundings. The allergic palate itches, and the patient soothes the itch by rubbing the tongue over the area. This action produces a pronounced "cluck," which may vary in volume depending on the age of the patient. It is an action that is often especially annoying to a parent.

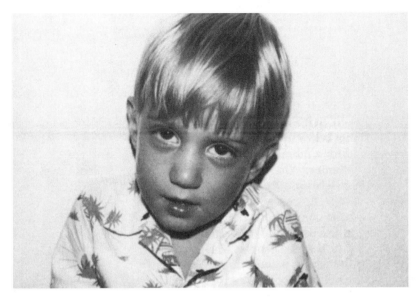

FIGURE 5–4. Allergic shiners: dark discoloration of the orbit resulting from venous stasis due to chronic nasal congestion. (From King HC. An Otolaryngologist's Guide to Allergy. New York: Thieme Medical Publishers; 1990:57.)

Facial Stigmata

Although the above gestures may be easily seen by an alert observer who has a good view of the office waiting room, in most cases the first good view of the patient will be obtained when the patient is in an examining room. At this point, the person making the initial clinical contact, be it the clinician, a nurse, physician's assistant, or other, has the opportunity to see the patient at fairly close hand. Certain facial appearances typical of the allergic patient immediately stand out.

Allergic Shiners

Probably the most outstanding feature of the allergic patient's face is the presence of dark staining below the lower eyelids (Fig. 5–4). This may appear in the very young patient, even in the toddler, and continue to be present throughout life. If the allergy is untreated, the discoloration may become permanent.

Dennie-Morgan Lines

Dennie-Morgan lines, or Dennie's lines (Fig. 5–5), are crescentic creases in the skin of the lower eyelid. These, like the allergic shiners, appear very early in life, and the two are usually present together.

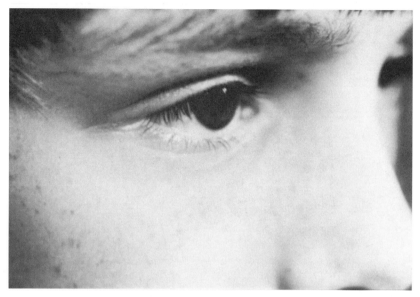

FIGURE 5–5. Dennie-Morgan lines: skin lines in the lower eyelid resulting from poor oxygenation of the unstriated muscle of Muller. This is the result of venous stasis in the orbit caused by chronic nasal congestion. Note also the long, irregular silky eyelashes typical of allergy. (From King HC. An Otolaryngologist's Guide to Allergy. New York: Thieme Medical Publishers; 1990:57.)

Both allergic shiners and Dennie's lines are the result of stagnation of venous blood in the orbital region. Venous drainage from the orbit begins in the marginal venous arcades and progresses through the angular veins, medial palpebral veins, inferior ophthalmic veins, and on into the sphenopalatine veins and the pterygoid plexus (Fig. 5–6). Congestion in the nose and paranasal sinuses results in pressure on the anterior complex of this group of veins, which run beneath the nasal and sinus mucosa. This in turn causes venous blood to back up in the orbit, resulting in darkening of the overlying tissue and eventually permanent staining of the skin caused by leakage of hemosiderin. In addition, the stagnating blood produces spasm in the unstriated muscle of Muller in the lower eyelid. This muscle is attached to the skin, and poor oxygenation and spasm result in the formation of creases in the skin that, like the discoloration, may well become permanent.

If the patient is a child and has been brought in by a parent, especially if a sibling is also present, it is interesting to observe the entire group. Allergy is a familial disease, and it is not unusual to see the same facial stigmata reflected in all members of the family (Fig. 5–7).

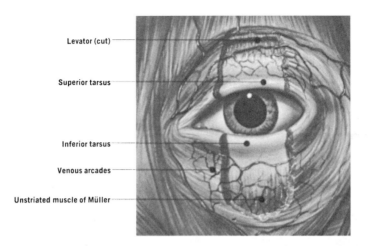

Levator (cut)

Superior tarsus

Inferior tarsus

Venous arcades

Unstriated muscle of Müller

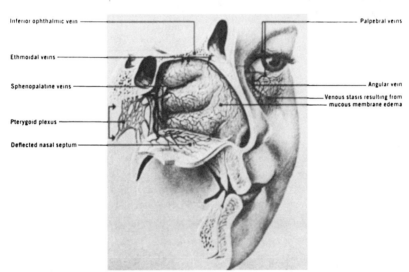

Inferior ophthalmic vein

Ethmoidal veins

Sphenopalatine veins

Pterygoid plexus

Deflected nasal septum

Palpebral veins

Angular vein

Venous stasis resulting from mucous membrane edema

FIGURE 5–6. Venous drainage of the orbit. The orbit is drained via venous arcades into the palpebral and angular veins, which in turn drain into the sphenopalatine plexus. Congestion in the nasal mucosa produces venous stasis in the orbit, resulting in allergic "shiners" and prolonged spasm of the unstriated muscle of Muller in the lower eyelid, producing Dennie-Morgan lines in the lower eyelid. (Courtesy of Upjohn Company, Kalamazoo, MI, Scopes Publications, "Stigmata of Inhalant Allergy.")

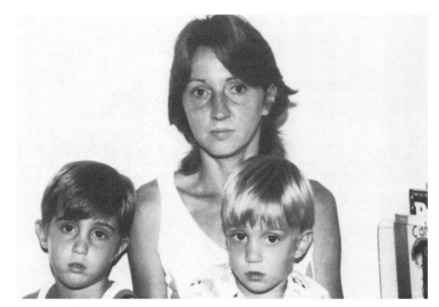

FIGURE 5–7. Familial allergy. A mother and two sons exhibiting similar allergic shiners and the typical facial signs of allergy. (From King HC. An Otolaryngologist's Guide to Allergy. New York: Thieme Medical Publishers; 1990:54.)

Supratip Crease

This requires a little closer observation than the previously mentioned findings, but is seen about as frequently. This does not appear as early in life as do the allergic shiners and Dennie's lines. It is represented by a clear crease in the skin of the nose between the mobile nasal tip and the more stable pyramid above (Fig. 5–8). The development of this crease requires about 2 years of repeated performance of the allergic salute at close intervals. When well established, the supratip crease may be extremely difficult to eradicate. Even during rhinoplasty, when access to the underside of the skin is available, extensive scoring of the skin may fail to eliminate the crease entirely. This crease is frequently quite annoying to teenagers, as it is often the nidus for unsightly pimples.

Crusting and Rawness in the Nostril Area

Excoriation in this area is primarily seen in children, and is by no means always present. When it does occur, however, it presents strong confirmation of an ongoing allergic condition. The allergic child has a chronically runny nose. This is a matter of degree. All children may be expected to have some degree of nasal drainage, more than is present in an adult. A normal adult nose will produce between 1 and 3 L of mucus in a day's time, and this amount may be greatly increased by allergy. A child is born with all the mucous glands the nose will ever have, confined in a considerably smaller structure than will be present later in life. More mucous drainage from the nose than will occur in adult life is quite normal, despite the mother's concern, and few children are well enough motivated or trained to concern themselves with the social implications of a mucus-laden nose. When the drainage is clear, it is not indicative of infection. However, when the drainage becomes markedly exaggerated and constant, as occurs in allergy, the area of the upper lip immediately below the nose and the nostril margins may become chronically irritated (Fig. 5–9). When present, this finding is strongly indicative of an ongoing allergic problem, even though allergic activity at the moment of examination may not be acute.

The above features of facial appearance may be seen by an alert observer before a more complete physical examination is performed. When present, they should provide a strong indication of allergy and place this diagnosis

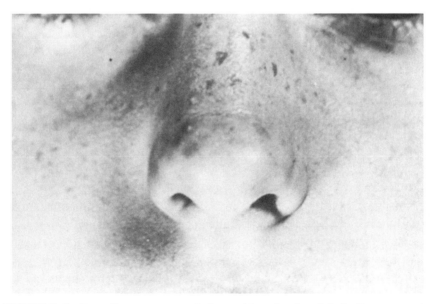

FIGURE 5–8. Supratip crease: repeated use of the allergic salute for 2 years or more may result in permanent creasing of the skin above the nasal tip. This may persist throughout life. (Courtesy of Upjohn Company, Kalamazoo, MI, Scopes Publications, "Stigmata of Inhalant Allergy.")

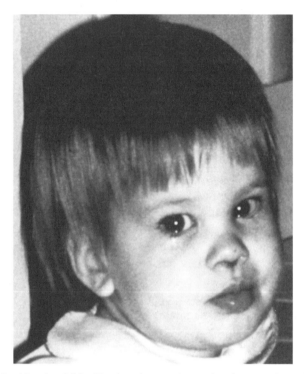

FIGURE 5–9. Allergic child with chronic nasal crusting from profuse rhinorrhea (in this case, caused by a food allergy to corn).

under consideration. The directing physician may now elect to perform a more detailed history and physical examination personally, or delegate this part of the procedure to the person designated as the regular allergy care giver.

INITIAL ALLERGIC HISTORY

The single most important aspect in allergy diagnosis, and in ongoing allergy care, is the allergic history. The physical examination is of importance in identifying the presence of allergy and in eliminating other conditions, such as structural defects, but it is the history that usually determines the overall condition, indicates the nature of the exposure, and leads to a suspicion of specific offenders. The restrictions placed by third-party payers on avoiding the extensive use of laboratory tests has made the history an even more important part of the diagnostic approach. The clinician practicing allergy is expected to have a broad understanding of the condition, and to use this knowledge to direct the studies necessary and not test at random.

It is an axiom of allergy that the history is never taken as a single entity or at a single sitting. The patient's memory is frequently undependable in regard to seasons and exposures, especially when an adequate amount of time has not been allowed to give these matters thought. Many patients have not considered allergy as a significant part of a presenting problem at the time of their initial visit, and they are too, surprised by the proposed diagnosis to recall details reliably. Often, a better background picture will be provided by family and associates than by the patient, as many patients who have been allergic for years consider this condition to be a normal state. Only when a complication occurs, or they are pressed by family or associates, do they seek medical care. A detailed background history cannot be expected at this point. The patient must be made aware of the type of symptoms and the pattern of onset and remission that will aid the physician in making a diagnosis, both of the basic nature of the disease and probable offenders. Because allergy is frequently not a dramatic condition, the events producing symptoms may not be at all obvious to patients until they have been made aware of the information necessary to provide a diagnosis, and have given considerable time and thought to the answers.

A large number of factors influence the allergic pattern, including such things as season, age, exposure, environment, and intercurrent disease. The more of these that can be identified, the better results may be expected from treatment. No matter how dedicated the person taking the history may be, it is impossible to obtain complete information covering all possibilities during a single session, especially with the time constraints necessary in the average office. Time is not normally allotted for an extensive and time-consuming history when the condition has not been identified. Nonetheless, certain aspects of history must be obtained and evaluated as early as possible to determine the direction further study and care should take.

No routine format can be presented for this evaluation, but certain approaches may serve as a guide to both the physician performing the initial evaluation and the designated allergy care giver, who will enlarge the history, and also indicate the steps to be followed in confirming the proposed diagnosis and instituting care. These two parts of the basic allergy history will not usually be taken at the same time. This division in history taking allows different approaches on the part of the directing physician and the ongoing care giver, which may be used to facilitate and streamline the overall evaluation.

History by the Physician

The first person to encounter the patient on a medical basis and to hear the patient's history is usually the treating physician. On occasion, because of the pressures of managed care to streamline practices, the first person encountering the patient may be a nurse or physician's assistant. However, when this is the case, the person selected for this important task should be highly competent and familiar with the technique of obtaining a history that will include consideration of allergy as a primary or contributory cause of the patient's symptoms.

Allergy should be considered on the basis of the initial complaint and initial physical observations, and the possibility should be weighed that this condition may be a major contributor to the complaint. The major limitation for this examiner is time. When the patient's initial visit is scheduled, it is not known that allergy will be the primary or at least a significant part of the complaint, and an insufficient amount of time may have been allotted for evaluation of the patient with so complex a problem. The patient must be accommodated if good care and a satisfactory ongoing relationship are going to be established, but at the same time an excessive amount of time cannot be spent with the allergy patient without delaying other patients unnecessarily. Adjusting to this dilemma is essential if the directing physician is to provide all aspects of care in an appropriate manner. As the physician (and other members of the allergy team) come to understand more about the disorder, less time is required to obtain essential information from patients with possible allergy.

It must be recognized when considering allergy that history is the most essential aspect of the initial evaluation. A detailed history is not necessary, however, to determine the direction needed to pursue an appropriate course of diagnosis and treatment. The physician involved in initial contact with the patient must determine certain critical factors indicating the presence of allergy and, in an overall way, the nature of the probable offenders. There are many possible routes to clarify this diagnosis, but one pattern of questions will usually provide the necessary information to direct the next step in diagnosis and treatment. Certain questions tend to go to the heart of the problem and allow the physician to feel relatively confident in the preliminary diagnosis. It should then be realistic to proceed with a more extensive diagnostic history and appropriate definitive tests.

Symptoms

The classic opening question "What brings you here?" is as good an initial approach as any. The patient will then normally present the primary complaint. This may have nothing to do with allergy, and if so may be treated on its own merits. If, however, the primary complaint suggests a good possibility of an underlying allergic condition, the physician may then explore this possibility with questions directed specifically to allergy. Taking this part of the history competently requires a broad knowledge of the problems that allergy can cause. Most of the more common ones have been enumerated in the preceding pages. Unfortunately, the complete list is almost endless and is complicated by the fact that other conditions may mimic allergy in much the same way that allergy mimics other conditions. Certain factors, however, tend to suggest allergy.

Onset

"When did the problem start?" Although the tendency to allergy is genetically determined, it is rare to see inhalant allergy appear in infancy. (Food hypersensitivity is a different situation, and will be discussed independently.) It is also rare to see true allergy appear in the geriatric patient as a new condition. Provided the environmental situation is stable, (i.e., the patient has not made a major geographic move or been exposed to new potential offenders, which will be discussed separately), inhalant allergy may begin to appear around the age of 2 or 3 and increase from that time to about the age of 30, when it usually peaks. The condition then tends to remain stable or decrease gradually into the 60s, at which time there is sometimes a small peak followed by a decline in sensitivity. Although many patients feel that such a situation has occurred, it is rare to have an elderly patient experience the onset of allergy after the usual retirement age. This is not impossible if the patient has coupled retirement with a major environmental change, but the possibility should be considered with caution. This situation would be an appropriate one for a limited inhalant allergy screen, largely to clarify the situation and satisfy the patient.

Fluctuation

"Is the condition constant, or does it change from time to time?" This can be a key indicator. If the condition is unchanged from season to season and from one location to another, it suggests perennial allergy, either mediated by mites, molds, or epidermals to which the patient is constantly exposed, or by foods that the patient eats regularly. As discussed in the various sections on foods, most people are habit eaters and consume the same foods day after day. The form may vary, but the basic food is the same. This may apply even during travel if the patient is able to select all the foods eaten. If, however, the symptoms change radically during travel, an investigation of the inhalant allergens in the various areas needs to be considered, and if these are not different from those at home, the food pattern deserves evaluation.

If a definite symptom change is seen from one season to another, the indication is strong that the patient has an inhalant allergy. Pollens have definite blooming seasons, as described in the section on selection of antigen for therapy in Chapter 4. For the patient in whom inhalant allergies are developing, it is not unusual to see symptoms appear in the early stages in only one or two seasons and then escalate during succeeding years until eventually they become a perennial problem. This pattern typifies an allergic pattern that usually responds well to immunotherapy.

Exposure

"Has anything changed in your environment?" This general question must usually be expanded on. However, by this point, time is becoming limited for an initial evaluation, so the patient must usually be prompted to bring forth significant changes without enumerating every possibility. Has the patient moved to this geographic area relatively recently? The move does not have to precede immediately the appearance of symptoms. It usually takes months or years for allergic symptoms to develop after the initial contact and continued exposure occur. Has there been a change of job or of workplace? Has the home been changed or redecorated? Have any new pets been brought into the home? Has the patient started any new medications or radical changes of diet? These last factors are often neglected, as both physician and patient are now thinking about environmental exposures.

Family History

"Does anyone in your family have allergies?" Allergy is a familial disease. It has already been noted that superficial allergic stigmata often appear in many family members. When inquiring about a family history of allergy, the physician should be sure to investigate the common euphemisms for allergy, such as catarrh, sinus, and bronchial conditions.

Previous Allergy Tests

"Have you ever been tested for allergy?" This question is the least likely to produce a positive answer, but if the patient has been tested and the form of testing is reliable, much may be learned. If the testing has been performed in the same geographic area in which the patient now resides and performed during adulthood, a totally negative or a strongly positive result of testing supports or makes less likely the presumptive diagnosis of allergy. Confirmatory tests are indicated, but the pattern of testing may be based to some degree on previous results with a considerable saving in time and procedure.

These questions and their answers will usually fill the time available during the initial visit and direct the ensuing history taking along the most productive lines. A more detailed history will be necessary, as is discussed below, but this will usually be taken after the complete physical examination for allergy has been accomplished, and it may not be always be taken by the directing physician.

FINDINGS ON PHYSICAL EXAMINATION

The previously noted items of facial appearance may be seen by any observer before a complete physical examination is performed. Such findings should alert the observer to the presence of allergy and indicate the potential benefit to be expected with appropriate treatment. Because of the constraints of managed care, with cost control a major concern, a good history and physical examination must replace or reduce the use of random, and at times excessive, laboratory testing. The main thrust of this section is the physical examination, after which a more complete history is needed to establish the relevance of the physical findings, avoid misinterpretation, and set the stage for appropriate treatment planning. This more specific and complete allergic history is discussed in the next section of the present at this point in the initial evaluation, a step-by-step progression through a complete ear, nose, and throat examination is required, with emphasis on findings that potentially indicate allergy.

Eyes

The eyes may show signs of allergy (e.g., edema of the conjunctivae, increased tearing, and vascularity) without nasal symptoms beyond the usual "hay fever" season. The presence of Dennie-Morgan lines in the eyelids of the allergic patient and the nature of allergic shiners have already been described. A typical finding on the allergic eye is long silky eyelashes of uneven length. This produces a very attractive eye appearance; however, the relationship to allergy should not be ignored (Fig. 5–10).

In addition to these findings, the eye itself frequently shows typical allergic stigmata. The conjunctivitis seen with hay fever is easily recognized. Tearing and itching are profuse, and the patient is miserable. Less easily identified

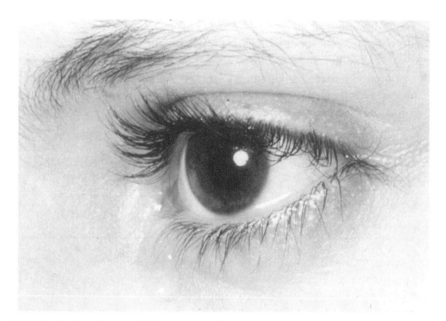

FIGURE 5–10. Allergic child, demonstrating frequent finding of long, silky eyelashes. (Courtesy of Upjohn Company, Kalamazoo, MI, Scopes Publications, Marks M, "Stigmata of Respiratory Allergies.")

is the edema that may affect the cornea, making wearing contact lenses difficult. This is often the result of sensitivity to airborne allergens, frequently the same as those causing hay fever, that is responsive to treatment. Questioning at this point often elicits a history of excess ocular itching that was not originally mentioned.

At times, exudates may be apparent beneath the eyelids or at the limbus. An area of marginal eczema involving the upper eyelid is a common finding in the allergic patient.

Ears

The ears are divided into three distinct parts, each representing a different organ system. Allergic manifestations for the most part are directed to a specific organ system, so it is not surprising that each part of the ear represents a different target organ and problems specific to that organ.

External Ear

The external ear canals in most allergic patients are quite normal. However, the external ear, being part of the skin, is a dark, warm area, often moist and easily colonized by either bacteria or fungi. These conditions, although not always easy to treat, may be expected to respond to the usual forms of antimicrobial therapy. In addition, however, the external ear is at times subject to a form of eczema that appears quite similar to the infections described (minus the presence of any pus) and is resistant to any form of antimicrobial therapy. Cultures routinely show no growth. Steroid creams of drops give only temporary relief, and the problem returns when the medications are stopped. This condition, relatively rare, may represent an allergic problem: an id reaction (from the term *dermatophytid*) to a fungal infection elsewhere in the body. These conditions are rarely mentioned in the literature, although they have been described since early in the century[1] and frequently respond well to appropriate allergy care. The common term for the problem is *T.O.E. reaction*, mnemonic for the skin fungi commonly invading the primary site: *Trichophyton*, Oidiomycetes, and *Epidermophyton*.

The treatment of T.O.E. hypersensitivity is a complex matter, not in wide use in the medical community and not appropriate for the novice allergist.[2] Bodily areas other than the ear, such as the inframammary and inguinal areas, are subject to the same condition, but the external ear canal is a common site.

Middle Ear

The middle ear is a branch of the respiratory system, with many of the same vulnerabilities as the nose, sinuses, and bronchial tree. In addition, the middle ear, connecting with the external world solely through the eustachian tube, is subject to obstruction from localized edema. The mucosa of the middle ear routinely absorbs air, producing a partial vacuum relieved by swallowing, which relaxes the eustachian tube musculature; it has been felt that middle ear effusions result purely from the developing vacuum when inflammation or edema produces congestion that obstructs the eustachian tube. Based on current studies, the mechanism described appears to be the cause of eustachian tube dysfunction in many circumstances.[3] It is known, however, that allergy may affect the middle ear mucosa directly, and that an effusion may result from a direct mucosal reaction in this area,[4] which may explain some of the instances of persistent drainage from a properly placed ear ventilation tube with negative microbial cultures. Effective treatment requires control of the underlying allergy; such treatment may also reduce the additional eustachian tube edema.

Concern for the possibility of occult middle ear disease should be heightened in the allergic patient, and attention should be paid to the possibility of nonpurulent middle ear fluid, even to the extent of performing tympanometry if any question of fluid exists. An effusion in the middle ear of an allergic patient may be yellow, but it may also be clear and practically invisible through the eardrum. In the child, otitis media with effusion (OME) may easily be overlooked. Erythema and bulging of the eardrum indicate infection, of course, and must be treated as such. This does not, however, eliminate the possibility of an underlying allergy strongly contributing to the problem. Repeated episodes of otitis media in a child, beginning before the age of 1 year, strongly suggest allergy and are often indicative of a sensitivity to foods.

Inner Ear

It has now come to be accepted that allergy (both inhalant allergy and food sensitivities) may contribute significantly to inner ear dysfunction, especially to the tetrad of ear fullness, hearing loss, tinnitus, and dysequilibrium that constitute Menière's syndrome.[5] Furthermore, appropriate allergic management may materially benefit these patients. As a general rule, this improvement (if it is to occur) will be evident within the first 3 months of treatment, although in some instances a longer time is necessary before benefits become evident.[6] Failure to recognize this concordance of allergy and inner ear disease may result in inadequate results of medical management and the performance of unnecessary surgery.

Nose

The external nasal stigmata of allergy have already been described. Internally, the nasal mucosa of the normal nose should have the appearance, both in color and moistness, of a freshly cut watermelon. Deviation from this appearance toward a pale, bluish tone with associated swelling of the mucosa and narrowing of the airway is typical of inhalant allergy. This will hold true in most cases; however, a predominantly dust-mediated sensitivity may produce a reddened, inflamed appearance strongly resembling that of a viral respiratory infection. In such a case, secretions are scant and yellowish, frequently associated with a small degree of crusting.

It is worthy to note here that a common misconception exists in the public mind that colored mucus always indicates infection. Copious yellow or white mucus does indeed usually indicate infection; however, any nasal mucus that dries or becomes crusty will gradually acquire a yellowish and eventually a greenish brown cast. Some of this color change may be the result of colonization by saprophytic bacteria, but some is a normal result of desiccation of mucus. Other indications of infection, such as fever and pharyngeal inflammation, should be sought before a diagnosis of infection is made based only on the appearance of nasal mucus.

Nasopharynx

The nasopharynx presents no findings unique to allergy. Lymphoid tissue is usually increased in allergy, and the adenoid mass may be larger than usual, but this is so variable that a size variation cannot be considered useful in diagnosing allergy.

Oropharynx

In this area, findings again are nonspecific but may be suggestive of allergy. Especially in food allergy, patchy, denuded areas may develop on the tongue that are migratory in nature ("geographic tongue"). At times, the entire tongue may become denuded and red. The condition is rarely associated with any great discomfort, but the tongue's appearance frequently concerns the patient. Such changes in the tongue's appearance are not unique to allergy, but allergy may cause the condition. The tonsils are frequently enlarged in the allergic patient, but as with the adenoids, the condition is so variable in the normal population that it cannot be considered a specific finding in patients with allergy. The posterior pharynx is prone to the development of enlarged lymphoid islands, which are much more noticeable if the tonsils have been removed. Prominent vascularity of this area is also a finding suggestive of allergy. The uvula is composed of extremely soft tissue and is prone to edema when exposed to any allergic insult. The most common allergic offender in this regard is a food, but the edema may also occur with inhalant exposure. At times, this edema may become massive and even dangerous. This situation is covered in greater detail in Chapter 12, Allergic Emergencies, and Chapter 14, Food Allergy.

Mouth

It has already been noted that the mouth of an allergic patient is frequently kept slightly open. This condition is more often noted in children than in adults. Mouth breathing and an open-mouthed countenance in an adult are often equated in the public mind with a low mentality, an unjustified assumption but one that pressures many adults consciously to avoid mouth breathing, even when afflicted with nasal congestion. Nevertheless, careful observation frequently reveals clandestine mouth breathing in the most sophisticated adult. Sometimes, slightly raw areas are visible at the mouth commisures from the constant moisture in the area.

The necessity of keeping the mouth open for comfortable breathing produces developmental changes in the teeth and dental arches of children. The growth of the mandible is usually limited, creating a receding chin. The palate frequently develops with a high central arch and a narrowed premaxilla, producing protruding front teeth and an overbite (Fig. 5–11). This results from a condition similar to, and in many cases actually an extension of, the condition in the orbits that produces allergic shiners; the veins draining the dental arches anastamose freely with the veins draining the nasal cavities and are also easily compromised in allergy (Fig. 5–12). When this situation, accompanied by the typical alteration in buccinator muscle activity and accompanying tongue thrust (which may also be partially caused by allergic irritation of the palate) is present for years, marked changes in the configuration of the mouth occur that are readily evident. The same open mouth and poor venous drainage alter the acidity of the saliva, resulting in more frequent dental caries in allergic children.

Larynx

In most cases, the larynx of the allergic patient is normal. Under some circumstances, the vocal cords may become edematous, resulting in husky speech. When somewhat swollen vocal cords are observed in the absence of any visible inflammation, allergy should be suspected. Pooling of excessive secretions in the hypopharynx may contribute to excessive throat clearing in allergic patients. As in the case of the uvula, massive, life-threatening edema of the larynx may occur, but this is usually diagnosed clinically well before a routine laryngeal examination is performed. This is discussed in Chapter 12, Allergic Emergencies.

Neck

The lymphocyte is the key cell of allergy, so it should not be surprising that lymphadenopathy may be a common finding in allergy. This reaction is not limited to the neck; it may occur elsewhere in the body or on a generalized basis. The neck is simply the first area to be encountered when the examiner is an otolaryngologist. Such findings may easily be caused by chronic infection or other disease, and unexplained lymphadenopathy deserves serious investigation. In the absence of other explanations, an allergic cause is a real possibility.

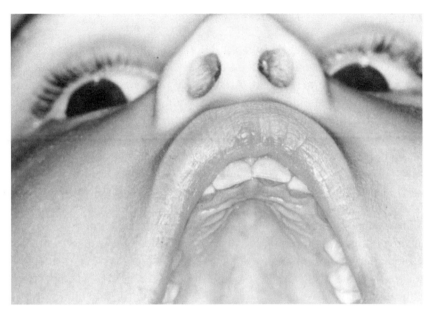

FIGURE 5–11. High dental arch in patient with nasal obstruction. (From Marks M. Stigmata of Respiratory Tract Allergy. Kalamazoo, MI: Upjohn; 1977; with permission.)

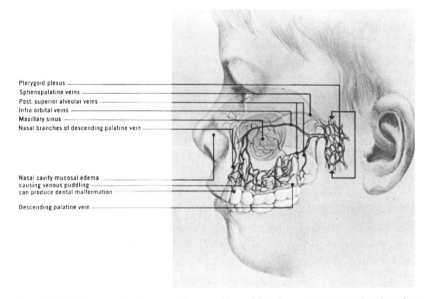

Pterygoid plexus
Sphenopalatine veins
Post. superior alveolar veins
Infra-orbital veins
Maxillary sinus
Nasal branches of descending palatine vein

Nasal cavity mucosal edema
causing venous puddling
can produce dental malformation

Descending palatine vein

FIGURE 5–12. Venous drainage of the maxillae. Allergic nasal congestion interferes with venous drainage, causing slowed circulation in the dental alveoli and adjacent tissues. The resultant tissue anoxia and acidosis may cause changes in dentition and the surrounding musculature of the dental arch. (From Marks M. Stigmata of Respiratory Tract Allergy. Kalamazoo, MI: Upjohn; 1977; with permission.)

Skin

The skin is a favorite target organ of allergy. Scaling eczema may occur in any part of the body, and although frequently allergic in origin, the condition is beyond the scope of this text. An example (although not related to inhalants) is contact dermatitis, which frequently involves areas of the face and neck and areas in contact with restrictive clothing. In many cases, a careful history followed by removal of specific items of jewelry, a change in cosmetics (including hair preparations), a change in specific articles of clothing (especially new ones still containing fresh dyes or sizing), or a change in laundry detergents may offer help. If this fails, specialist help is indicated.

Allergic urticaria is another matter. Whereas skin itching may result from airborne contacts, including pollens and dust, generalized urticaria, especially that involving areas normally covered by clothing, is frequently mediated by food allergy. Not too many years ago, it was reported that about 15% of urticaria was the result of allergy, and the remaining 85% was not. Recent publications have reversed the percentage: 85% is probably allergy-related, and 15% is not. Few allergic problems are more frustrating to decipher than urticaria. Despite the knowledge that a large number of such cases are the result of food sensitivity, this type of response is usually a delayed one, and hours or even days may have passed since the causative food was consumed, so that innumerable other foods have been consumed since ingestion of the offender. The percentage of successes in analyzing and correcting the problem is not high. Nonetheless, when the attempt is successful, the result is an extremely happy patient, justifying the effort directed at dietary manipulation. Approaches to such analysis are discussed in Chapter 14, Food Allergy.

EXPANDED ALLERGIC HISTORY

The directing physician or the representative of the physician will by now have completed and recorded the results of the physical examination and such additional parts of the history as are brought forth as a direct result of physical findings. It has already been stated that the history is more critical in the pursuit of proper allergy diagnosis and care than is the physical examination. The initial history, taken at the time of the patient's first visit, should have directed the physician (and the allergy team members) to consider allergy as a significant part of the patient's problem. At this point, the next step is the gathering of data for a more extensive allergy history. This process will not only be more time-consuming, and more detailed, but will also be more specifically directed to the factors bearing on proper allergy diagnosis and treatment.

A major factor influencing the result of this portion of the evaluation is the time available between the patient's first office visit, when allergy has not necessarily even been considered by the patient, and the patient's subsequent re-evaluation to acquire the necessary information. This gives the patient an opportunity to think over background aspects of the complaint and begin to place them in perspective. To make this self-evaluation advantageous, the patient must be provided with an explanation of what information is necessary for the physician and/or allergy care giver to make at least a preliminary diagnosis. The explanation should include, first, the material indicating that the problem is indeed allergic and, second, information that points to specific possible offenders. As noted, random testing for allergenic contacts is no longer acceptable. If allergy testing is to be performed, as is necessary to confirm a diagnosis, the field must be narrowed down by history to a reasonable number of possible offenders, this number varying by the geographic area, identified exposures, and the limitations placed on such specific studies by third-party payers.

The initial history described in the preceding section may prove surprisingly indicative of an allergic diathesis. The physical findings will usually confirm this, as completely as possible without the benefit of specific inhalant testing. Inhalant allergy is usually the result of direct airborne exposure, and the comprehensive history may provide most of the necessary information for such specific testing.

A printed history form, completed by filling in the blanks, will never provide all the information needed to establish a firm diagnosis. Nonetheless, it is a valuable adjunct to history taking. Most patients, on leaving the office after their initial visit, are confused. They have not only suffered the stress always engendered by a visit to a physician's office, but they have also been presented with a problem with which they are often unprepared to deal. They are now being asked to provide detailed information that they have not previously even considered. They need time. A well-prepared allergy history form will provide them with this time, and also direct their thinking in directions that will aid the history taker as the situation unfolds. Even the more definitive history taken at this stage of evaluation will be altered by subsequent changes in lifestyle, employment, and stress. The allergy history is always an ongoing procedure, subject to constant change as the patient's exposures change!

NURSE'S NOTE

The allergy history never ends, and the allergy care giver, as the person in weekly or biweekly contact with the patient, must constantly update the history. Patients move to a new home or apartment, change places of employment, acquire (or lose) pets, change the medications they take, give up or begin smoking (or have their exposure to smoke changed by some other factor), and undergo numerous other changes in their lives. All this should be elucidated during continuing contacts with the allergy nurse or assistant, documented in the chart, and brought to the attention of the physician as necessary.

Symptoms may develop during a season that patients had previously considered "safe," or patients may simply have forgotten to mention symptoms that later surface. In all these cases, their conduit to the physician is the allergy team member who sees them most regularly.

The conclusion of the initial office visit is usually a good time to provide the patient with an initial allergy history form, to be filled out at leisure and after appropriate thought. The importance of this information to planning the subsequent testing and therapy should be stressed when the form is presented. The patient needs to know that this is not "busywork" but will be a major factor in directing care. This form should be brought to the office at the time of the next visit and discussed, if possible, with the patient present. The basic confirmatory tests will usually be determined at that time.

Although the printed form is a fine initial guideline, it is usually not beneficial to expect the patient to fill out too extensive a history form between the first and second visits. Such a demand tends to precipitate an attitude of "I can't do it!" and the form is either not filled out at all, or the answers are all reported the same, indicating that no consideration has been given to the questions. In any practice, history must be tailored to the individual. Appendix 3 includes a simple initial history form that provides the physician with directions in which to pursue further questions. Most patients will fill out such a form without complaint. The physician or allergy care giver may than go over the form with the patient, clarify any questionable points, and then direct further questions initially within the fields indicated by the patient's responses.

Although the original history form is fairly easy for the patient to fill out, expanding on such forms for a more detailed history may not prove to be practical. The direction indicated by the initial history should serve to guide the person following up with more specific questions, but in many cases too many possibilities exist to be included in a checklist type of form. After a number of patients have been questioned, it may be possible for the history taker to develop a bank of questions that are useful in identifying specific problems. Such a question bank, however, will usually prove too large for the patient to manage if asked to go over each question and enter the appropriate reply. Most patients have been asked to fill out too many surveys, and balk at more. It often becomes the responsibility of the allergy care provider to do the appropriate screening and sift the information provided in the interview to determine the important information. History taking will be an ongoing procedure for however long the patient is in therapy, so missing some points in the early stages is not critical. The questions may be asked (and reasked) at a later date if necessary, and in many cases the patient will bring forth useful information without stimulation as a better understanding of the situation develops.

Although filling out an additional history form may meet with resistance on the part of the patient, this is not always the case. Some patients prefer to use such forms in the interest of saving time in the physician's office, and also because they are able to consider the answers more carefully, sometimes with the help of other family members. The use of such a form may vary between offices, depending somewhat on the patient population. What is almost always self-defeating is to give the patient a large number of forms at the same time and request that they all be filled out and returned. This is basically a ''shotgun'' approach and is not conducive to patient confidence. It implies that the patient is being fed into a mill and not treated as an individual. It is also not necessary, at least initially. The first information form should direct the examiner in the proper direction. The answers should indicate the likelihood of inhalant allergy and identify the probably class of the leading offenders. The examiner may then elect to ask specific questions from their information bank, or, if the history form option is elected, provide the patient with a form covering only the conditions that appear to represent the specific problem. In either case, certain information is especially valuable in guiding necessary testing.

Questions for All Patients

Symptom Pattern and Fluctuation

At what age did symptoms appear? How did the symptom pattern progress? Are there now, or have there been in the past, major seasonal or location variables? How long has the patient lived in this area? Inquire whether conditions are better during the week or on weekends.

Occupation

This includes not only the job designation, but the physical location of the job and type of possible job-related exposures, such as chemicals (e.g., copying fluid, cleaning solvents, beauty shop aerosols, paint). Is the work performed largely indoors or outdoors, mostly in one area or in a wide range of locations (e.g., making deliveries)? In what type of building is most of the work performed? Is industrial pollution close by, to which the patient may be exposed? Is animal exposure involved? How stressful is the job? (This may be directly related, as stress may aggravate allergic symptoms, but the question frequently stimulates the patient to describe other exposure factors that may not previously have been reported.) Are the symptoms particularly bad at one part of the workplace?

This is a limited list, to which other questions may be added as patient replies indicate common problems. This may be especially true in a town where most of the patients work for the same employer. Such answers may indicate a trend that may be amenable to environmental control.

Living Conditions

These include the type of home, presence of pets, type of heating, age of the home, recent redecoration, type and age of beds and pillows, type of floors and carpeting. Are symptoms worse in certain rooms of the house?

Questions for Pollen Sufferers: Season

Many patients will report that they have symptoms ''during the pollen season.'' This requires clarification. Trees habitually bloom in the spring, the starting dates varying with the geographic location. This may be altered to a degree by the presence of nonnative trees, but it is a good general rule. Grass blooms in summer, weeds in the fall. All these seasons vary from year to year to some degree, and some overlap is always present. In addition, the majority of pollen-sensitive patients are, or become, sensitive to additional pollens as exposure is prolonged. Many patients relate their symptoms to the presence of visible pollen, such as pine pollen, which tends to coat autos and driveways. Such pollens are rarely major allergens, and patients should be made aware of this fact, so that they do not attempt to alter their environment to no avail. The same consideration applies to colorful flowers, which are primarily insect-pollinated. When the patient is made aware that the major offenders are rarely noticed by anyone other than botanists, attention is paid to the potential true offenders in the patient's immediate vicinity.

These may be identified by any nursery, or in most cases by checking a book on local plants. If a large collection of offending pollinators is near the house or on the property, and if the pollinating season coincides with the patient's symptoms, some real benefit may be obtained by environmental control.

Questions for Mold Sufferers: Exposure

Mold is actually more of a perennial offender than a seasonal one, and mold is ubiquitous, as discussed briefly in the section on antigen selection in Chapter 4. When the initial history suggests a mold problem, the questions should be directed primarily to sources of mold exposure, many of which may be unsuspected. Patients should be questioned about the age of their dwelling, areas of dampness, including the garage or basement, and type of air conditioning, including condensation pans if window units are used. Has the plumbing been examined for condensation? How about the condensation pan under the refrigerator? The patient should also be questioned about damp areas in the workplace, as much time is spent there. At home, are there many indoor house plants? Is there heavy foliage against the house or large, overhanging trees? Does the patient spend time clearing overgrown areas of the property? What is the geographic relationship of the dwelling to ponds, swamps, or other water sources? How much watering or irrigation goes on, and at what times? Questions regarding mold exposure may go on almost ad infinitum in humid areas of the country, and indoor mold sources cannot be ignored, even in the desert.

The patient should be asked how symptoms are affected by cold fronts, which tend to carry heavy loads of mold. Are the symptoms better or worse in the evening? Mold spores, being light, are often carried by even very faint wind currents above the level at which they may be inhaled until the cool of the evening allows them to descend.

These questions usually identify a mold sensitivity. Unfortunately, a seasonal pattern for mold is not predictable, nor is an individual mold easy to identify by either history or examination of the area. The best approach is usually to depend on any available mold surveys and to test for the most prevalent molds in the area. It is possible to have individual mold surveys performed by purchasing appropriate kits from some of the major allergy supply houses and sending the plates for analysis, but this is rarely necessary.

Questions for Dust Sufferers: Season

Traditionally, the dust season was said to be winter, when the house was closed up tightly. When spring arrived, the house was opened up and the airborne dust allowed to dissipate. Actually, today the dust season is a year-round condition, varying with locations and under specific conditions. The determining factor is usually the degree of environmental conditioning and control. Constant air conditioning, frequent in public buildings, results in a fairly constant dust level throughout the year. In tropical areas, the dust season may peak in midsummer. The patient should be questioned about the presence of dust catchers around the house, such as heavy carpeting and draperies, as well as the age of the house. (Old houses accumulate dust no matter how much cleaning is done.) How often is the house cleaned, and how? Is the dust-sensitive patient present when the cleaning is going on?

There is an inevitable overlap between the various types of allergen exposure, and this will be reflected in the answers to the questions posed in taking the expanded history. In addition, few allergic patients are sensitive to only one or two offenders, and further sensitivities tend to develop with time. It is not practical to present a generic list of questions to be asked of every patient. There is too much variation between different geographic areas and types of practice. The above pattern of history taking, however, should allow the person taking the more specific history to develop a practical list of questions that may be used as a reference source, or if desired used to construct a specific history form to be given to the patient at the appropriate time. If more than one group of offenders is suspected, additional specific questions may be brought forth. An extensive mass of information may be eventually accumulated, but it has been the author's experience that dividing it into individual segments results in better patient cooperation and more accurate information.

Consideration of Allergic Symptoms Beyond the Ear, Nose, and Throat Area

Pulmonary Symptoms

Although allergy is by nature a highly individualized response, certain organs tend to be especially common targets. These include, more or less in order, the upper respiratory tract, lower respiratory tract, gastrointestinal tract, and skin. In the field of allergy, the lungs may be considered essentially a branch of the respiratory tree, as are the nose, paranasal sinuses, eustachian tubes, and middle ears. This does not imply a similar function for these structures, but simply that allergy affects the mucosal lining of all in a very similar manner. Increased production of mucus and mucosal congestion and irritation are common to all. Those structures, such as the bronchial tree, that contain musculature capable of constricting or dilating passages show an additional overall effect. In most cases, appropriate treatment for one part of the respiratory tree will be effective to a large degree in all parts, subject to the limitations of the structural makeup of the individual organ. In other words, proper allergy care will generally benefit the lungs in the presence of allergic bronchitis or asthma. Additional treatment may be required for the nonallergic elements of the problem.

Not all asthma or asthmatic bronchitis is allergic in nature; however, allergy is a major factor in many, if not most, cases of asthma. The inciting agent may be either an inhalant or food. Detailed examination of the lungs may or may not be an integral part of the initial physical examination, but observation of shortness of breath, wheezing, or coughing should be routine. Although the classic picture of asthma is the expiratory wheeze, it has been well established that about 50% of asthmatic patients wheeze, whereas the other 50% cough. Cough-variant asthma (CVA) is frequently overlooked, however, in the evaluation of the patient with a chronic dry cough. So much concern has been expended over other causes of such a cough, like gastrointestinal reflex disease (GERD), drugs such as angiotensin-converting enzyme (ACE) inhibitors, and other, more esoteric conditions, that the simple diagnosis of CVA is often not even considered. Asthma, particularly in the child, is a very frequent result of food sensitivity. Although much of the diagnosis is made by a more detailed history, considered further in a later chapter, recognition of the possibility may open the door to a more effective evaluation.

Gastrointestinal Symptoms

Although not normally considered a target organ for inhalant allergy, the gastrointestinal tract is the chief portal of entry for foods. In addition, several studies have identified significant portions of inhaled allergens appearing in the digestive tract after having cleared the nose and been swallowed. Although the portal of entry does not necessarily reflect the target organ in any way, the most common target organs for food sensitivity are, roughly in order, the upper digestive tract, lower digestive tract, lower respiratory tract, upper respiratory tract, and skin.

Gastrointestinal allergy is especially prone to masquerade as other diseases. Stomach upsets, recurrent diarrhea, specific food intolerances, and even ulcers may be the result of allergic insult. Unfortunately, these same conditions may result from infection, enzyme deficiency, simple irritation, or a wide variety of other situations. It is only prudent to consider first the possibility of nonallergic causes of these complaints, as these conditions may threaten the overall health of the patient more seriously than true allergy. (The controversy regarding the difference between food "allergy," food "hypersensitivity," and "adverse reactions to foods" will be discussed in more detail in Chapter 14.) For now, a persistent recurrence of the complaint, especially accompanied by negative findings on other studies, should raise a question of a specific adverse reaction to food, regardless of the location of the target organ.

CONFIRMING THE DIAGNOSIS OF ALLERGY

The factors already discussed should raise a strong suspicion that the patient is allergic, and in a general way provide a due to the identity of the offenders. It is now necessary, however, to confirm these findings. It is an axiom that the diagnosis of allergy is made by the history and physical examination, but to this should be added the caveat that not all that appears originally to be allergy is in fact allergy. In the case of inhalant allergy, it may safely be said that nearly half the cases in which allergy appears to be present will not be confirmed by testing. If the nose alone is considered, there are numerous forms of nonallergic rhinitis that will initially appear to be allergy. For the initial approach, it is necessary to bear this in mind and alert the patient to the fact. It is embarrassing to prepare the patient fully for a treatment program, only to find that the condition is one masquerading as allergy. (As frequently as allergy masquerades as other conditions, it is not surprising that the reverse is also true.) The details of testing for inhalant allergy are covered in Chapter 6, but some basic tests are discussed here that can confirm the diagnosis and maintain the patient's confidence.

Screen Testing for Inhalant Allergy

Let us assume at this point that the physician has not yet decided to what extent the office should become involved with definitive allergy care. This is a good opportunity to explore the patient volume that will make up an ongoing treatment load if the patients desire this approach rather than symptomatic care only. It also allows the physician and staff to see how accurate their presumptive diagnosis of allergy may be. Sorting out the truly allergic from the nonallergic patient is not difficult, especially if only inhalant allergy is to be considered.

It would be unusual at this early stage of the practice of allergy to begin skin testing, as this requires a considerable investment in both personnel and equipment, discussed in the section on getting started in Chapter 4. Testing alone, without setting up a treatment program, can be done by in vitro methods with minimal equipment, and will identify the presence of allergy with considerable accuracy. If the decision is then to provide ongoing care, based on practice evaluation, patient desires, and load identification, one can order supplies and arrange for the training of personnel necessary to administer treatment with no harm having resulted from the wait. Allergy care is rarely an emergency situation, and if a good rapport exists between physician and patient, this will usually override any resistance to a slight delay in treatment.

In Vitro Screens

The first need is to determine that the patient is truly allergic. Numerous in vitro screening methods are available for this purpose. The simplest such screening test is known in general as the *dipstick test*. Several laboratories now supply the test equipment, which comes in a kit with full instructions. The kits, like the screening radioallergosorbent test (RAST) disks, are regionally selected. As for the disk tests, both seasonal and perennial kits are usually available. The selection of the allergens in the kits is usually made clear, and may be compared with the actual allergens known to be present in the area. (This is covered in the section on antigen selection in Chapter 4.)

Like the more sophisticated RAST, described later, the dipstick test is performed on the patient's serum. The serum is separated from the whole blood and placed in a test tube. According to directions in the kit, a paper dipstick impregnated with the various antigens to be tested, arranged in bands on the stick, is inserted in the test tube containing the serum. After an appropriate interval, it is passed through a series of rinses and insertions in other test tubes containing various chemicals to induce a colorometric reaction. The exact details of the procedure are included in instructions that come with the kit. Finally, the dipstick, now containing bands of color of varying depths, is compared with a chart (Fig. 5–13). The comparison of color depth with the chart gives a rough idea of the degree of sensitivity to the antigens on the band.

In a sense, the dipstick test is more quantitative than the multiantigen disk screen described below, as each antigen is represented by an identifiable separate band. At the present stage of its development, however, the dipstick allergy test must be considered only semiquantitative, and more testing is needed to determine the exact sensitivity of the patient to the antigens incriminated. The greatest advantage of this test is that the equipment (in the form of the kits) is not expensive, and the test is not difficult to perform. Although immunotherapy cannot be based on the results of the test, it is an excellent

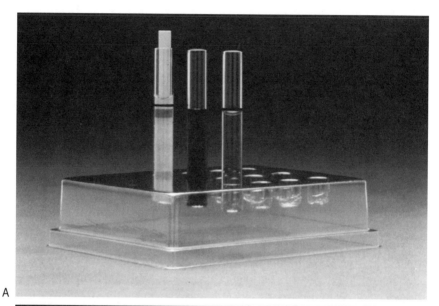

A

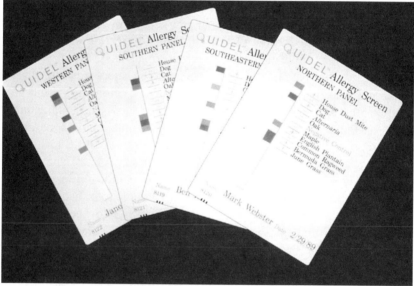

B

FIGURE 5–13. (A,B). A dipstick screening test for inhalant allergy. The dipstick is incubated with the patient's serum, then a series of chemicals. This produces gradations of color in areas on the dipstick representing specific antigens. Dipsticks are available that contain key antigens for different areas of the country. (Courtesy of Quidel Co., San Diego, CA.)

tool for practitioners who wish to determine how many allergic patients are seen in their practice from day to day, and to begin consideration of more definitive treatment.

More complete information to diagnose inhalant allergy may be obtained from allergen-specific quantitative in vitro assays. The simplest way for the novice practitioner to acquire this information is to utilize the services of a reference laboratory performing RAST or enzyme-linked immunosorbent assay (ELISA). These are both in vitro (''in glass'') tests, performed on the patient's blood and not requiring the presence of the patient during the actual test procedure. This is in distinction to in vivo (''in the living'') tests, such as skin tests, which require the patient to be present throughout the entire test procedure. It is important to understand these terms and the categories of tests they encompass. The principles and range of such tests are discussed in detail in Chapter 6, *Testing Methods for Inhalant Allergy.*

A wide range of allergy testing reference laboratories are available throughout the country, and any practitioner who has been involved with allergy care can easily direct the physician developing a new practice to such a laboratory, and usually provide a fair picture of the degree of cooperation and accuracy of results that can be expected. The laboratory will supply a list of available tests, instructions for preparing and sending serum, and usually the necessary equipment for mailing serum for allergy testing. If the physician's office does not have a centrifuge, any local laboratory or hospital can generally be prevailed on to separate the serum. (The centrifuge will be one of the items needed if allergy care is to be pursued through the office, but this can come later.)

Some testing laboratories offer a screening test in which a single test disk contains several regional allergens. Usually, two tests are required, one for seasonal allergens and one for perennial allergens. This is an inexpensive means of identifying the truly inhalant-allergic patient and obtaining an idea of the particular offenders. For the novice, the rating levels of response are usually printed on the report. The test has definite weaknesses, in that of necessity the various antigens included on the disk represent a mix, which dilutes the strength of each individual antigen to some degree. This is usually not enough of a problem to make the overall test unreliable. Also, not all significant, relevant antigens may be represented on the disk. Most importantly, it must be understood that should the test result be positive, individual antigens will have to be tested again to confirm the degree of sensitivity to each individual allergen and to determine a proper initial dose for treatment. As a screen, however, the test is rapid, accurate, and inexpensive. It may be combined with a measurement of the total immunoglobulin E (IgE) level if further information is desired.

The single- or two-disk screen is usually effective in determining the presence or absence of inhalant allergy, but it provides little direction in identifying the individual offenders. A slightly more extensive approach, still not by any means excessive, will provide more exact information and may reduce the amount of retesting necessary when the single disk containing multiple allergens is employed as a screen. This is the RAST miniscreen. To use this approach, a group of "index" allergens, those predominant in the area, are selected for testing. This usually includes two trees, two weeds, one or two grasses depending on the area, house dust mite, and one or two epidermals if indicated. Most third-party payers designate the number of allergens that will be covered in preliminary testing, the usual number ranging from eight to 15 depending on the area. It has been shown that if a "miniscreen" composed of one grass, one weed, one tree, two molds, and one dust mite is tested, the sensitivity of such a screen is 94% (only 6% of allergic patients are missed), with a 96% specificity (4% possible false-positives).[7] The sensitivity and specificity may be further increased to almost 100% by the use of a "midscreen" of two grasses, one weed, two trees, three molds, and one dust mite.[8] If any of the test results are significantly positive, this indicates the presence of an allergic entity and also directs the subsequent testing in a particular direction. In the demonstrated presence of allergy, third-party payers may be more cooperative in allowing the necessary additional testing. An additional benefit is that the tests already performed in doing the screen do not need to be repeated. The results for those antigens have already been provided.

The RAST screen need not present an inflexible pattern. It may be blended effectively with the detailed history already taken. The basic pattern is an extremely reliable one, but if the history is strongly indicative of a particular allergen or group of allergens, an allergen may be added to the screen or one may be substituted. This approach is quite effective for any allergy practice, new or established, and aids in promoting credibility and providing immediately useful information.

In Vivo Screens

Although novice practitioners may wish only to determine the number of allergic patients in their practice, utilizing an outside reference laboratory to perform in vitro determinations, some may choose to utilize skin test screening methods. However, to perform these tests, the physician must have a trained staff, and the office must be equipped to manage a possible anaphylactic reaction. Probably the most efficient screening skin test, although by no means the only available such method, is the Multi-Test skin prick testing technique. This employs a device consisting of two parallel rows of four test heads, each of which contains nine plastic points arranged in a square pattern. Test antigen is applied to the points, and the device is used to puncture the skin in a uniform fashion. The details of the technique, and of other skin test methods, are found in Chapter 6.

Screening for Food Allergy

It is suspected that inhalant allergy is considerably more common than food hypersensitivity, but this has by no means been conclusively proved. It may well be that the incidence of some forms of food hypersensitivity eclipses that of inhalant allergy. The medical morass of food allergy occupies several chapters later in the book. At the present initial stage, it need be considered only that patients who appear by all physical signs to have allergies, but have negative results on all inhalant tests, may in fact be victims of food hypersensitivity. Before the condition is diagnosed as nonallergic, with symptomatic treatment available, some basic consideration should be given to the possibility of food hypersensitivity.

Diagnosing food hypersensitivity is much more difficult than diagnosing inhalant allergy. First, it must be stated that there is at present no single test that will establish or rule out the presence of food hypersensitivity. There are too many routes by which food may adversely affect the body. In addition, the range of target organs is virtually unlimited. These factors have led many practitioners of allergy to abandon all but the most obvious indications of food hypersensitivity, and thereby deprive many patients of the possibility of relief from a multitude of symptoms.

The full details of food allergy investigation require prolonged discussion. There are, however, certain factors that suggest food sensitivity and justify a further search. Almost all these indications come from the patient's history and require patient, probing questioning. The original history will not be complete, and only suggestive factors will probably surface in the initial interview. Even these will often be missed unless the investigator pursues them.

Food hypersensitivity may affect almost any organ of the body. A routine system review will usually pinpoint an involved area, although it may not identify the cause of the problem. Initially, the usual course of evaluation will be to check out the typical nonallergic causes of such a complaint, and this is as it should be. The suspicion of allergy arises when the usual studies yield negative results, or when the history becomes suggestive.

In some cases of food allergy, symptoms are constantly present. These usually indicate a diet that varies little from day to day, a condition that is not truly rare. Many people are habit eaters, even though they are not aware of it. The body recognizes only basic foods, not in most cases the preparation involved. Beef is beef, whether it is in a roast, bouillon, or hamburger. Milk is milk, whether plain, in yogurt or cheese, or as the base of multiple prepared food dishes. The patient who is a strong habit eater and is suspected of being food-allergic may be tested quite simply. The best route is to have the patient prepare a food diary, listing all foods eaten in their basic form. (Example: There is no such thing as a salad. There is lettuce, onion, and tomato, but not simply ''salad.'') The clinician going over this list will often be struck by certain foods consumed on a daily basis, and often several times a day. Milk and coffee are common examples. In screening, it may be necessary only to provide the patient with a list of major sources of the food in question and request that it not be eaten for a week in any form, watching the symptomatic result. Many times the result will be clear enough to convince both the patient and the examiner, and appropriate elimination regimens may be prescribed. This approach, although the simplest, is far from consistently practical. The initial impression might well be that no food would appear as a possible culprit with so many food options available, but surprisingly a single food is often readily identified. The first tenet in tracing the offender is that if it is not in the body, it cannot cause a problem. If the problem is relatively constant, it then follows that the patient is consuming the food on a regular basis. There is an adage in the diagnosis of food allergy: ''Find out what they like and take it away from them.'' There is more than a little accuracy in the statement. If the patient does not like the food, it will certainly not be consumed, at least on a regular basis. Food regularly eaten has a better opportunity of inducing an allergic reaction than food eaten only at infrequent intervals. It is not unusual, when patients are requested to keep a food diary and are advised that after the diary has been completed, they may well be asked to eliminate a few specific foods during a test period, for the reaction to be, ''Don't take my coffee away! I can't function without my coffee!'' The same reaction may be expressed about ice cream, chocolate, or any other food. This will not always be the case, but it occurs with enough frequency to make it a worthwhile initial approach, if only to see the reaction.

Requesting the patient to eliminate the food for a week has a practical purpose. It takes the body 5 to 7 days to metabolize a food completely and eliminate it from the body. (This process will normally be complete in 5 days, but allowing for the patient following directions imperfectly and consuming some traces of the food, and also for variations in digestive speed, a week is safer and easier to remember.) Results may not be perfect within a week, but if the primary offender has been correctly selected, there should be considerable improvement.

Not all persons are habit eaters, and many have widely varied diets with much in the way of sauces and dressings added to their food. The presence of food sensitivity in these persons requires a little more dedication on their part. Starting with the food diary, even if imperfectly kept, a temporary diet may be designed. This should be a version of the so-called "caveman diet," consisting of very plainly prepared meats such as roasts cooked without additives, berries, fruits, and nongrain vegetables that are raw, boiled, or steamed. The diet should not contain any of the foods commonly eaten by the patient. Another way to put it is "Eat all you want of everything you don't like." It is necessary to impress on the patient at this time that this is not designed to be an ongoing plan, but simply will be used as a test. A week is again the recommended duration, and it is often valuable to suggest to the patient that a week's supply of the appropriate food be purchased and prepared in advance, allowing only for heating or cooking appropriately before eating. This simply aids compliance by reducing the urge to cheat. Again, if food sensitivity is involved, there should be a significant improvement in symptoms, and further specific evaluation may be arranged. This is discussed in Chapter 14. Because no laboratory test is reliable today, the elimination and challenge format is still considered the "gold standard" of food testing, and the above procedures present a simple shortcut to establish or rule out for the most part the presence of the disease. Furthermore, this method does not involve food skin testing, which is often as feared by the treating physician as by the patient.

For the novice, this approach to allergy may both introduce the program to the practice and provide the necessary information concerning the impact that may be expected. Of course, if the practitioners have already accepted the need for allergy care as a part of the practice, the shortcuts are unnecessary. The preceding chapters have provided the basic information required to add allergy to a general clinical practice, including necessary basic knowledge (reduced to a "need-to-know" pattern) and a format for selecting the equipment needed to proceed with allergy care. Subsequent chapters deal with the material and information needed as the practice enlarges.

REFERENCES

1. Jessner M, Hoffman H. Untersuchungen uber subcutane trichophyton innokulationen. Arch Dermatol Syph 1926;151:98.

2. King HC. An Otolaryngologist's Guide to Allergy. New York, NY: Thieme; 1990: 210–212.
3. Fireman P. Otitis media and eustachian tube dysfunction: connection to allergic rhinitis. J Allergy Clin Immunol 1997;99:S787–S797.
4. Hurst DS. Association of otitis media with effusion and allergy as demonstrated by intradermal skin testing and eosinophil cationic protein levels in both middle ear effusions and mucosal biopsies. Laryngoscope 1996;106:1128–1137.
5. Derebery MJ, Valenzuela S. Menière's syndrome and allergy. Otolaryngol Clin North Am 1992;25:213–224.
6. Howard BK, Mabry RL, Meyerhoff WL, Mabry CS. Utility of a screening RAST in a large neurologic practice. Otolaryngol Head Neck Surg (in press).
7. King WP. Efficacy of a screening radioallergosorbent test. Arch Otolaryngol 1982;108: 781–786.
8. Lehr AJ, Mabry RL, Mabry CS. The screening RAST: is it a valid concept? Otolaryngol Head Neck Surg 1997;117:54–55.

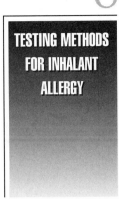

6

TESTING METHODS FOR INHALANT ALLERGY

It must be assumed at this point that the directing physician has made the decision that both the practice and the patients will benefit if the office provides allergy care. The earlier chapters have emphasized the importance of allergy as a medical problem, outlined the basic material necessary for diagnosing the condition, and set the stage for proceeding into providing therapy.

In previous chapters, basic screening procedures for inhalant allergy, and even an initial limited screening procedure for food sensitivity, have been described. Although such screening provides an adequate initial approach to determining the patient's overall status, more definitive studies are needed before treatment that includes immunotherapy is undertaken.

COMPLETING THE TESTING FOR INHALANT ALLERGY

Although it is axiomatic that the initial diagnosis of allergy is made by history and physical examination, the findings must be confirmed by tests that identify the specific causative antigens if the investigator wishes to be certain of the diagnosis and proceed to treat the patient effectively. Another condition, or group of conditions, known collectively as *nonallergic rhinitis*, may mimic true allergy so well that even an experienced examiner can be misled. This is discussed in more detail in Chapter 13. Because proper treatment depends on proper diagnosis, definitive allergy tests are appropriate at this point.

In this era of cost control, ordering or performing a nearly unlimited number of tests for allergy is to be studiously avoided. (Actually, the approach, pursued at times throughout history, of performing an immense range of tests and then sorting out those truly appropriate has never been a truly good one. It is wasteful, unnecessarily expensive, and hard on the patient.) Before the specific test methods to be used are considered, therefore, it is well to consider the patient and the plan of approach to treatment.

This chapter deals with techniques for completing the identification of inhalant allergens initiated with the limited screening tests previously described. Most clinicians adding allergy to their practice will begin with the treatment of inhalant allergy only, as this is the best-understood form of allergy at present and offers the best possibility of a clear diagnosis and good treatment results.

Before any tests are initiated, however, the patient's motivation must be considered. How persistent are the symptoms, and how severe? If the symptoms are of brief duration and limited to a certain location or a particular season, specific testing may not be necessary. Although immunotherapy offers the only possible "cure" for allergy, and although environmental control is the ideal (although often unattainable) means of management, as a rule any control of symptoms that can be obtained by either of these means can also be obtained by proper medication. Thus, if no specific treatment by immunotherapy is planned, it may not be necessary to identify specific offenders. Here, the patient must be consulted. If the patient wants to know the offender, regardless of the treatment plan, reliable testing is available. It is always nice to know where one stands in regard to offenders, but it is difficult to explain to the patient (or insurer) why a wide range of expensive tests were ordered so that offenders could be identified, and then an antihistamine was prescribed. This could have been done by history alone, without the tests. Specific testing is indicated when the patient wishes to know the offender, when treatment by environmental control is to be undertaken (so as to practice effective avoidance measures), or when immunotherapy is to be considered. The indications for each of these selections will be considered in the chapters on therapy. One indication, for example, would be intolerance to ordinary pharmacotherapeutic measures.

At this point, we can assume that specific testing is to be performed. Today, a wide range of testing modalities pertaining to inhalant allergy are available to the physician. Parenthetically, it may be clearly stated that no laboratory test today is reliable for food sensitivity, although some may be useful for screening. Reliable tests are available for inhalant allergy alone. (Even these are not 100% reliable, but very nearly so.) Because unlimited testing is not an option, how should the situation be approached?

SCREENING: THE FIRST STEP

A good history is the key for selecting allergens to be tested. Usually, third-party payers will accept only a limited number of allergens in an initial battery, anywhere from eight to 15 being a typical number. If the patient's symptoms are of pollinosis and present only in the fall, an appropriate initial battery of allergens would be a selection of local weeds. (Preparing a proper antigen selection is discussed in another chapter.) If the problems occur in an old house, dust, mold, and probably epidermals should be tested. This allows the physician to customize testing to maximize the range with the best possibility of obtaining positive results. The main purpose of a screen is to establish the presence of allergy in the patient's makeup. It is not expected to catch all significant allergens. Once the presence of allergy has been established, additional testing is indicated. Again, the selection of tests should be dictated by the history. At times, additional tests performed after a positive screening examination will incriminate antigens not initially suspected.

Although a number of individual methods are in use today to identify specific inhalant allergens, they all fall into one of two basic types: "in vivo" tests (for all practical purposes these are skin tests, although provocation tests are used in research centers) and "in vitro" tests (tests performed on the patient's blood, usually by a reference laboratory). Most clinicians adding allergy to an already active practice will probably initially opt for in vitro tests, as little or no equipment is required (if a reference laboratory is utilized) and the results are easily applicable to patient treatment. It must be understood that if the treatment to be used is immunotherapy, a certain amount of skin testing will still be needed at some point, but this is not an immediate requirement. The necessary equipment for various forms of therapy is discussed in the section on getting started in Chapter 4.

The simplest form of office-based in vitro testing is the so-called "dipstick test." This has been described under screening testing for inhalant allergy in the section on confirming the diagnosis of allergy in Chapter 5. At its present level of quantitative sophistication, the test can be considered only a screen, but it is semiquantitative, easy to perform, and inexpensive, and it does provide some immediate information. The test may be the only study needed if all that is necessary is to establish the presence of allergy, and if the therapeutic procedures are to be limited to environmental control or pharmacotherapy. Modifications and refinements are constantly being developed for the test, and in time it may be fully quantitative. In its present stage, it will accurately identify the inhalant allergic patient, identify some of the offending allergens, and give a rough idea of the degree of sensitivity. It is not yet accurate enough to be used as a therapeutic tool, especially if immunotherapy is to be considered. Other in vitro screening methods include the use of disks containing multiple antigens, or specific testing for only a selected number of antigens initially.

Although most new allergy practices may benefit from the initial use of in vitro tests, this is not always the case. Many practices have thrived from the beginning using skin testing alone. In addition, in many regions of the country third-party payers may provide a strong incentive not to perform in vitro testing, despite the fact that it has been shown to be cost-effective when screening is done properly. All these factors may influence the type of testing selected.

In vivo screening skin tests may consist of skin endpoint titration (SET) performed for a limited number of antigens, with expansion of the testing panel based on the initial results. Another convenient skin test screen involves the Multi-Test, which is a type of multiple prick-puncture test that allows testing to be performed for several antigens with a minimum of effort. Specific details of these tests are presented later in this chapter.

It is worthwhile to mention that although allergy testing as a preliminary step to immunotherapy is not by any means always an ideal approach from the physician's point of view, as a practical matter most patients seeking allergy care are prepared for immunotherapy. Because a large percentage of antiallergic medical products have become available over the counter, and because the public has been bombarded with information regarding allergy in the literature, most patients have already tried and rejected, or at least felt dissatisfied with, this approach and wish something more definitive. It must be granted that their use of such products and information has frequently been less than ideal, but a clarification of proper use of products already tried frequently results only in the patient's consulting another physician. Patients consulting a doctor usually want a significantly different approach.

Regardless of the initial type of screening test for allergy, an understanding of the underlying principles involved and of the risks and benefits of both in vitro and in vivo tests is necessary to make proper decisions and to apply the correct test in a proper manner. There is a close scientific relationship between the two types of test. In the early days of in vitro testing, a popular belief was fostered that the tests were basically completely different in nature, and therefore not comparable. This is not accurate. A simple way to compare the two types of test is to think of the in vitro test as an advanced technologic means of performing the in vivo test. This may be an oversimplification, but is a useful approach in understanding the principles involved.

IN VIVO TESTS

In vivo testing, or skin tests, are considered first, as these were the first allergy tests to come into practical use. They have been refined and upgraded through the years, and various degrees of quantification have been added. The in vivo tests are the best known and best understood type of allergy test, and once the in vivo test is understood, it is fairly easy to make the jump to understanding the in vitro test. The underlying physiologic principle of the two types of test is the same. All that differs is the method of measurement.

Essentially, all inhalant allergy is produced by immunoglobulin E (IgE), a bodily substance present in more than trace amounts in only about 20% of the population. IgE is present in the skin, serum, and most bodily organs. Because the skin contains IgE (including the specific form for all antigens to which the patient is allergic), applying an allergen to an abraded spot on the skin will result in a wheal-and-flare reaction in the patient sensitive to that allergen. (For those unfamiliar with the terminology involved in skin testing, the wheal is the raised area in the center of the test site, whereas the flare is the erythematous area surrounding the site.) The specificity and sensitivity depend on the strength of the antigen preparation applied and on the method of application. Skin testing is the oldest form of allergy testing, and actually was first described in 1865. Accurately controlled skin testing that includes some degree of quantitation dates to about 1910.[1]

Factors Affecting Skin Test Results

The size of a skin test reaction is influenced by a number of factors, including the volume and potency of the antigen injected, the depth to which it is introduced (epidermal or intradermal), the degree of sensitization of mast cells in the skin, and the reactivity of the skin to histamine and other mediators released as a part of the allergic reaction. Furthermore, the response may be modified by drugs, the presence of blocking antibodies (from previous immunotherapy), the age and race of the patient, the area of the body injected, the distance separating individual skin test sites, and the time of day of testing.

Intradermal testing introduces antigen in a much more quantified way than do scratch and prick tests. In intradermal testing, the size of the initial wheal is related directly to the volume injected. For example. 0.01 mL is said to produce a wheal of about 4 mm in diameter, which enlarges to about 5 mm because of physical spreading. If the volume injected is increased to about 0.05 mL, the resulting wheal size is about 7 to 9 mm.

Because intradermal tests introduce much more antigen than do prick tests, intradermal tests should either be preceded by a screening prick test or (as in SET) be performed with sequentially more concentrated antigen solutions, starting with a weak and anticipated nonreacting concentration.

The reactivity of the sensitized skin mast cells and the degree of antigenicity of the solution injected affect the amount of histamine and other vasoactive amines liberated as a result of the skin test, and ultimately affect the size of the resultant wheal. The skin of some individuals is overly responsive to trauma, and a wheal-and-flare response (called dermatographs) will be seen in these patients even following the injection of an inert substance. For this reason, a negative control of an inert substance, such as diluent, is always necessary in skin testing.

Increasing amounts of allergen exposure have the same effect on skin reactivity as the use of stronger testing antigen solutions; both result in the production of a more intense skin reaction. Thus, patients will usually be found to be more sensitive to skin testing carried out during the season of their offending pollen, or after increased exposure to a perennial antigen. The results obtained during this "coseasonal" testing may often indicate a higher degree of sensitivity than those obtained when testing is performed out of season.

Patients who have undergone previous treatment may have altered skin test responses, resulting from changes in both IgE and IgG formation. As a practical matter, the existing state of the patient's immune system is generally accurately reflected in the response to skin testing. In vitro studies, which measure only IgE, fail to take into account the effect of IgG "blocking antibody" formed as a response to prior allergy injections.

The skin of some patients, especially infants and the elderly, is said to be less reactive to skin testing than that of the population as a whole. A general decline of skin reactivity after the age of 50 has been described, although in vitro tests have shown that allergy continues to exist unabated in this age group.

The area of the body where skin tests are applied may affect the responses obtained. Decreasing reactivity of skin occurs in the following order: mid and upper back > lower back > upper arm > forearm (ulnar > radial) > wrist. The reason that intradermal testing is performed on the upper arm, rather than the back, is to allow the placement of a tourniquet above the injection site in case of a reaction. Because prick tests are less likely to result in a systemic reaction, they are often carried out on the back.

Axonal reflexes may affect the results of a skin test. Positive skin tests (or positive reactions to histamine controls), if placed too near other skin tests, can initiate axonal reflexes that drive the wheal-and-flare response. Thus, the histamine control should be placed well away from other tests, and individual skin tests should be separated by at least 2 cm.

The skin is said to be up to 2 1/2 times more responsive to tests applied between 7:00 and 11:00 PM than to those applied at 7:00 AM. This variable will affect only the most conscientious allergist.

Antihistamines suppress the wheal-and-flare response. With almost all common antihistamines, this effect for all practical purposes ceases within 24 hours or less of the delivery of the last medication to the body, and skin testing may be carried out if the patient has taken no such drugs for 36 to 48 hours. Short-acting antihistamines such as diphenhydramine (Benadryl) and triprolidine (Actifed) can sometimes be taken even the day before testing without affecting skin test responses. A notable exception is astemizole (Hismanal); clearance of this drug and its metabolites from the body is extremely slow. If tissue saturation has occurred by prolonged therapy, from 3 to 6 weeks must elapse after cessation of astemizole before skin testing may be accurately performed. A return to normal skin reactivity should be confirmed by a positive histamine control before further testing is carried out. It is important to remember (and to remind patients) that antihistamines are also contained in or include soporifics, cough syrups, "cold" remedies, antipruritics, and anxiolytics.

Tricyclic antidepressants, such as doxepin (Sinequan) and amitryptiline (Elavil), have been observed to suppress skin test responses for from 2 to 4 days after the last dose of the compound has been administered.

Decongestants, cromolyn, corticosteroids, and bronchodilators do not affect skin test results.

As a practical matter, patients should be advised to omit antihistamines for 48 hours before allergy testing (except astemizole, which requires prolonged omission). Patients on tricyclic antidepressants should discontinue them for 4 days before testing, if at all possible.

Forms of Skin Testing

Several forms of skin testing are in common use today. In many cases, a combination of methodologies is used to produce better results. These methods are reviewed individually.

Scratch Test

This is one of the older forms of skin testing. A small drop of a fairly concentrated extract of an allergen is applied to the skin, and the drop is scratched through with a sharp instrument, breaking only the surface layer of skin. In a variation of this technique, the scratch is made first and the drop of allergenic extract is applied to the scratched area. Results are read on a 0 to 4 + scale of reactivity. This test has been evaluated by the American Medical Association's Council on Scientific Affairs, which in 1987 advised that scratch testing resulted in too many false-positive and false-negative responses to be considered a reliable diagnostic test. Although scratch testing is still performed by some practitioners, use of the test has declined precipitously since the late 1980s and will probably be replaced entirely by more reliable tests as time goes on. One specific problem with the scratch test has been that the mechanism of the test is to induce the release of histamine from the skin, and histamine has a triple reaction, one of which is to produce an axon reflex. When several negative tests are performed close together, followed by a strongly positive test, the axon reflex from the positive test may ignite a false-positive reaction in the nearby tests previously read as negative.[2] This contributes to the unreliability of the test. Furthermore, in scratch testing, quantification of the amount of antigen introduced is extremely poor. As it can be completely replaced by more comprehensive tests, the scratch test will not be missed.

One invalid use of the scratch test has been in small children. For some time, it has been common practice to perform scratch tests in children under the age of 4 to determine sensitivity to both inhalants and foods. It is rare, but not impossible, to see inhalant allergy in a child of this age. On the other hand, food sensitivity is common in this age range, but it is rarely IgE-mediated. Because scratch testing is generally not considered reliable for other than IgE-mediated disease, scratch tests for food sensitivity that did not produce a positive wheal-and-flare reaction were interpreted as negative and the parent was informed that the child was not sensitive to foods. These negative skin reactions often discouraged the parent and the physician from further investigation to show that an adverse reaction to foods might be based on other than IgE production. This in turn often led to a failure to identify a real problem that, had it been identified and corrected, could have prevented future difficulties.

Prick Test

The prick test has been in use since about 1910, and today it remains the standard method employed by a large percentage of allergists. In many ways similar to the scratch test, the prick test is nonetheless much more reproducible.

In performing the test, the upper layer of the skin is lifted with the point of a sharp instrument, most frequently a needle, and allowed to drop back. The goal is not to penetrate the skin but to produce a small prick in the upper skin layers (Fig. 6–1). A drop of antigen extract, at a concentration of 1:10 to 1:20 weight/volume (w/v), is then placed on the pricked spot, and after 15 to 20 minutes the result is read. A variation in this technique, which has become more popular, is to place the antigen on marked areas of

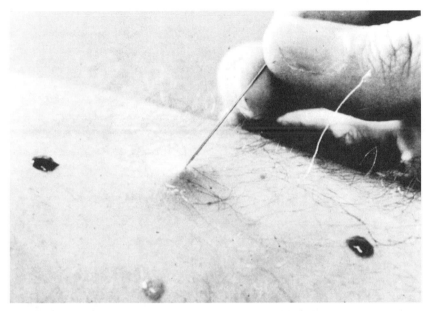

FIGURE 6–1. Prick test. In the earliest forms of prick testing, almost any sharp instrument, most frequently a needle, was used to prick only into the upper layers of skin, as shown. Before or after the prick, a drop of antigen was placed on the pricked area, and the skin reaction interpreted after 10 to 15 minutes. Accuracy was limited by the variability of skin penetration.

the skin first, then prick through the drop of antigen. Results are rated on a scale of 0 to 4 +, comparing the responses with a positive (histamine) and negative (diluent or glycerine) control.[3] In prick testing, the size of both the wheal and the flare produced by the test are measured and recorded.

A problem associated with the mechanics of prick testing has been the use of the "prick and wipe" technique. For speed, the test has often been applied with one needle per patient, wiping any antigen off the point between sticks. Of course, cross-contamination with antigens is possible if the needle is not adequately cleaned between pricks. Fears of personnel suffering needle sticks using this prick and wipe method has led to a recommendation by the Occupational Health and Safety Administration that the technique be changed, so that each stick is performed with a needle that is then discarded into a sharps container before a new needle is used for the next stick.[4] Although some proponents of the prick and wipe technique continue to use this method, other methods are gaining in popularity.

In the early days of allergy testing, the prick test suffered from a lack of

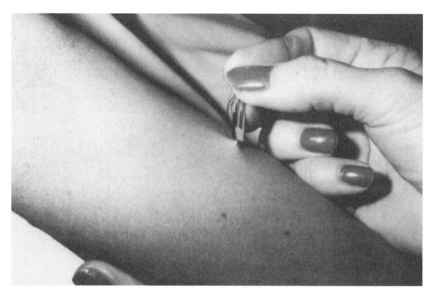

FIGURE 6–2. The prick test, administered manually. A drop of test antigen is placed on the skin and the skin is "picked" with a sharp instrument, lifting the skin and releasing it without penetrating through it. The results are more reliable than the scratch test, but still subject to variables ranging from proficiency of administration to individual skin reactivity.

uniformity, both in testing and results. Through the years, the variability inherent in performing a test of this type became evident, and newer and better means of administering the prick were developed. Today, instruments are available to administer the prick in a uniform manner each time, based on a controlled depth of penetration, usually 1 mm (Fig. 6–2). Further advances have produced instruments that apply the antigen at the same time the prick is administered; the drop of antigen is carried in a rosette of tiny needles (Fig. 6–3). These instruments penetrate the skin to a somewhat deeper level than do the single-pointed instruments, delivering a somewhat larger, although uniform, amount of antigen into the skin. This produces a reaction closer to that seen in an intradermal test than with the single-pointed instrument (Fig. 6–4).

Unfortunately, there is still no uniformity in designating a single method for reading and reporting the results of prick tests. Table 6–1 shows one of the accepted formats for interpreting the prick test results. Another alternative is simply to compare test wheal-and-flare reactions with those obtained from the positive (histamine) control (Fig. 6–5). In this system, a 2 + reaction is half the size of the histamine control, a 3 + reaction is the same size as the

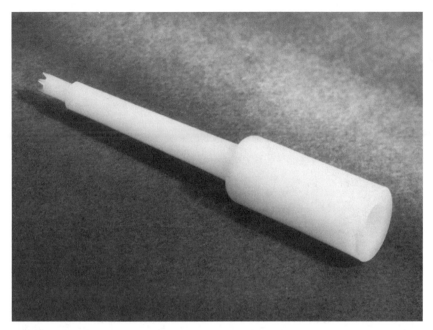

FIGURE 6–3. Multiple-point, single-antigen "pricker": the Greer Pik (Greer Laboratories, P.O. Box 800, 639 Nuway Circle, Lenoir, NC 28645-0800). Further refinements in the prick test format resulted in the development of an instrument carrying a larger amount of antigen and containing six points of measured depth. This yields much more reproducible prick test results.

control, and a 4+ result is twice that size. A third suggestion has been to measure the resulting wheal in two dimensions, add the diameters, and divide by two, expressing the result in millimeters, or outlining the wheal in ball-point pen and transferring the marking to paper using clear tape.[5] The exact grading system is probably not so important as consistency and familiarity with the system chosen, which should be indicated on any test results.

TABLE 6–1. Typical grading system for skin prick test*

Grade	Wheal size	Erythema size
0	<3 mm	0–5 mm
1+	3–5 mm	0–10 mm
2+	5–10 mm	5–10 mm
3+	10–15 mm	10–20 mm
4+	>15 mm or pseudopods	>20 mm

* Readings of 3+ and 4+ are considered positive. Wheal and erythema size are the average diameter of the reactions, measured in two axes.

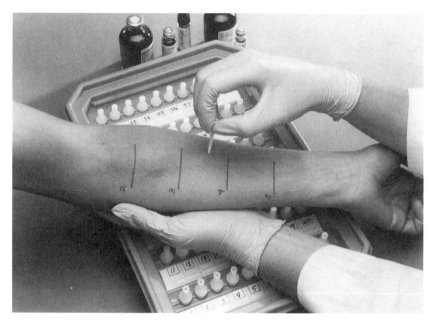

FIGURE 6–4. Wheal production from the prick test, which characteristically produces both a central area of induration (wheal) and a surrounding area of erythema (flare). Note the responses to the tests already placed.

Clearly, although the uniformity of prick testing has greatly improved, interpreting the test results still allows considerable latitude. Attempts to rate the magnitude of a response to a single prick test continue to be open to serious question.

A variant of the prick test involves a multiple prick-puncture apparatus, the Multi-Test device, which consists of two parallel rows of four test heads. Each head contains nine plastic points that are 1.9 mm in length and arranged in a 2 × 2-mm square pattern (Fig. 6–6). Test antigen is applied to the points by a patented applicator and is held to the test head by capillary action. When the device is firmly applied to the skin (with pressure followed by a gentle rolling action), a uniform amount of antigen is delivered to the epidermis and superficial dermis. Positive and negative controls (histamine and glycerine) are applied along with test antigens, and the results are graded on a 0 to 4 + scale as with the prick test. Because of the reproducibility of the amount of antigen delivered, as well as the depth of penetration involved, the Multi-Test may be more comparable with intradermal testing than with a true prick test. Prior studies have confirmed its reproducibility[6] and validity as a screening test.[7]

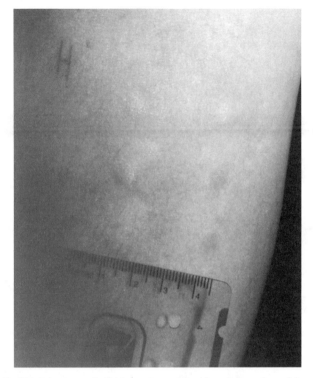

FIGURE 6–5. Prick test result. A histamine control has been placed (*upper left*), and the wheal and flare produced by testing with each antigen are compared with the positive control.

Most allergists do not depend on a single prick test for diagnosis. In the interest of safety as well as accuracy, many initially administer a prick test, which delivers a very small total amount of antigen in comparison with intradermal testing. This initial use of the prick test is a very safe means of screening to identify patients with high degrees of sensitivity. If the prick test result is negative, it is safe to progress to an intradermal test, if indicated. It should be emphasized that stopping testing after a negative prick test result may result in failure to identify patients with lower degrees of hypersensitivity that may materially contribute to symptom production. To screen fully for inhalant allergy using the prick test requires a follow-up intradermal test for patients who are negative prick reactors.

Intradermal Test

The intradermal test is a more definitive means of evaluating specific allergic sensitivity. General allergists usually utilize antigen at a 1 : 100 w/v concen-

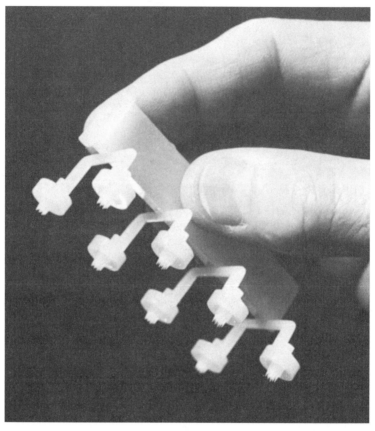

FIGURE 6–6. The Multi-Test device. This instrument produces more uniform and reproducible results in comparison with standard prick tests. Testing can generally be performed more rapidly using this device, especially the most recent modification. However, quantification is more limited than with intradermal titration or RAST. (Courtesy of Lincoln Diagnostics, P.O. Box 1128, Decatur, IL 62525.)

tration for single-dilution intradermal testing, testing only with this concentration and only after a negative prick test result for that same antigen. A special testing syringe with an incorporated fine needle and an intradermal bevel is used. The antigen is introduced into the outermost level of the skin to produce a skin wheal, generally 1 to 3 mm in diameter (Fig. 6–7). Control wheals of histamine (positive control) and diluent (negative control) are also placed. The results are read after 15 to 20 minutes, with both the size of the wheal and the surrounding erythema measured. The measurement most commonly used is the average of the maximum and minimum diameter of

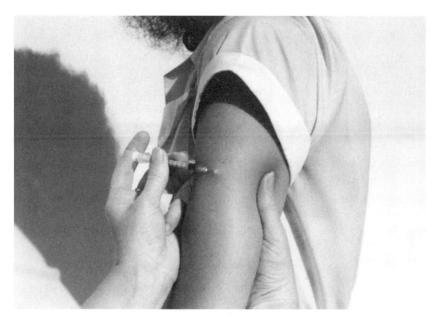

FIGURE 6–7. Intradermal testing: proper technique. The material is deposited in the outer layers of the skin; the wheal produced should be regular and firm.

the reaction produced. The presence of pseudopods is also noted. Grading on a 0 to 4+ scale, in comparison with controls, is carried out.[8] Unfortunately, as with prick testing, more than one schema for reporting single-dilution intradermal test results is in use.

The antigen described above for single-dilution intradermal testing was a 1 : 100 w/v solution. Today, most antigens may be purchased in the traditional weight/volume (w/v) form. This indicates the weight of the antigen in milligrams per milliliter of diluting fluid. This older designation of antigen strength is being replaced by the allergy unit as standardized vaccines become available. To date, the number of antigens for which standardized extract is available is limited, but as it becomes available the standardized form is replacing the w/v form by government regulation. Details in this are presented in Chapter 10; however, for comparison of testing techniques, only the older w/v measurement is used to avoid confusion.

Like the single prick test, a single intradermal test may present difficulty in interpretation. Furthermore, as in prick testing, several methods of reporting intradermal test results exist. The responses to a prick test followed (if negative) with an intradermal test indicate either a high degree of sensitivity (positive prick test), a low degree of sensitivity (only a positive intradermal test), or no demonstrable sensitivity. This is generally quite adequate if the mode of therapy is to be environmental control, in which case only the major offenders need to be identified, or if pharmacotherapy is to be the treatment approach. (In this case, however, it is reasonable to question the need for specific testing at all.) For immunotherapy, this approach is acceptable and has been in use for many decades, but it is far from optimal. Most otolaryngologists, and many other practicing physicians, have felt dissatisfied with the approach described and wished for greater accuracy and quantification of sensitivity to treat effectively by immunotherapy. This desire led to the development of *skin endpoint titration* (SET), once called *serial dilution endpoint titration* (SDET), and more recently termed *dilutional intradermal testing*. In this text, we utilize the generally accepted term, SET.

Skin Endpoint Titration

SET evolved progressively from the 1930s through the early 1960s. In principle, it is not a different approach to skin testing, but rather a refinement of the format described above, in which testing involves introducing small quantities of antigen initially, followed by larger amounts if necessary. In the SET method, quantification of the various allergens tested is accomplished by serially diluting concentrated extracts on a 1:5 basis (i.e., 1 mL of antigen diluted with 4 mL of diluent) and administering them in a sequential fashion, starting with an anticipated nonreactive strength. The fivefold dilutions advocated by Rinkel, the father of SET, were found to provide much more highly reproducible results than the 1:10 dilutional system in general use at the time.

One of the advantages of SET is that regardless of the source of any given concentrate, a bioassay for sensitivity is performed in each individual patient for that antigen, and the antigens for treatment come from the same material used in testing. The results of SET testing indicate a safe starting dose for immunotherapy. The technique of SET involves testing the individual patient with specific antigens, starting with a test dose anticipated to be both safe and nonreactive. This is generally a #6 (1:312,500) dilution, although in specific circumstances (detailed later in this chapter), an experienced and skilled tester may begin at a #4 dilution (1:12,500). Testing involves progressively applying stronger concentrations of the antigen in a controlled manner until evidence of sensitivity is demonstrated. At the point at which a definite sensitivity to the allergen is demonstrated, the testing may stop, this point indicating a safe level at which to initiate immunotherapy.

NURSE'S NOTE

Several factors influence the dilution at which SET may be begun. These include the following:

1. Experience of the tester.

2. Season and circumstances affecting current antigen exposure (the greater the exposure, the greater the expected sensitivity).

3. Antigen involved (grass is especially potent).

4. Status of the patient. A "brittle" patient, such as an asthmatic person or a patient with a history of prior severe reactions, should always be started with a very dilute (#6) antigen.

Antigen Variability and the Benefits of SET

In a few instances, commercially prepared extracts for some unusual allergenic offenders cannot be purchased. When such extracts are available, the potency may vary significantly between different suppliers and at times between different batches of extract prepared by the same supplier. Two or three decades ago, this variability was the rule rather than the exception. Such variability was often the cause of adverse reactions in patients undergoing skin testing and/or immunotherapy. Because at that time the number of commercially available extracts was much more limited than today, many active clinicians were forced to depend on antigen suppliers with less than optimal quality control, or even to prepare their own extracts. Inevitably, the uniformity of the antigens produced suffered greatly, but with SET, it was possible to compensate for this by comparing the product, regardless of uniformity, with the patient's own skin response and initiating therapy based on this response level. Provided that the allergenic extract, regardless of the source, had been adequately tested for safety, the results were still successful.

The preceding historical note puts into perspective ongoing new developments affecting available concentrations of allergenic extracts, which may in turn have a major effect on established treatment programs. The switch from w/v to standardized extracts is still in progress, and will probably remain so for a prolonged period of time. Converting established immunotherapy maintenance programs to new formats and initiating new treatment programs will present a problem for quite a while. Until the situation is stable, however, no simple conversion pattern can be useful. More about handling the current and immediately ongoing situation is discussed in Chapter 10. To apply the conversion factors as they become available and understand the changes that must be made as this occurs, it is necessary to understand the previously uniform format of SET, as all such changes must be applied to this format.

NURSE'S NOTE

Antigen manufacturers are frequently able to be of great help in the conversion from w/v to standardized extracts (from the same antigen supplier). They have information available that indicates the relationship of the previous and new antigens, and generally will share this to assist in the transition.

As discussed under the historical section on SET, variability among concentrates was for a time the rule, and communication between allergists when a patient had to move to a new area or receive care from a new allergist usually necessitated complete retesting and institution of a new immunotherapy pattern. Because of the lack of a uniform starting point, translation was essentially impossible. For reasons as yet unclear, the new regimen was frequently less effective than the previously successful one. Acknowledging this situation and the increasing mobility of the American public, the American Academy of Otolaryngic Allergy (AAOA) in 1983 began a program designed to make SET, the preferred treatment format, as uniform as possible, so that all those opting for the approach would be able to communicate with their peers and approach problems cooperatively. To achieve this end, all dilutions were to be calculated on a w/v basis, the standard of the time, and all were to be made uniform throughout the dilution format. This format blended with the modified radioallergosorbent test (mRAST) format of in vitro testing, as is discussed in Chapter 11. Since the institution of this format, many changes have taken place, and many more are scheduled to take place in the future, all with a view to producing better standardization of testing and treatment patterns. At present, however, a variety of different extract concentrations are available, and more come and go on an unpredictable basis. These changes will eventually produce antigen concentrations that will supercede the currently available ones that have traditionally been used in testing and treatment. Until stability arrives, interim adjustments will have to be made to cope with the ongoing changes. The best way to deal with these variabilities appears to be to acquire an understanding of the simple serial dilution pattern developed by the AAOA before the start of standardization for preparing and utilizing SET dilutions. The necessary conversions can then be made from these measurements as the changing patterns become stabilized.

Antigens in various concentrations are purchased from a reputable provider. Antigen may be purchased in different concentrations from commercial supply houses, but if the benefits of SET are to be realized, every attempt should be made to establish uniformity in all the testing and treatment dilutions, so that other physicians using the same technique will have as little difficulty as possible in interpreting results. To this end, an attempt is made to convert all concentrates purchased to stock antigen bottles that are as close to the same strength as possible, so that all subsequent dilutions will be the same for all antigens. Because of availability and the gradual conversion of w/v measurements to allergy units, this is not something that lends itself to a simple interim solution. Changes are occurring constantly in the form in which antigen extracts can be purchased, making a conversion scale between the different concentrations something that is subject to constant revision. This will be discussed later in the chapter. For the sake of understanding and clarifying the concept, it will be considered that all antigens may still be purchased in the more traditional w/v form, which is still the case for the majority of antigens at this present time. As noted, the 1:20 w/v concentration is more or less considered a standard "concentrate."

Some antigens are available in 1:10 w/v concentrations, and if these are chosen, they may be converted to 1:20 by diluting the concentrate with an equal quantity of diluent, keeping in mind that this also effectively halves the amount of glycerine in the resulting 1:20 solution. However, it is still highly recommended that the novice start with all antigens at the 1:20 concentration, as to do otherwise simply presents one more possibility for an error in compounding.

Performing Skin Endpoint Titration, the Otolaryngologist's Standard

The technique of SET has been taught to otolaryngologists in courses for more than 30 years. These seminars have been attended by increasing numbers of physicians of other specialties, who in turn have adopted the technique for use in their practice. Although more time-consuming in application, the format is easy to understand and reduces the subjective element present in other forms of in vivo testing. Unlike a screening prick test, followed if necessary by intradermal testing at a single dilution, all SET testing is carried out by carefully measured intradermal injection. Testing starts with the weakest dilution and progresses to the use of more concentrated antigens in five-fold increments, each increment representing one "dilution," ranging from dilution #6 (1:312,500) to dilution #1 (1:100) if skin reactions remain negative. Each skin wheal is carefully measured after it is placed, insuring that the same amount of extract has been injected each time. Wheal enlargement is measured after 10 minutes. Erythema, which is reported in prick or single-dilution skin test results, is ignored. If a wheal shows irregularity or pseudopods, it is crossed out and another test dose of the same strength is applied. This makes the test interpretation completely objective. Because all the test measurements are objective, the novice may compare results with those of a more experienced practitioner for clarification. Although not a substitute for hands-on experience at an appropriate course, for the benefit of the novice, a step-by-step introduction to SET follows.

Preparation of Equipment for Testing   The antigens initially needed for testing and treatment have been discussed under selection of antigens for therapy in Chapter 4. After these have been purchased, any that are not 1:20 are brought to this concentration. The purpose of using a uniform "concentrate" is to provide uniformity in progressive dilutions. Because of this uniformity, the allergist need not be concerned with varying degrees of sensitivity to different antigens on the part of the patient, as this variation is adjusted for automatically in the serial titration, which indicates the level at which each antigen produces an immunologic response on the part of the patient.

The various dilutions of antigen used in testing are placed in boards constructed specifically for SET. These normally accomodate 5-mL vials, a fairly standard size for testing. Testing boards may be purchased in one of a variety of standard sizes, or may be custom-made. Many allergy supply houses have their own variations available. The ideal board accommodates all the antigens likely to be needed for testing the usual number of the allergens in the area (allowing for cross-reactivity) in progressive dilutions from #1 (1:100) to #6 (1:312,500) (Fig. 6–8). Concentrates should not be placed on the testing and treatment board (even when purchased in a small enough vial to be accommodated in this space), to avoid inadvertent injection with concentrate material.

NURSE'S NOTE

Skin testing and injection is *never* performed with concentrate material. Fortunately, concentrates in the 30-mL size will not fit the holes in most boards. Even if smaller-size vials of concentrate are available, they should never be placed on the testing or treatment board, to minimize the risk for such an error. The concentrates should be kept in a separate container and brought out only for mixing vials or making a new board.

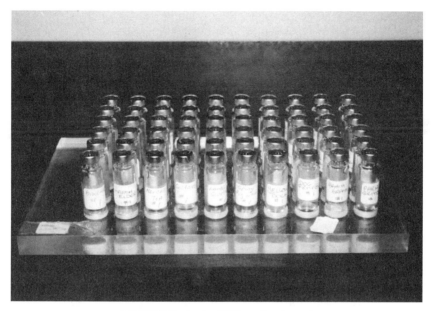

FIGURE 6–8. An SET testing board.

Serial dilutions must now be made. As discussed in the section on preparing the office, 5-mL vials should have been purchased, each containing 4 mL of buffered saline solution. These vials are labeled with the name of the antigen prepared and numbered from 1 through 6. They will eventually be placed in the holes in the board designated for that specific antigen in descending order of strength, #1 being first and #6 being last. However, for purposes of making the dilutions, it is more efficient, at this point to line the vials up from #1 to #6 on the counter and, after each dilution is made, place the vial into the proper position on the board. The allergy assistant or nurse is now prepared to make the serial dilutions.

One milliliter of concentrate is withdrawn from the concentrate vial for the antigen in question. This is injected into the vial that has been labeled with the antigen name and designated #1. Without withdrawing the needle, a series of two or three slow injections and withdrawals of the solution is performed to mix the diluted antigen thoroughly. Tilting the vial further assists in the mixing process. Next, an identical procedure is performed on the #1 dilution. That is, 1 mL of the #1 dilution is withdrawn and injected into the #2 vial. This is then gently mixed in the same manner. The same procedure is again carried out with the next vial, withdrawing from the #2 vial and injecting into the #3 vial, mixing, and proceeding in the same manner until a final injection into the #6 vial has been performed. This procedure is carried out until six serial dilutions of each antigen are present in the testing board. *It is a time-consuming procedure, requiring careful measurements and intense concentration, and must be performed when patients are not present and no interruptions are expected.* When the ''board has been made,'' the nurse or assistant is ready to perform SET.

NURSE'S NOTE

It is important to point out here that the higher number indicates that the antigen has been diluted more times, and thus is less concentrated (e.g., a #5 dilution is five times weaker than a #4 dilution). It is also confusing that otolaryngic allergists refer to ''dilutions'' #1 through #6 when they are actually speaking of varying ''concentrations.'' This is a historical precedent and unlikely to change, but it represents yet another potential pitfall and source of confusion for the novice.

If the concentrate is $1:20$ w/v, then

1 mL of concentrate $+$ 4 mL of diluent $=$ 5 mL of #1 dilution $(1:100)$
1 mL of #1 dilution $+$ 4 mL of diluent $=$ 5 mL of #2 dilution $(1:500)$
1 mL of #2 dilution $+$ 4 mL of diluent $=$ 5 mL of #3 dilution $(1:2500)$
1 mL of #3 dilution $+$ 4 mL of diluent $=$ 5 mL of #4 dilution $(1:12,500)$
1 mL of #4 dilution $+$ 4 mL of diluent $=$ 5 mL of #5 dilution $(1:62,500)$
1 mL of #5 dilution $+$ 4 mL of diluent $=$ 5 mL of #6 dilution $(1:312,500)$

One additional step is necessary to ensure the validity of the ensuing tests. This is the preparation, and subsequent application, of positive and negative control tests. Although the skin of the allergic patient is responsive to allergenic exposure, it is also subject to external influences unrelated to the allergenic sensitivity. The skin of some patients is poorly responsive to stimulation of any sort, and some patients have decreased skin responsiveness resulting from various medications, most especially antihistamines. Other patients have skin that is overly sensitive, as in dermatographia, and reacts to nonspecific stimulation unrelated to allergy. A small group of patients will demonstrate a skin reaction to the buffered saline diluent alone in a manner suggesting a positive response. To be sure that none of these conditions is affecting the validity of the skin test, negative and positive control tests should be applied before the specific tests for allergy are administered. These controls need not be placed immediately adjacent to the allergenic skin tests if space on the arm is at a premium, but if the space is available on the patient's arm, there is some benefit to be derived in the convenience of a side-by-side comparison.

The controls needed are histamine, glycerine, and buffered saline solution. Histamine is the body substance producing the majority of allergenic skin reactions. If an injection of histamine into the skin at a concentration known normally to produce a wheal comparable with that of a positive allergen response does not produce a typical wheal- and-flare reaction, there is little point in pursuing a controlled test for allergy. For one reason or another, the skin is not reactive at that time. This may be a temporary situation, as in the presence of a drug inhibiting skin reactions, which is the most common cause of skin nonreactivity. Patients should always be warned about medications that should be avoided before testing, but frequently the warnings are not successful in preventing the problem. A few patients have skin that simply reacts poorly. These patients are not good subjects for skin testing. In these cases, in vitro testing is the best option.

Histamine, used in skin testing for decades, is now available mainly in strengths more suited to producing a positive control for prick testing rather than SET. To perform the appropriate test for skin reactivity to histamine, histamine phosphate must first be purchased in the only available concentrations, 0.0275 mg/mL. To make a dilution to be used as a positive control in SET, start with a vial containing 4 mL of buffered saline diluent. One milliliter is withdrawn from the vial. To the remaining 3 mL of diluent, add 2 mL of the 0.0275 mg/mL preparation bringing the total volume to 5 mL. This is a histamine concentration comparable with a #2 allergenic extract dilution. This concentration of histamine is then diluted fivefold (#3 dilution), using the same technique outlined in the preparation of a treatment board. This #3 dilution of histamine is the test dose used to identify potential reactivity of the skin. An intradermal injection using this concentration of histamine should result in a 7-mm or larger wheal in 10 minutes, exactly as is seen in antigen testing. If this does not occur, the skin may be considered nonreactive, and further skin testing at this time must be considered unreliable. Details for preparing and using the histamine control are found in Table 6–2.

Antigen extracts are available without glycerine added as a preservative, but their shelf life is greatly reduced, and the potency of solutions for both testing and treatment declines rapidly. The use of nonglycerinated extracts causes a variability in extracts that is difficult to quantify and potentially dangerous. As the potency declines, injections for both testing and treatment decline in strength, producing unreliable information. When a new batch of extract is brought into use, the strength of the new antigen is greatly enhanced, presenting the risk for a precipitous increase in potency and a possi-

TABLE 6–2. Steps in making histamine dilutions for skin test control*

To make histamine #2 from the currently available concentration:			
Histamine, 0.0275 mg/mL	0.2 mL	1.0 mL	2.0 mL
Saline solution	0.3 mL	1.5 mL	3.0 mL
Total amount	0.5 mL	2.5 mL	5.0 mL

* Note that any amount of this material can be prepared, depending on the situation. The end product is a #2 dilution of histamine, which is then diluted fivefold in the same fashion as antigens are to make a #3 dilution. The skin test control is a wheal from the #3 dilution, and in a positive response, a 4-mm wheal should enlarge to at least 7 mm in 10 minutes. If it does not, the patient is not reacting appropriately to skin test challenge. Be certain the patient has not taken an antihistamine or tricyclic antidepressant, which suppresses skin whealing.

The histamine control begins to lose some potency after about 2 weeks and must be remade at least every 6 weeks.

ble adverse systemic reaction. A few patients are sensitive to glycerine per se, and they are usually not appropriate treatment candidates for the inexperienced allergist. In all but the rarest of cases, glycerinated extracts are indicated.

For reasons detailed earlier, glycerine in a concentration of 50% is used as a preservative in almost all commercially prepared allergenic concentrates. Although an excellent preserver of potency, glycerine itself is quite capable of inducing a significant skin reaction. In addition to skin reactions, patients receiving antigen mixes containing significant amounts of glycerine often complain of pain at the injection sites.

Skin reactivity to glycerine must be considered during skin testing. Extracts are purchased in 50% glycerine, and a skin test with this material (which is *never* recommended) would induce a strong skin rection in almost every patient, from the glycerine if not the antigen. When the 50% glycerine of the stock bottle is diluted in a ratio of 1:5, as occurs in going from a concentrate to a #1 dilution in SET, the glycerine concentration drops to 10%. In most patients, this concentration alone will still induce a significant skin reaction. A #2 dilution of extract contains 2% glycerine. This may or may not induce a skin reaction strong enough to mimic a true allergic response. Below this level, glycerine alone is not likely to affect the skin.

The skin is so variable a responder that it is not possible to make arbitrary judgments about its reactivity to glycerine. Thus, one or more glycerine control tests are placed. To prepare these, 50% glycerine (available in bulk from allergy supply houses) is diluted fivefold (#1 dilution) and again 1:5 (#2 dilution), following the format of the serial dilution of the true antigen. A test dose of a #2 dilution of glycerine (which contains 2% glycerin) is placed. If this does not cause a reaction in 10 minutes, responses to antigen tests at a #2 dilution can be assumed to be unaffected by the glycerine content at that dilution. If antigen at a #1 concentration is to be administered, a test dose of a #1 dilution of glycerine should be administered. If this does not cause a reaction in 10 minutes, it may safely be assumed that even at the #1 level test responses will not be caused by glycerine alone. If a reaction occurs to one or more dilutions of glycerine, all tests with allergenic extract must be compared with the glycerine response. Those matching the response seen to glycerine alone at the corresponding concentration must be considered no more responsive than the control, and hence negative. Responses to tests with allergen may be compared with the response to glycerine alone in the same manner as responses to other dilutions of antigen.

Buffered phenolated saline solution is used in all standard antigen dilutions. When this diluent produces a reaction, a hyperreactive condition of the skin, such as dermatographia, is usually demonstrated; in rare instances the reactivity may be caused by the phenol. Changing the diluent rarely prevents this problem. These rare patients are not usually appropriate candidates for testing by any skin test format, as reliable results cannot be expected. They require in vitro testing.

Unbuffered saline solution containing phenol as a bacteriostatic and viricidal agent is also available. Its use is rarely indicated, but the novice should appreciate the difference and be certain to obtain the buffered, phenolated saline solution.

Rare instances are said to occur in which patients are felt to be hypersensitive to phenol. As a practical matter, this is such a rarity that the novice may never see such a patient. Because the bacteriostatic and viricidal properties of phenol are important the authors feel that it should not be omitted from testing and treatment sets, and have successfully continued this practice for many decades with no adverse reactions observed.

Technique of Testing   Prick tests may be applied in almost any uniform arrangement, but SET requires the use of a clearly established test pattern because of the number of individual test injection sites and reactions that must be read. This pattern has for many years been taught to virtually all those using the SET approach, and deviation from it in current practice is minimal.

Before allergen testing is performed, the controls should have already been applied and the results of that testing read in the same fashion as is described below for the allergen skin tests (Fig. 6–9).

The test wheals are applied on the outer surface of the patient's upper

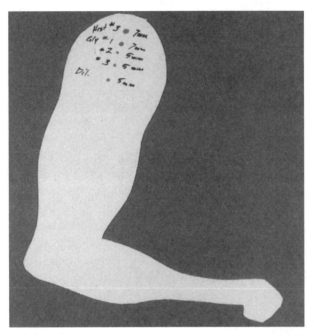

FIGURE 6–9. SET testing technique. After the arm to be used in SET testing has been cleaned with alcohol, 4-mm control wheals of histamine, diluent, and glycerine are applied as described in the text.

arm. Both arms may be used if necessary because of the number of tests applied. The arm is first cleaned with alcohol, after which the location of the tests to be performed is indicated with the use of a skin-marking pen. Numbers are placed from 6 through 1 horizontally at the top of the testing area. The marks are placed at least 2 cm apart. This is to allow for enlargement of test wheals and to minimize wheal enlargement caused by an axonal reflex stemming from an adjacent positive response. Next, the designations for the various antigens to be tested are marked along the left side of the testing area, one above the other, with the same spacing between them as between the horizontal numbers (Fig. 6–10). Intradermal skin tests are performed in the following manner: The arm is grasped from behind with the left hand (assuming the tester is right-handed), and the skin is drawn tight (Fig. 6–11). First with a #6 dilution, a small amount of antigen is drawn up into the testing syringe. Although only 0.01 mL will be injected, no attempt need be made to draw up only this amount. Such a small amount cannot be accurately premeasured in

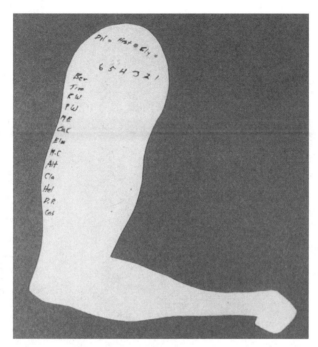

FIGURE 6–10. SET testing technique. The arm to be used in testing is now marked horizontally across the top of the testing area with the numbers 6 through 1, representing the dilutions to be tested, and vertically with abbreviations of antigens to be tested. (The controls are not shown here because of limited space.)

the syringe, as some will inevitably be lost in performing the injection. Instead, about 0.02 to 0.05 mL is drawn up. The novice will find that it is better to draw up a bit too much and waste the excess than to find an insufficient amount in the syringe should some of the material be lost in unsuccessful wheal placement.

There is a benefit in using an allergy testing syringe (rather than an injection syringe) for intradermal testing. The needle attached to the testing syringe has a short bevel. The skin test should be performed with the bevel facing downward, as this allows the needle opening to enter the skin completely in the shortest distance from the point of insertion. The less distance the needle must pass within the upper layers of skin, the less opportunity exists for damaging the skin layers; such damage makes the formation of a clear wheal impossible. In actual testing, it is frequently useful to start exerting a gentle pressure on the plunger of the syringe even before the tester is completely sure that the needle bevel is entirely

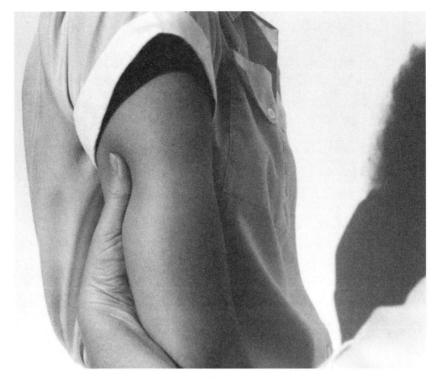

FIGURE 6–11. SET testing technique. To apply a proper intradermal wheal, the arm is grasped from behind and the skin of the upper arm stretched tight.

beneath the skin. If the bevel of the needle is down, the wheal will start to form as soon as the bevel completely enters the skin. If a slight leak occurs, it indicates that a portion of the bevel is still not beneath the surface of the skin. This is harmless. The syringe is simply advanced a little further until the leak stops and the wheal appears. The antigen solution that leaked is wiped off the arm with an alcohol sponge. A small warning is necessary at this point. If the procedure as outlined is followed with the bevel up and the insertion is incomplete when pressure is applied to the plunger, the antigen will be squirted directly upward, frequently into the eyes of the tester.

The point of the needle is introduced into the most superficial layers of the skin, while an attempt is made to keep the bevel of the needle as close to parallel to the bulge of the skin surface as possible (Fig. 6–7). Enough fluid is injected into the skin to produce a skin wheal of

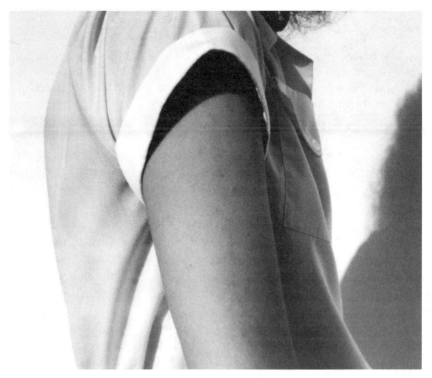

FIGURE 6–12. SET testing technique. The wheal formed by the intradermal injection should be firm and regular. If pseudopods occur, or the wheal created is not 4 mm in diameter, it should be crossed out and another applied.

4 mm in diameter. It is important after placing the wheal to measure it, to confirm that the diameter is 4 mm. Such a wheal contains almost exactly 0.01 mL of antigen solution. When properly performed, the wheal is raised, white, and round, with distinct margins and no pseudopods (Fig. 6–12). It is helpful for the beginner in visualizing the proper wheal size to remember that a 4-mm wheal is about the diameter of a saccharine tablet. This same method of wheal production is used both in testing all antigens and in forming control test sites.

It must be emphasized that it is impossible to measure 0.01 mL in a syringe and inject all of it into the skin in such a way as to form a perfect wheal. Years of experimenting have shown that the 4-mm wheal contains almost exactly 0.01 mL of antigen solution. This measurement is accurate enough to provide a basis for all subsequent treatment calculations, and clinical results have validated the concept.

NURSE'S NOTE

The tension of patients undergoing skin testing is frequently reflected in the tension of their skin. If the patient is able to relax, it is possible to create the wheal with less pressure, resulting in more accurate wheal placement and less patient discomfort.

Similar injections of #6 dilutions of each antigen to be tested are placed in a vertical row to the right of their designated positions on the arm and beneath the #6 in the top horizontal column. The entire battery of #6 antigen dilutions is placed as rapidly as is consistant with accuracy, after which a timer is set for 10 minutes. After this length of time, the injection sites are examined. It is expected that each wheal will have expanded to at least 5 mm simply from hydrostatic pressure, and if negative will also have lost firmness and some definition. When this occurs, and no other changes are evident, the reaction is considered negative; that is, the patient is not sensitive to that antigen at the weak dilution tested.

Let us consider negative reactions first. If all the #6 dilution wheals show no evidence of progression, the same format may be used to place #5 and #4 dilutions, also in vertical rows, beneath the #5 and #4 in the top horizontal line and to the right of the #6 test sites. These two rows of injections may be placed at the same time if the reaction to the #6 injection is negative. The safety of this incremental increase has been confirmed by decades of testing using this format. The reason that both #5 and #4 dilutions must be tested will become apparent when the interpretation of results is discussed; the concept of both an endpoint wheal and a confirming wheal is involved. After the #5 and #4 wheals are placed, the timer is again set for 10 minutes, after which the injection sites are examined. If both the #5 and #4 dilutions produce negative reactions, #3 and #2 dilutions are injected in the same manner and the results read after 10 minutes. If all reactions are negative, #1 dilutions may be placed, but for these to be read reliably they must be compared with #1 dilutions of the glycerine control. If the injection sites match the control, and if all #1 wheals are the same, it must be assumed that the reaction is caused by the glycerine alone, and the responses must be considered negative. (Actually, if all #2 sites are positive, they must be compared with the glycerine control, as this is more likely to indicate a more pronounced sensitivity to glycerine than a reaction at this level to all antigens. A positive reaction to all antigens would be most unusual, at least at the same level.)

Negative test results may indicate a nonallergic cause of the patient's problems or may suggest the need for additional tests of other antigens. This is discussed in Chapter 13, Nonallergic Rhinitis. If the test results are positive, they must be interpreted to determine the presence and degree of sensitivity for each antigen.

A negative wheal is an initial 4-mm-diameter wheal that enlarges to no more than 5 mm in a 10-minute period, usually also becoming soft and less well defined. By definition, a positive wheal is one that enlarges to a size at least 2 mm greater in diameter than that of the preceding negative wheal, and that initiates a similar pattern of progression in size in succeeding wheals of increasing strength. In the usual case, if additional wheals of increasing strength are placed on the patient's arm, each shows a similar progression in size. A typical pattern of wheal size is 5 mm, 7 mm, and 9 mm (Fig. 6–13). Although additional growth in 2-mm increments would be expected of wheals placed with progressively stronger antigens, it is important to realize that in practice, only two wheals showing a positive progression are applied after the last negative wheal. This is in the interest of safety; adverse reactions are extremely rare when this pattern is followed.

The first positive wheal does not provide a definite diagnosis. It may herald one of the patterns of bizarre whealing to be discussed later. However, two successive positive wheals, each increasing in size as described, establish a pattern of allergic sensitivity that may be relied on. Following this testing format produces a pattern on the patient's arm that may easily be read, and indicates not only the presence of allergy but the degree of sensitivity to each allergen tested. It also indicates an "endpoint" of titration: the point at which negative testing becomes positive. The importance of this level of response will be made clear when immunotherapy is discussed. Because determining the endpoint for each antigen is the goal of all titration testing, it may be well at this point to define the endpoint clearly. This definition should be kept in mind when any questionable result is interpreted. The endpoint is the first positive wheal that follows a series of negative wheals and that initiates progressive whealing. The wheal marking the endpoint must be at least 2 mm larger than the preceding negative wheal, and each subsequent wheal in the progression must be at least 2 mm larger than the wheal that precedes it. This definition may be applied to both the standard progression and to the bizarre whealing reactions to be described. For example, a whealing sequence of 5 mm, 7 mm, and 9 mm would have the 7-mm wheal as the endpoint. If the sequence were 5 mm, 6 mm, and 8 mm, the endpoint would be the 8-mm wheal, as the 6-mm wheal is not 2 mm larger than the preceding 5-mm, negative wheal. In this case, an additional wheal

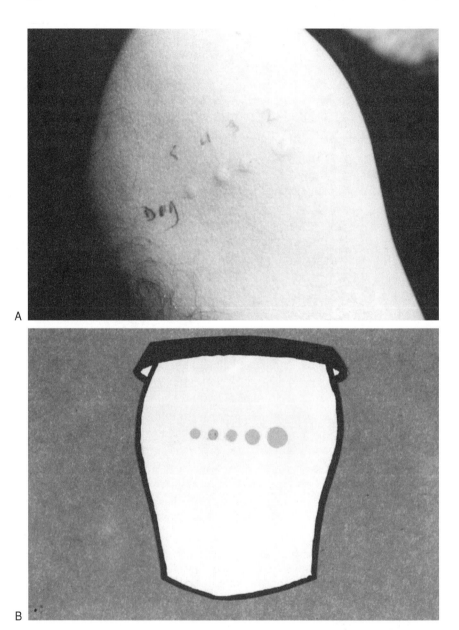

A

B

FIGURE 6–13. (A,B). Typical SET result. As progressively stronger concentrations of antigen are applied, the negative wheals on the left are followed by a positive wheal, then by a confirming wheal, which is even larger.

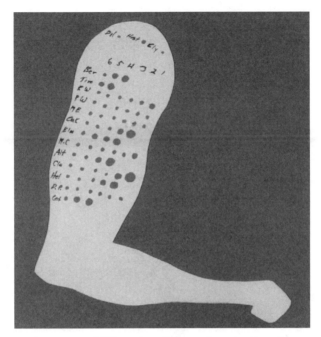

FIGURE 6–14. Completed SET testing. When all testing has been completed as described in the text, each positive antigen should show a definite endpoint. Testing is stopped after the confirming wheal has been applied. The endpoints are recorded on the titration sheet.

at the next stronger concentration would have to be applied, as one confirming wheal above the endpoint is needed to validate the progression.

Vertical Testing: A Shortcut The above format, representing the classic testing pattern for SET, is known as *linear testing* (Fig. 6–14). It is recommended for all novices, and must be completed if any variation in responses appears probable. Its only disadvantage is that it is relatively time-consuming, and patients do not relish all the intradermal injections that may be needed to establish reliable endpoints. A shortcut, known as *vertical testing*, may reduce both the testing time necessary and the number of intradermal injections, without compromising the result. For these reasons, most experienced skin-testing practitioners utilize vertical testing, but those who wish to employ this shortcut must be aware that confirmation of results obtained with limited linear testing will be necessary.

In the description of the method used in performing linear testing, it was noted that if the #6 dilution produces a negative wheal, the #5 and #4 dilutions

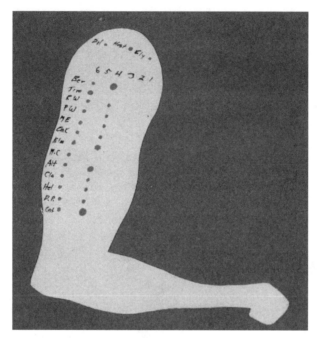

FIGURE 6–15. Vertical testing. Vertical testing is a shortcut that saves time and reduces the number of injections needed. After a #6 dilution is applied, if the result is negative, a #4 dilution may be applied, with #5 skipped temporarily. When a positive wheal appears, linear testing for the endpoint of this antigen must be completed.

may be applied at the same time. This is a safe procedure, because if the #5 dilution were to be, applying a #4 dilution would be necessary in any case to confirm the progression. With this borne in mind, if the #6 dilution is negative, the #5 dilution may be skipped at least temporarily, and only the #4 dilution applied. If the #4 dilution is also negative, the #2 dilution may be applied, with the #3 dilution temporarily skipped until the response has been determined (Fig. 6–15). This application of every other dilution saves time for the person performing the tests, and spares the patient a few injections. However, when one of the test results is positive, the skipped injections above and/or below it must be applied until a clear progression over three strengths (one negative followed by a positive wheal and a confirming, larger wheal) has been demonstrated. This establishment of a definite progression is necessary to prevent an inaccurate reading of the endpoint in the instances in which an unusual form of whealing occurs.

Unusual Whealing Reactions As has been stressed previously, the human body does not always follow prescribed patterns exactly. When the format described for administering SET is followed, most often a normal progression of wheals will occur: a series of negative wheals followed by increments in diameter of 2 mm or more for each stronger wheal. In a small percentage of cases, however, the whealing pattern deviates from normal. Fortunately, most of these deviations follow a predictable pattern, and the endpoint can still be determined reliably once the deviation has been recognized.

The most common form of bizarre whealing is the "flash response." This is characterized by the appearance of an exceptionally large wheal, frequently 10 to 15 mm in diameter, following a succession of negative wheals. An example would be wheals of 5 mm, 5 mm, 5 mm, and 12 mm (Fig. 6–16). The flash response does not represent an endpoint. Why it occurs is not known, although it has been postulated that it caused by the presence of a food to which the patient is allergic in the patient's system at the time of testing. The best approach to a flash response is to terminate testing of the antigen involved and have the patient return the following day (or later), at which time that particular test is repeated. The flash will rarely appear again. In most cases, a classic whealing pattern will appear, and a clear endpoint may be identified in the usual manner. This endpoint will usually be at a considerably higher level (i.e., a more concentrated level of antigen) than the level at which the flash response occurred, allowing the treatment to be started safely at a higher level and thereby speeding the results obtained from immunotherapy.

The second most common type of bizarre whealing seen is the "plateau response," in which a series of negative wheals is followed by two, three, or more positive wheals of the same size before a progression is established. An example would be wheals of 5 mm, 5 mm, 7 mm, 7 mm, 7 mm, and 9 mm (Fig. 6–17). The plateau response provides a good example of the advantages of arbitrarily following the definition of the endpoint. The first 7-mm wheal is 2 mm larger than the preceding negative wheal, but it does not initiate progressive whealing. The third 7-mm wheal is followed by a 9-mm wheal, and therefore represents the endpoint. It has been shown that if the sequence of injections is continued in the usual fashion, after the plateau, progressive wheal enlargement almost always occurs. However, as with all SET, testing beyond the formation of a confirming wheal is not normally continued, as once the endpoint has been identified, further testing only risks the possibility of an adverse reaction.

The third most common form of bizarre reaction is the "hourglass response." This is rarely seen today, as it has become standard practice to start testing at a #6 dilution. Before the level of antigen necessary to produce

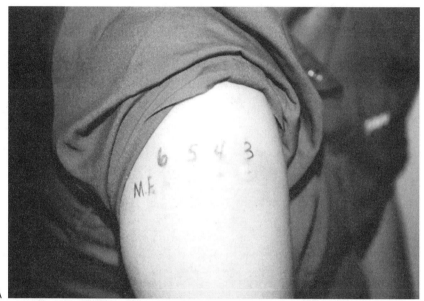

A

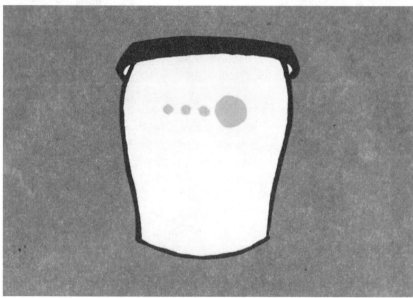

B

FIGURE 6–16. (A,B). Unusual whealing responses. Flash response, the most common form of bizarre whealing. Several negative wheals are followed by an extremely large wheal. This is not a true endpoint, and usually indicates a concomitant food sensitivity. Testing for this antigen should be stopped, and the test repeated in a day or so. The endpoint will usually be considerably higher.

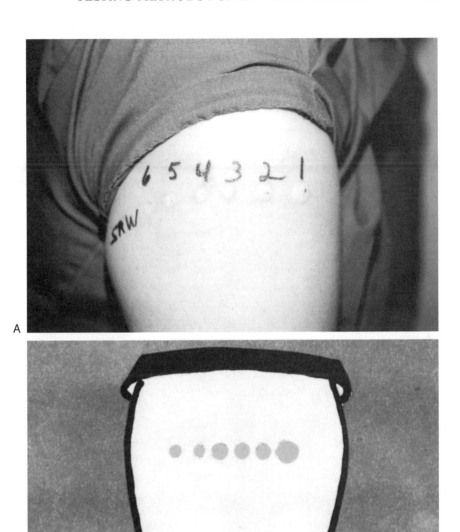

FIGURE 6–17. (A,B). Unusual whealing responses. Plateau response. Negative wheals are followed by a series of endpoint-sized wheals before a confirming wheal initiates further progression. The final wheal before the confirming wheal represents the true endpoint.

an immunologic reaction was accurately determined, it was common practice to begin testing at a #10 dilution (almost a 1 : 200,000,000 w/v concentration of antigen). Under this format, hourglass responses were common. In the hourglass response, a weak test dilution may produce a larger wheal than the succeeding stronger dilution, which in turn is followed by a still smaller wheal with the next stronger dilution. There may then appear negative wheals, followed by a usual sequence of progressively larger wheals. An example would be wheals of 9 mm, 7 mm, 5 mm, 5 mm, 7 mm, and 9 mm (Fig. 6–18). Here again, according to the complete definition of the endpoint, the true endpoint would be the second 7-mm wheal (followed by the 9-mm wheal).

It has become evident after years of experience with SET and variations on this format that skin reactivity may be present and progressive well below the level at which systemic immunologic responses can occur. Hourglass responses have been documented as appearing below a #20 dilution, expanding and contracting repeatedly. The reason for these skin responses is not understood; however, the fact is well established that immunologic effects on the body do not occur without stronger doses of antigen. Treating skin reactions produced by antigens tested at a level weaker than a #6 dilution is generally of little or no value, although it poses no significant risk. On occasion, a wheal appearing on a #6 dilution may show significant enlargement. The person performing the test must now determine which of several possibilities is causing this reaction: First, the reaction could be legitimate, indicating an endpoint. Although it is generally accepted that it is usually unnecessary to begin therapy at a concentration of antigen below a #6 level, this does not eliminate positive skin responses below that level. It simply means that treatment may safely be started in all cases at a #6 level. Reactions at strengths weaker than this will not induce immunologic activity in the patient as a rule. Second, the reaction could be part of an hourglass response, in which the true endpoint will be at a much stronger dilution. Third, the reaction could be a flash response, in which case the true endpoint will usually also be at a much stronger level. What procedure may be used to determine safely which reaction is actually occurring?

The simplest way to proceed is to make up a #7 dilution, diluting the #6 dilution fivefold as for all the previous dilutions. This will not occur frequently, so maintaining the #7 dilution on the testing board will not be necessary except for this particular test (and it will probably be out of date before it is used again). The patient is asked to return on another day, and at that time a wheal is raised using the #7 dilution. If the wheal grows larger than that from the #6 dilution, the original #6 response represents part of an

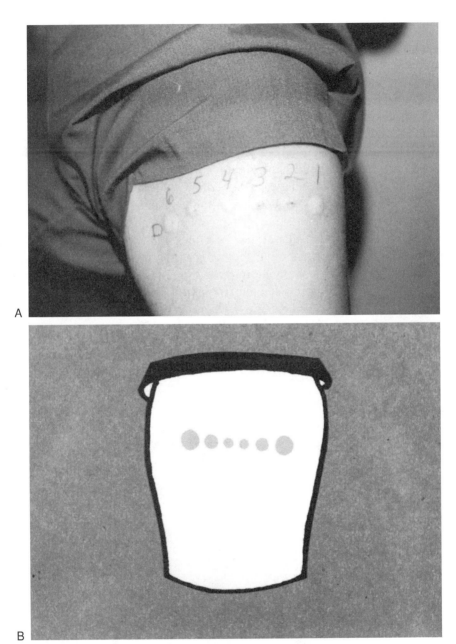

FIGURE 6–18. (A,B). Unusual whealing responses. Hourglass response. In this pattern, large wheals produced by testing with weak dilutions are followed by smaller wheals progressing to negative wheals as the antigen strength increases. These negative wheals are in turn followed by wheals of increasing size in a normal pattern, which will determine the true endpoint.

hourglass, and dilutions #5 and #4 may be applied as described. The usual pattern will be a reduction in the size of each succeeding test until a negative response is reached, after which successively larger test wheals will appear; the endpoint may then be determined as described previously for hourglass reactions. If the #7 dilution wheal is negative, the response is almost certainly a flash, and testing for this antigen may be continued in a normal fashion. If the #7 dilution wheal is slightly smaller than the #6, indicating a normal whealing progression, it may represent a true endpoint. If there is a question, RAST may prove helpful in clarifying the skin response. It should be borne in mind that experience has repeatedly shown that treatment may safely be started at a #6 dilution, even with the whealing response described. However, some practitioners prefer a cautious approach and choose to start treatment at the #7 dilution, and this cannot be criticized, although it is not really necessary. The discrepancy will be corrected as the doses escalate. What should be avoided is continuing to prepare and test even weaker dilutions, as this may lead to starting treatment at impossibly low doses that provide no benefit. Starting treatment at a #6 dilution, considering this an endpoint under the circumstances described, is safe. Dropping back one more dilution may relieve the therapist of anxiety. Diluting the treatment further is not productive.

Advantages of SET   The advantages of SET are multiple. First, uniformity of interpretation is greatly improved. The test pattern shows a definite scale, progressing from clearly negative reactions to progressively positive reactions as increasing strengths of the same antigen are applied, a sequence that is easy to interpret. Second, the format has proved extremely safe, as the starting test dose has been shown to be too weak to initiate an adverse immunologic response. Third, the quantitative approach identifies the strongest safe dose at which to initiate immunotherapy, hastening the production of symptom relief. Injections may be safely started at the level of the first test wheal showing a positive reaction, as this wheal and the confirming wheal contain the antigenic equivalent of the first treatment dose. These are unique characteristics of SET.

Through the years, various misinformation has been generated regarding SET, primarily by those who do not understand the procedure. Some of this misinformation results from a confusion between SET-based therapy and the earlier, very low-dose immunotherapy advocated by Hansel. In other instances, a misinterpretation of the technique resulted in erroneous assumptions. Unfortunately, some adverse remarks about the technique stemmed from physicians concerned that practitioners using SET might lure patients from their practice. For those who intend to use this approach to diagnosis and therapy, it is important that the true, unique characteristics of SET be known and understood. The approach is not different from the other skin test approaches already described, but is rather a refinement and quantification of the testing procedures in use since the advent of inhalant allergy testing.

The fivefold dilution format for testing was developed as a compromise alternative to the decimal dilution that was initially attempted by the originators of titration testing but proved difficult to replicate regularly. Tenfold dilutional testing and treatment based on it were more likely to produce adverse test reactions. Even narrower spacing of dilutions is more specific and is used in research settings for standardization and quantification. For example, the Bureau of Biologics uses a threefold dilution to standardize extracts. However, calculations based on these numbers are excessively time-consuming and clumsy for the clinician. Most physicians are familiar with the decimal format used in most medical measurements, but it has already been shown that a decimal system of extract dilution provides a high risk for reactions. A fivefold dilution system is almost as easy to use as a decimal system, and certainly less cumbersome than a threefold or sevenfold system. Fortuitously, the fivefold system used in SET also correlates well with the steps between classes of the Fadal-Nalebuff mRAST system.

Extracts Although as much accuracy as possible is desirable, allergy is an inexact science at best. The key to obtaining satisfactory results is a combination of concern and flexibility. The clinician should demand the most uniform extracts available for testing and treatment, so as to provide the most uniform point from which to start. With Food and Drug Administration control, and especially with the move to standardized extracts, it is unlikely that any licensed commercial laboratory will produce and market a truly inferior extract. The extracts must then be handled with care in the office; they must not be exposed to excessive heat or temperature fluctuation, and not kept past their expiration dates. Mixing for testing should be done every 6 weeks, and if one or two dilutions of an antigen run low, the entire sequence (#1 through #6) should be remade for that antigen. Concentrated bulk antigens preserved in 50% glycerine have a long shelf life. Treatment vials mixed to contain 10% glycerine are potent for 3 months. Antigens not containing this amount of glycerine as a preservative expire within 4 to 6 weeks after the time they are made. Following these directions should keep testing material adequately reliable. Even so, some variations may occur. Fortunately, these should be minor in nature, and such minor variables will be corrected automatically during immunotherapy as dose advancement is pursued. SET is the most quantified approach to allergy care in use at present, but it is not perfect. Outside influences affect the accuracy of testing, but not enough to invalidate the studies. Concerned clinicians who wish the best results for their patients and who opt for the use of SET should make every effort to keep the testing material as accurately prepared and uniform as possible. At the same time, it must be realized that allergy skin testing, even with SET, is perhaps not as well quantified as we would like. Antigens, even standardized antigens, may vary in antigenic potency by up to 400% between batches. Fortunately for the clinician, some leeway is allowable. When appropriate antigens for testing are purchased, and when these are prepared and handled properly in the office, the end results of testing and subsequent treatment should be highly satisfactory. Limiting the variables as much as possible aids in this. Accepting the compromise between perfection and practicality is necessary at this stage. The approach to testing described provides an excellent starting point for therapy. Adjustments may be made later as the need becomes apparent.

IN VITRO TESTS

The amount of space devoted in this chapter to in vitro tests is less than that given to skin tests. This is for the simple reason that skin tests can be performed by any office practitioner of allergy, but they demand a careful adherence to technique and interpretation to ensure safety and effectiveness. On the other hand, it is unusual for the practitioner to perform laboratory tests in the office, instead utilizing reference laboratories for this purpose. Therefore, only a general discussion of the actual technique of these tests is included, centering primarily on their interpretation and proper use.

Unlike the in vivo tests previously described, in vitro (literally, "in glass") tests are performed on the patient's blood. Once the blood has been drawn, the patient need not be present while the tests are being performed. This difference in format has made in vitro testing extremely popular with a majority of patients, owing to the substitution of a single venipuncture for multiple skin tests; although properly performed skin tests are not truly painful, they are undeniably uncomfortable. In addition, the use of the in vitro test greatly reduces the time the patient need spend in the physician's office. In vivo testing may take a matter of hours, requiring time away from work, or the services of a baby-sitter. In today's market, in which time may be a major factor in evaluating cost, in vitro testing presents a distinct advantage.

The in vitro tests most widely used today are the RAST (radio-allergosorbent test) and the ELISA (enzyme-linked immunosorbent assay). These tests are based on the same general principles, and understanding the RAST makes understanding the ELISA and its variations relatively simple. A basic understanding of the principles involved in RAST and ELISA makes interpretation more meaningful and aids in the evaluation of other in vitro tests, some of which are already available and others in preparation for the market. No extensive immunologic background is necessary for the clinician to order these tests and understand how they are performed and interpreted.

NURSE'S NOTE

The in vitro tests in common use are run on serum. Blood samples must be obtained in a tube that does not contain a clot inhibitor, and then allowed to clot. They are next centrifuged, and the serum is decanted. The use of a separator-type tube aids in the separation of serum from the clot in this process. If a centrifuge is unavailable or inoperative, the blood can be allowed to stand overnight; generally, separation of the clot from serum is sufficient to allow enough serum to be decanted for testing. Generally, the serum is withdrawn using a bulb pipette and transferred into an appropriate screw-top, break-resistant container. Individual reference laboratories will provide information on sample preparation and material to assist in shipping samples.

Although the samples do not normally suffer significant deterioration at ambient temperatures during shipping, they should be kept refrigerated (or frozen) if shipping is to be delayed, and during summer months they should never be left in a hot mailbox for prolonged periods before being picked up.

The RAST and ELISA depend on the identification of allergen-specific IgE in the patient's serum. As noted earlier, IgE is present in 20 to 30% of the population in greater than trace amounts. This increase, a genetically determined abnormality of the immune system, is the source of essentially all inhalant allergy and a small segment of food allergy. IgE in the allergic patient is present in the blood, and is also fixed to mast cells in the skin and many other organs. Except for the skin, the most common location of mast cells is in the mucosa of the respiratory tract, although some are present in the heart and gastrointestinal tract. Measuring the amount of serum IgE specific to a particular allergen gives a direct, quantitative measurement of the degree of sensitivity to that allergen. This measurement is comparable with the quantitative measurement of IgE made on the skin by SET. In most cases, the degree of sensitivity indicated by specific IgE levels tends to parallel the severity of the patient's symptoms, but it is important to note that this is not always the case.

The first test for allergy to be developed based on IgE measurement was the PRIST (paper radioimmunosorbent test). This test measured the total amount of IgE in the patient's serum rather than the amount of IgE specific to an individual allergen. It was hoped that this test would separate the allergic patient from the nonallergic patient, opening the way for additional testing on the allergic patient alone, but this did not prove to be the case. Although there was a general tendency for the patient with high IgE levels to be allergic, a significant number of patients with low levels of total IgE proved to be highly sensitive to a limited number of allergens, and it was also possible for various pathogens, such as parasites, to produce a high level of IgE in the absence of allergy. PRIST is one of the more costly of the in vitro allergy tests, and despite the fact that it is still frequently used, it is not of enough value to be recommended as a routine test today. Understanding the principles of the PRIST, however, may make the RAST and ELISA easier to understand.

PRIST

The PRIST is performed with a test tube containing a paper disk to which anti-IgE (produced in laboratory animals) is bound. The patient's serum is placed in the test tube and allowed to incubate with the anti-IgE on the disk. In time, if IgE is present in the patient's serum, it binds to the anti-IgE on the disk. After appropriate washing to remove the serum and substances that are not IgE, a solution is added to the test tube containing additional anti-IgE bound to a radioactive marker. After further incubation, this radioactive anti-IgE binds to the already bound IgE, creating a complex consisting of the anti-IgE bound to the disk, the IgE from the patient's serum bound to the anti-IgE, and the radioactively labeled anti-IgE, now bound to the patient's IgE. The excess, unbound radioactive anti-IgE is washed off, leaving a complex in which IgE is firmly fixed between two layers of anti-IgE. This arrangement is referred to as the "sandwich technique." The most important portion of this complex is the IgE, the "meat" of the sandwich. The disk is placed in a gamma counter, and the amount of radioactivity present indicates the amount of radioactive anti-IgE present, which provides a quantitative measure of the total amount of IgE that is firmly bound on an exactly determined basis to the anti-IgE (Fig. 6–19).

The PRIST is not used extensively in clinical practice, but it remains of historic interest. The PRIST is the original test from which the RAST and ELISA were derived.

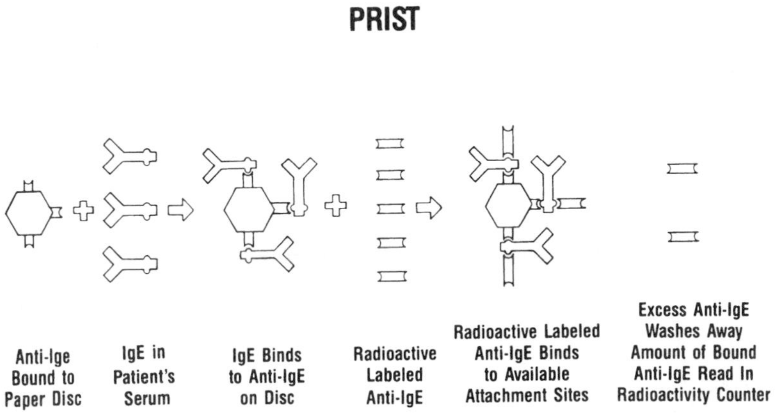

PRIST

Anti-IgE Bound to Paper Disc	IgE in Patient's Serum	IgE Binds to Anti-IgE on Disc	Radioactive Labeled Anti-IgE	Radioactive Labeled Anti-IgE Binds to Available Attachment Sites	Excess Anti-IgE Washes Away Amount of Bound Anti-IgE Read In Radioactivity Counter

FIGURE 6–19. Paper radioimmunosorbent test (PRIST). The original in vitro test, the PRIST measures the total amount of IgE in the patient's serum. It was hoped that this test would be a decisive indication of the presence or absence of inhalant allergy. Unfortunately, this was not the case and the uses of the test today are limited. (From King HC. An Otolaryngologist's Guide to Allergy. New York: Thieme Medical Publishers;1990:87.)

RAST

The RAST is considered the ''gold standard'' of in vitro testing, in that all other such tests are usually compared with the RAST. In the RAST, as in the PRIST, a matrix is used, usually a paper disk placed in a test tube. To this disk is bound a specific antigen (e.g., ragweed). The patient's serum is allowed to incubate with the disk, and allergen-specific IgE in the serum binds to the particular antigen on the disk. Note that IgE specific for other antigens (e.g., cat) will not form any attachments. When the disk is washed by rinsing the tube containing it, IgE specific to other allergens (and thus not bound to the disk) is removed from the test tube. After this washing, a solution containing radioactively labeled anti-IgE is added and allowed to incubate with the disk in the tube. The radiolabeled anti-IgE binds to the existing complex of allergen-specific IgE from the patient's serum and the antigen on the disk. A second washing is performed, removing the unbound and excess radioactively labeled anti-IgE. The disk is then transferred to a clean test tube, where the bound, allergen-specific IgE level is measured by determining the degree of radioactivity using a gamma counter (Fig. 6–20). This gives an accurate measurement of the IgE specific to the antigen selected.

Types of RAST

When originally developed, the RAST was felt to be an interesting laboratory study but of little clinical use. The original developers were concerned with

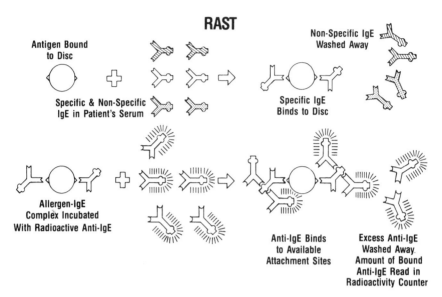

FIGURE 6–20. Radioallergosorbent test (RAST). The first allergen-specific in vitro test, the RAST indicates the amount of IgE in the patient's serum reacting directly to the individual allergen under investigation. (From King HC. An Otolaryngologist's Guide to Allergy. New York: Thieme Medical Publishers;1990:86.)

designing a test a high degree of specificity. To obtain specificity, a degree of sensitivity was sacrificed. In fact, the original Phadebas RAST was highly specific, but so insensitive that a large percentage of patients with negative test scores were proved to be clinically allergic by their response to direct exposure to the allergens being tested. This situation was addressed by two clinicians, Richard Fadal and Donald Nalebuff. They modified the technique for the test and adjusted the scale by which results were graded. The result was the Fadal-Nalebuff modified RAST (F/N mRAST). This version gave results that correlated well with SET, and results from the two forms of testing could be interchanged with only moderate adjustment. It is important to differentiate between the F/N mRAST and the original Phadebas RAST, which is also routinely available from reference laboratories (Fig. 6–21). The clinician should be aware of the difference and specify the form desired. If the test is to be used for clinical care, the mRAST is the version that closely parallels SET.

ELISA

Even in the earliest days of RAST, it was felt by many that RAST would not be the final stage in the evolution of in vitro analysis. The equipment

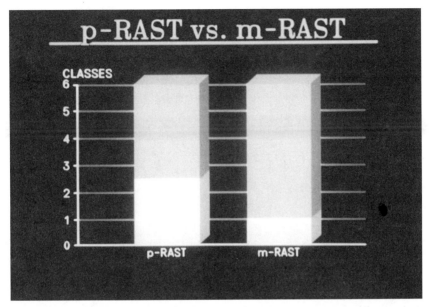

FIGURE 6–21. Comparison of original RAST and Fadal-Nalebuff mRAST. It is evident that a significant differences exists between the two, mainly in regard to the "cut-off" point of clinical significance. The mRAST has been shown to correlate well with SET.

was large and expensive, and there was governmental concern about the disposal of radioactive waste, even though the degree of radioactivity involved was minimal. RAST was also noted to be slightly less sensitive than skin testing, even with the mRAST refinements. Based on RAST technology, a second form of in vitro testing was developed. This testing format is very similar to RAST, with the exception that it uses an enzyme-activated marker rather than a radioactive marker for measuring the amount of bound IgE. This enzyme produces a reaction resulting in changes in the test solution that may be colorimetric, fluorometric, or even chemoluminescent in nature. The amount of the marking material, and therefore the amount of bound specific IgE, can then be assayed in an appropriate reader. For the colorimetric markers, the reader is a colorimeter. For the fluorometric markers, the reader is a fluorometer. Chemoluminescent markers are exposed to Polaroid film and the density of the film exposure is measured. The testing modality that uses such markers is known as *enzyme-linked immunosorbent assay* (ELISA) (Fig. 6–22).

Although the principle of the ELISA is essentially identical to that of the RAST, in many ways the ELISA is more versatile than the RAST. Many

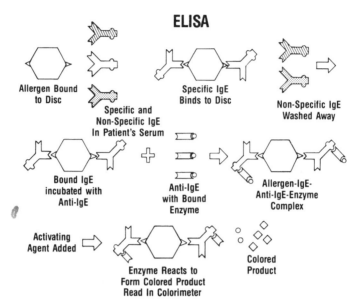

FIGURE 6–22. Enzyme-linked immunosorbent assay (ELISA). The in vitro test succeeding the RAST, the ELISA uses the same principles but uses an enzymatic marker rather than a radioactive marker. (From King HC. An Otolaryngologist's Guide to Allergy. New York: Thieme Medical Publishers;1990:91.)

variations on the technology are possible, and more are appearing constantly. The equipment necessary to perform ELISA is also much less expensive than RAST equipment, making it more affordable for the physician's office laboratory. However, one caveat is necessary in this regard: At the present time, governmental regulations (the Clinical Laboratory Improvement Act of 1988, or CLIA '88) have so restricted in-office laboratories that the required quality controls and restrictions are nearly prohibitive. It is accepted that quality control of laboratory results is necessary. Nevertheless, allergy testing is an inexact science at best. Skin testing, not subject to the same controls as in vitro testing, is far more variable. However, governmental regulations are always subject to change, and socioeconomic or medical pressure to return in vitro allergy tests to the physician's office laboratory may well alter this situation in the future.

Although the principle of the ELISA remains similar for all technologies, the amount of equipment available for performing the tests varies extensively. Basic testing may require only the use of a centrifuge to separate blood cells from serum, an appropriate incubator and washer, and a reader. This may be expanded to major automation, in which almost everything is done automatically. One of the simplest ELISA has been the one utilizing chemoluminescence as a marker; it requires very little equipment. However, even that test can be automated to a greater degree if the practitioner so desires. The ELISA system, then, is available in almost any degree of complexity the clinician wishes and is prepared to pay for.

ELISA also have a wide range of other uses (including testing for AIDS), but these are outside the range of a text on allergy.

The technologies already mentioned are those most often used for ELISA at the present time. Other methodologies are available. The simplest of these, as a group, are the dipstick tests. These also are based on the determination of IgE and follow the same format as the more definitive ELISA. At present, they are semiquantitative, but the potential exists for these tests to approach the quantification level seen in the more complex ELISA. At present, they are most appropriate for the primary care physician who is not interested in administering allergy immunotherapy, but who wishes only to determine the presence or absence of true allergy, identify some of the major offenders, and make an appropriate referral to someone prepared to treat the problem definitively. The ability to do this improves the image of the referring physician, who demonstrates a degree of understanding of another, pertinent field, even though not choosing to render specific immunotherapy.

The dipstick test comes in a kit. It is not expensive, requires no special equipment, and may be ordered from the manufacturer in a format containing representative index inhalant antigens appropriate to the region of the country in which the patient resides. All directions for performing the test are included in the kit. More than one manufacturer produces the tests, but the format is similar for all. The patient's blood is drawn, and the serum is separated from the cells by centrifuge. The serum is then placed in a test tube supplied, and a "dipstick" is placed in the serum. This dipstick, usually of paper, consists of a series of bands containing the appropriate allergens to be assayed, plus a control. After incubation with the serum, the dipstick is passed through a series of incubations and tap water rinses, and finally compared with a test card showing the allergen bands and the possible degrees of colorimetric response (Fig. 6–23). The test is quite reliable, although only semiquantitative at best, as the technology is basically the same as that of other ELISA formats. More exact quantification may be available in the future.

RAST and ELISA technology may be used to test for inhalant allergy, insect sting allergy, and the limited number of food sensitivities produced by IgE. Testing for drug allergy by these formats may eventually be possible, but at the present time this application is quite limited. It is hoped that reliable in vitro drug allergy testing will be perfected in the near future, allowing

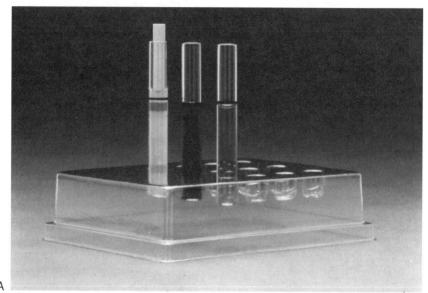

A

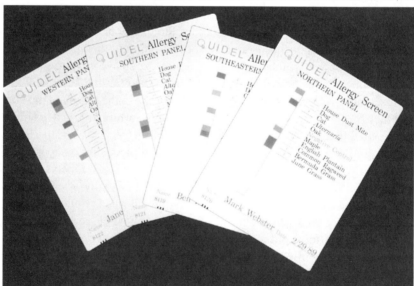

B

FIGURE 6–23. (A,B) A dipstick screening test for inhalant allergy. The dipstick is incubated with the patient's serum, then a series of chemicals. This produces gradation of color in areas on the dipstick representing specific antigens. Dipstick are available that contain key antigens for different areas of the country. (Courtesy of Quidel Co., San Diego, CA.)

differentiation of adverse reactions (e.g., diarrhea, vague rash) from true drug allergy.

Basophil Histamine Release Test

One additional test for inhalant allergy deserves special mention, as it employs a completely different method of operation from those previously described. This is the basophil histamine release test (BHRT). This test permits assaying the degree of sensitivity to specific allergens without regard to the production and/or presence of IgE. Like other in vitro tests, the BHRT is performed on the patient's blood. Unlike the RAST and ELISA, which measure the amount of allergen-specific IgE in the serum, the BHRT measures the amount of histamine released into the serum by the blood basophils after specific antigen exposure. The test depends on an affinity of histamine for glass microfibrils, to which the histamine attaches so that it can then be measured. The advantage of the test is that it opens up to analysis hypersensitivity reactions that result in the release of histamine by means other than the production of IgE. This includes some food reactions, and other responses that result in the release of histamine without directly involving the immune system. This type of reaction is discussed in more detail in Chapter 14. For example, the ingestion of certain foods, such as strawberries and tomatoes, results in the production of vasoactive amines, and susceptible persons may react to them in a fashion sometimes perceived as ''food allergy.'' Other foods, such as red wine, chocolate, and red meat, may cause the release of histamine in susceptible individuals without involving the immune system. Such nonimmunologic reactions, as well as those mediated by IgE, may be appropriately analyzed by BHRT.

A major disadvantage of the BHRT is that, to date, the results do not correlate with SET, RAST, or ELISA determinations. This means that although offenders may be identified, the results cannot be used in the administration of immunotherapy. For food hypersensitivity, elimination may be the most appropriate means of treatment, so that the inability to use the results for immunotherapy may not be of great importance. Another drawback, unfortunately, is that all food reactions do not occur through the release of histamine, so BHRT is of limited value even in food testing. In inhalant testing, if immunotherapy is the course desired, any use of BHRT to determine allergenic offenders must be followed by specific testing using SET, RAST, or ELISA to determine a safe starting dose for immunotherapy.

At present, although some applications are already practical (such as investigation of food hypersensitivity), the application of BHRT is limited for the average clinician. Despite these drawbacks, the BHRT appears to have great potential, and if correlation with SET and RAST is achieved in the future, the test may come into much wider use.

REFERENCES

1. King HC. Skin endpoint titration: still the standard? Otolaryngol Clin North Am 1992; 25:13–25.
2. Nelson HS. Diagnostic procedures in allergy. I. Allergy skin testing. Ann Allergy 1983; 51:411–418.
3. Lawlor GJ Jr, Fischer TJ, Adelman DC. Manual of Clinical Allergy. 3rd ed. Boston: Little, Brown; 1995:33–37.
4. Kniker WT. Choosing a skin test device. Ann Allergy Asthma Immunol 1997;78:524.
5. Mygind N. Essential Allergy. London: Blackwell Scientific Publications; 1986:121.
6. Kniker WR. Multi-Test Skin Testing in Allergy: a Review of Published Findings. Ann Allergy 1993;71:485–491.
7. Levine JL, Mabry RL, Mabry CS. A comparison of Multi-Test skin testing and modified RAST results. Otolaryngol Head Neck Surg 1998 (in press).
8. Lawlor GJ Jr, Fischer TJ, Adelman DC. Manual of Clinical Allergy. 3rd ed. Boston: Little, Brown; 1995:33–37.

7

ENVIRONMENTAL CONTROL (AVOIDANCE)

Up to this point, the information given has been nearly all concerned with various aspects of inhalant allergy. This is the most practical approach, as most new practitioners of allergy begin with the diagnosis and treatment of inhalant problems. Many experienced allergists also restrict their practice largely to the diagnosis and treatment of inhalant allergies, but we hope to guide the reader beyond this point. There will be failures in allergy diagnosis and treatment no matter how carefully problems are researched. Investigations into other aspects of allergy, discussed in later chapters, may reduce the frequency of such failures. Inhalant allergy, the best-understood aspect of allergy and the form most responsive to therapy, is the logical place for the novice to start both diagnosis and therapy.

Practical means of reaching a definitive identification of offenders in inhalant allergy have already been discussed. This is a necessary precursor to treatment in the majority of cases and a valuable step in all cases, regardless of the form, or combination of forms, of treatment finally selected. It now becomes incumbent on the directing physician to discuss with the patient the various approaches to therapy available, and to select the most appropriate method or methods for each specific case.

This decision is not as complex as it might seem at first. Despite the advances in allergy care during the past several decades, there are still only three basic, accepted approaches to allergy care: (1) avoidance; (2) pharmacotherapy; (3) immunotherapy. In the not-too-distant future, other approaches may merit consideration as mainstream therapy if future studies substantiate the efficacy of the primarily anecdotal results reported thus far. Most of these new approaches are directed toward reprogramming the immune system to avoid the defect that occurs in the allergic patient, but such methods are not currently in general use. Today's patient must opt for one or more of the established approaches presently available.

Every allergist agrees that the ideal approach to the control of allergy is simply to have the patient avoid contact with the allergenic offender. If the patient never comes in contact with the allergen, no sensitization can occur. Although allergenic attachment sites are genetically determined and cannot be altered, even if the potential for sensitization is present, the site cannot

155

NURSE'S NOTE

Environmental control is a prime teaching area for the allergy assistant. Education in this area requires more than one session. During multiple sessions with the patient, the opportunity exists for the allergy care giver to repeat and clarify instructions, emphasize the importance of avoidance, and remind patients of simple control measures. The allergy department should be well stocked with printed information regarding environmental control, and these should be given out freely. Avoidance is obviously most important in the case of patients who are sensitive to dust mites, mold, and animal danders, but it can also be emphasized to the pollen-allergic individual. In this area, the allergy nurse or assistant is always the most important source of information and encouragement for the patient.

---

be activated without several contacts with the potential allergen. Even if sensitization becomes established through a series of allergenic exposures, producing allergic symptoms, further symptoms will not appear until additional contact with the allergen occurs. If, through conscious avoidance or lack of opportunity, the patient is not exposed to the allergen for a prolonged period of time, the immunologic progression that caused symptoms will gradually subside, so that future brief contacts with the allergen may not induce symptoms. This situation may lead to a false sense of security on the part of the patient. Nevertheless, it is always possible for full-blown allergic symptoms to develop in the sensitized patient if sufficient allergen exposure occurs. Consider the immune system to be acting as a computer, not an unreasonable comparison. A previous contact, repeated frequently enough to establish a predictable allergic reaction, has not appeared for a prolonged period of time. The response is still in the memory banks, but deeply buried. When a new exposure to the inciting allergen occurs, it may be insufficient to trigger that memory. If the exposure is repeated at frequent intervals, however, the immune system's computer will eventually recall the previous adverse reaction and reactivate the progression, leading to allergic symptoms. The memory is never lost, simply buried. The number of exposures required to reactivate the immune reaction is quite variable. Sometimes reactivation is almost immediate, whereas at other times it may require weeks or months. The time involved may also be affected by additional exposure to antigens that have allergenic combining sites (epitopes) in common with those to which the patient is allergic. The speed and severity of the development of an allergic reaction may also be increased by exposure to other allergens to which the patient is sensitive, producing a "priming effect." This effect is simply the result of the immune system's becoming more sensitive to all stimulation, and reacting more rapidly and violently even when the primary offender is present in amounts normally too small to produce an allergic reaction. This response can even be triggered by nonantigenic stimuli, such as air pollution and cigarette smoke.

As is well recognized, the ideal approach to inhalant allergy care is to avoid the offending allergen. Like most ideals, this approach is very difficult to achieve. Effective control of multiple airborne allergens by avoidance is an almost impossible task. This limitation should not preclude an attempt to reduce allergenic exposures as much as possible, however, as any degree of reduction makes whatever additional form of treatment is elected more effective. Several approaches to environmental control are possible, all able to limit the degree of patient exposure, none likely to eliminate the problem effectively. Certain exceptions to this rule occur, most notably when the number of allergens involved is truly limited and when these are confined to a small and predictable area. Unfortunately, this situation applies in a very small number of cases.

GEOGRAPHIC MOVE

It is common for the patient in whom allergies have developed and increased through successive years to broach the subject of a possible move to a different climate. This time-honored and usually impractical approach dates to the 19th century, was common during the 1930s and 1940s, and is still recommended at times today. The patient may hold out hope for this solution, but the physician should regard it with caution. It may work, it may not. If a radical change of climate is involved, as in a move from the northeastern to the southwestern United States, a significant degree of improvement may well appear immediately after the move. This improvement is frequently temporary, however. Most allergic patients harbor a large number of immunologic attachment sites for potential allergens on their mast cells, and these may be activated by repeated exposures. The fact that such exposures have never occurred in the northeast is no guarantee that they will not occur in the southwest, where different potential allergens are present. As far as the future is concerned, only time will tell.

Some help can be obtained by consulting various vegetation maps of regional flora, which provide information about potential allergens. Some of the best of these are available through governmental agencies, such as the U.S. Geological Survey, Washington, DC 20244. These maps cover the flora of a limited region and should be available for the section of the country the patient has under consideration. It is certainly worthwhile to consult such maps in advance if the patient is seriously considering a relocation. It would be of little value to advise a patient to move from one area of the country to another to reduce allergic exposure if the same allergens are present in the new area. It might surprise the physician as well as the patient to discover the wide distribution of a large number of major allergens throughout a large portion of the continental United States, a situation that would make a geographic relocation useless for most patients.

Whether or not the distribution of allergens has been a significant factor in migration over much of the country, a major change in the distribution of the population of the continental United States has occurred in the past few decades. This in turn has resulted in some important changes in the ecology of various parts of the country. Arizona, for example, has had a great increase in population. This in turn has resulted in the irrigation of large areas of desert that, although previously extremely dry, are now able to produce significant crops. All this change has benefited the population. On the down side, these areas now grow many crops with the same allergens previously present only in less arid areas, as well as quite a few new allergens, all of which may affect the allergic patient adversely. The end result of these changes in the ecology created by human ingenuity is that no area may be considered safe for the allergy patient on a long-term basis. The country is growing and changing constantly. These changes, by and large, are beneficial to the economy and to the comfort of residents. The allergic patient, however, is an anomoly, representing a relatively small segment of the population. Although allergy represents one of the largest medical problems in the country, there is to date no accurate means of determining the future allergic potential of any particular location. A major geographic relocation is not a move to be undertaken lightly. An entire lifestyle may be expected to change, family and friends may be left behind, and a whole series of new challenges must be faced. Although the patient may be anticipating major lifestyle changes in any case, such as relocation for better employment opportunities or retirement, it would be unwise for a physician today to encourage such a move purely as a means of controlling allergic problems. The various factors affecting the allergic problem that may be influenced by a geographic relocation should be discussed with the patient, so that these factors may be considered realistically in relationship to the other reasons for the move. The physician cannot then be accused of recommending such an action for medical reasons and creating in the patient the hope of receiving benefits that may prove to be unrealistic.

It is sometimes helpful to inquire whether the patient contemplating a geographic move has in fact lived in the area under consideration at some time in the past, and if so, for how long a period of time. Not infrequently, this will prove to be the case, with the patient weighing the benefits of returning to a familiar area that is remembered fondly. If the patient lived in the area for several years without allergic symptoms, the odds are better that the allergies will be less severe in that location. Even in this case, however, it is wise to advise the patient to check the degree to which the ecology of the region has been altered since the last time the patient resided there. Industrial or urban development over a previously pastoral area may affect the allergens present to a major degree. The best approach is to advise the patient to make a trial move if possible, renting rather than buying, to see if the climate is as beneficial as hoped.

It must be acknowledged that even considering a geographic move in an attempt to control allergy is something that may be appropriate only for the allergic cripple. Such people are rare, but they do exist. They are sensitive to multiple airborne allergens, have major symptoms throughout the year, and respond poorly to antiallergic medication. They also have usually tried immunotherapy with unsatisfactory results. In such cases, a carefully planned geographic relocation may truly be of major benefit. Even when this is pursued with the most careful investigation of the area beforehand, however, it is likely that the patient will continue to require some additional treatment. What can be hoped for is that routine treatment, previously inadequate, will now provide the relief sought, as the allergic load has been greatly reduced.

ENVIRONMENTAL CONTROL WITHOUT GEOGRAPHIC RELOCATION

The vast majority of patients are ill-equipped to embark on a geographic relocation to pursue allergy benefits, even if the results are predictable. Allergy is an annoyance and a major burden, but it rarely produces a pronounced functional disability. Other lifestyle considerations, such as employment, education, and living conditions, usually take precedence over allergy relief, at least until all other avenues of relief have been exhausted. Although environmental control is rarely completely effective in an area in which allergens to which the patient is sensitive abound, many measures are available to reduce the total allergenic impact. These measures may be categorized in a general way as *control of indoor allergens* and *control of outdoor allergens*, or under specific approaches to control of allergens to which the patient has been demonstrated to be sensitive. The former is the more widely used approach. However, understanding the way in which limiting exposure to specific allergens affects the effectiveness of approaches to overall inhalant allergen control may make the entire concept more understandable and allow the formulation of a plan appropriate for individual circumstances.

It is important to note here that environmental control represents an area in which repetitive teaching is required. The allergy care giver has the opportunity, through recurring contacts, to instruct patients continually in the appropriate measures for their particular situation, and re-emphasize the need for environmental control and avoidance. Although immunotherapy is beneficial, it is never as helpful when the patient continues to be exposed to the offending allergens as when avoidance (within reason) is practiced.

Pollen Control

The control of exposure to seasonal pollens can be relatively simple, although not especially practical. The seasons in which pollination reaches its peak also represent the times of year most conductive to outdoor activity. To review the seasonal pattern of pollination discussed previously, trees primarily pollinate in the spring, starting as early as late January or early February in some parts of the country. One species of tree may pollinate for a few weeks, but other species will have started to pollinate during this period of time, so that the overall tree pollination season may last into May or June, depending on the geographic area, temperature, and rainfall. Grasses pollinate primarily in summer, but the grass pollination season frequently overlaps the tree pollination season to some degree, and at times also extends into the fall weed pollination season. In some areas, grasses pollinate throughout the year, although the peak season is still the summer. Weeds primarily pollinate in the fall, starting in August and continuing into the period of the first frost, again depending on the area of the country concerned. There are exceptions to these rules, such as the winter pollination of mountain cedar in the southwest, and these regional variations should be clarified before any program of allergy control is undertaken, regardless of the approach or approaches decided on.

Filtration Devices

Allergenic pollens usually fit into the size range of 15 to 50 μm, as described under Thommen's postulates. (Table 7–1) These are usually filtered out by almost any efficient air-conditioner filter. The members of the allergy team

---

NURSE'S NOTE

Principles of environmental control:

1. Take preventive measures. Avoid exposure by using filtering devices (e.g., dust mask, electrostatic filters). Avoid the allergic reaction by using nasal cromolyn or taking an antihistamine before an anticipated exposure.

2. Reduce unavoidable exposure. After allergen exposure, rinse the nose with saline solution. After mowing or gardening, dirty clothes should go directly into the washer, and the patient should shower and shampoo hair. During periods of high pollen exposure (or air pollution), stay indoors in a controlled environment. Use the "recirculate" setting for automatic air conditioner. Keep windows closed at home, and use an effective filtration system.

---

should have a good general understanding of various types of air conditioner filters, as well as filtration systems in general. First, it must be recognized that the standard fiberglass filter provided with most air conditioners is not appropriate for the allergic patient. This filter may reduce the amount of debris being brought into the house through the air conditioner's intake and further reduce the amount recirculated within the house, but the filtration properties are not adequate to remove the airborne particles that produce allergic reactions. For the allergic patient, three basic types of filter may bear consideration.

The first is the high-efficiency particulate arresting (HEPA) filter. This is probably the most efficient type of filter available, but like all such items, the HEPA filter has its good and bad aspects. The filter is essentially an accordion-pleated sheet of paper, interposed between the air intake and output, incorporated into a three- or four-stage arrangement. Most such HEPA filters capture particles to 0.3 μm in diameter. This pore size effectively

TABLE 7–1. Thommen's postulates

For the pollen of a plant to be an important allergen, it must satisfy the criteria listed below, which were originally set forth by A. A. Thommen in 1931.

1. The pollen must be wind-borne (anemophilous). This requirement rules out showy flowered plants with sticky pollen, which are insect-pollinated.
2. The pollen must be produced in large quantities. This is characteristic of wind-pollinated plants.
3. The pollen must be sufficiently buoyant to be carried considerable distances. This would include plants producing pollen grains in the size range of 15 to 58 μm.
4. The plant producing the pollen must be widely and abundantly distributed.
5. The pollen must contain specific excitants or antigens to produce hypersensitivity.

filters out pollen grains, dust mite, mold spores, and animal danders (including cat dander, which has an average diameter of 2 μm).

The filter's advantage is its efficiency. Its disadvantage is the fact that filtered material builds up on the filtering surface fairly rapidly. This increases the efficiency of the filter, straining out more airborne particles, but puts an increasing strain on the mechanics of the filtration system. Manufacturers of the HEPA filter generally recommend the installation of an additional air-handling system so that the filter does not place enough strain on the regular air-conditioning system to burn out the motors. This entails additional duct work, more electrical connections, and additional motors. In addition, the filter must be changed frequently, both to preserve good function and to prevent the increasing back pressure of the filtered material from damaging the ancillary system.

Changing the filter should not present a major problem. Access to the filter, on the other hand, often becomes quite difficult. For the patient electing to make use of an HEPA filter, easy access to the filter and simplicity of changing the filter as necessary should be discussed in detail with the person installing the necessary additional duct work and connections. No one wishes to need the services of an air-conditioning service person several times a year, simply to change an HEPA filter.

For patients unable or unwilling to invest in a central filtering system, a portable HEPA filtration system should be considered (Fig. 7–1). These portable room air cleaners are generally equipped with an HEPA filter and a charcoal prefilter, and they incorporate a blower system that draws air through the filters and circulates it. Such room air cleaners are available in several sizes from various commercial suppliers of environmental control devices; they are especially beneficial when placed in the bedroom and/or living room, creating "safe havens" for the allergy sufferer.

Another filtering system designed to remove allergenic material from indoor air is the electronic precipitator. This equipment has been in use for many years. The principle involved is the passage of indoor air over a series of electronically charged plates, which attract the passing air particles. When functioning efficiently, the machine induces the charged particles to deposit on the plates, thereby removing them from the ambient air (Fig. 7–2). The principle on which this filtration system is based has been tested by long experience, and when the equipment is operated properly, such filters are quite effective. The difficulty with the electronic precipitator is that, although the principle of operation is completely different, the same servicing problems that arise with the HEPA filter apply. If the precipitator is integrated into the household air-conditioning system, additional electric connections

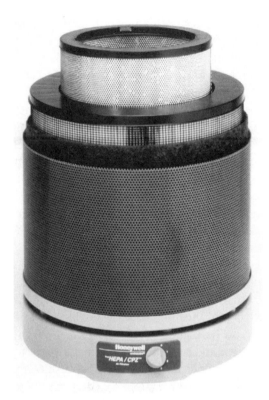

FIGURE 7–1. Room-size HEPA filtering system. This self-contained system features a circulating fan and an HEPA filter, plus a charcoal prefilter. The use of such a room-size system may allow patients to turn their bedrooms into "safe havens" when they are unable to install central HEPA filtration systems. (Courtesy of Allergy Control Products, Inc, 96 Danbury Rd, Ridgefield, CT 06877.)

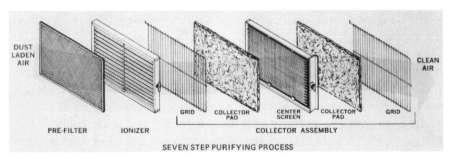

FIGURE 7–2. Electronic filter. Particles are first passed over electronically charged grids, and then deposited on special collector pads. This filter is installed in a heating/air-conditioning system, requires electrical wiring, and must be cleaned on a regular basis. It has not been shown to be a significant source of ozone and is very efficient.

are needed, frequently the duct work may require modification, and convenient access to the filter is essential.

The electronic precipitator has certain unique properties. First, if the filtering portion is less than 2 in. in depth, little particulate material is removed by the plates. This means that access to a fairly large filtering module is necessary. If the electronic precipitator is not cleaned frequently, the particulate deposits build up on the plates, gradually producing the same problem that affected the older sand and gravel swimming pool filters. With time, the plates are unable to accumulate more material, and passages develop through the filter that allow the ambient air, containing the particles that should be removed by the filter, to pass on into the living space. Although not removed from the air, these particles are now electronically charged and tend to adhere to the ceiling, walls, and upholstery of the living area. This often results in the accumulation of dark greasy deposits on the surfaces involved. The problem may be prevented by regularly removing the filters and cleaning the plates with a garden hose or in the dishwasher; such cleaning cannot be neglected without inviting the appearance of the problems described. The frequency of cleaning necessary will vary with the area, but a competent installer of the equipment should be able to provide the homeowner with a good idea of the frequency involved.

A third approach to indoor air purification is the electrostatic filter (Fig. 7–3). It is not truly possible to give a reliable comparison of the effectiveness of various types of air filtration systems on indoor air in normal living spaces, as the degree of closure of homes in different locations is highly variable. The probability is that this type of filter is somewhat less effective in removing particulate matter from the air than the HEPA or electronic filters, but it is by far the simplest and most practical to install. This filter is still far superior to the standard fiberglass filter supplied with most air-conditioning systems. The electrostatic filter requires no special duct work and no electrical connections. The filter is tailored to fit in the same space as a fiberglass filter, and it removes particulate material from the air by electrostatic attraction. Like both previously mentioned filters, the electrostatic filter must be cleaned with a garden hose every month if full efficiency is to be obtained, but if such cleaning is not performed on time, the only common complication is a reduction in filtration efficiency. The recommendation described in the previous filtration options regarding easy access to the filter continues to be important. Although failure to clean the electrostatic filter at frequent intervals is less likely to produce any damage to the overall air-conditioning system, the efficiency of filtration still suffers. If this filter is to be used, it should be cleaned regularly. If this is not done, it is a waste of money to

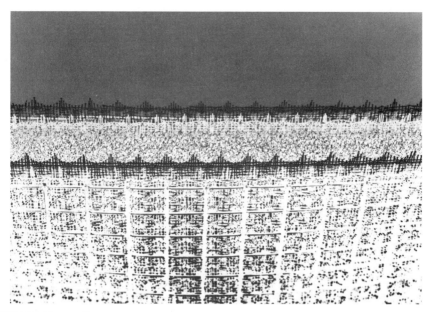

FIGURE 7–3. Electrostatic filter. This filter replaces the usual disposable filter in a heating/air-conditioning system. Air passes over layers of polypropylene (outer black layer, inner white layer), and the electrostatic charge caused by this passage enhances the deposition of the particles on the central foam layer. These filters must be cleaned on a regular basis but can be reused for many years. (Courtesy of Dust Free, Inc, 1112 Industrial Park, Royse City, TX 75189.)

install the filter at all. If the filter is to be cleaned regularly, easy access is essential. All of us are human, and if an item is difficult to reach, it is only a matter of time before its maintenance becomes neglected.

There are many variations, but at the present time, most filtration systems in general use fall within the categories described. The allergic patient must decide whether the problems encountered are severe enough that any of these methods of indoor environmental control should be considered, and if so, how extensive the control should be. It is unlikely that any adult patient will be able to remain in a controlled environment at all times, even through the most severe season of allergenic exposure. However, a haven in which allergens are drastically reduced, and in which the patient may spend many hours daily, greatly reduces the overall allergic load. This haven is usually the bedroom. Such an allergen-free living area provides the patient, even if unable to avoid allergen exposure throughout the day, with a reduction in the overall level of allergic mediators of inflammation accumulating in the system for several hours each day. Although by no means providing a cure, this period of relief often aids the patient in coping with the daily total allergic load.

The question of commercial cleaning of air ducts often arises. If the patient is known to be sensitive to dust mite and molds, an initial cleaning of the air ducts in the home can significantly lighten the exposure to these allergens. However, this must be combined with the use of a filtration system to prevent their buildup in the future. Air duct cleaning is of lesser benefit if the patient's allergies do not include these perennial triggers.

Other Pollen Control Measures

The pollen-sensitive patient may be able to reduce indoor allergenic exposure by filtration of various types, and to some degree may reduce outdoor exposure by avoiding the presence of major allergens immediately adjacent to the house. These precautions may reduce the severity of the problem, but rarely present a complete solution.

If pollen-allergic patients are willing to stay indoors when the pollens to which they are sensitive are in the air, considerable relief may be expected. Preventing, or at least reducing, symptoms by this means is quite possible, but only at the expense of staying indoors during some of the most pleasant seasons of the year. For the patient sensitive to pollens prevalent during only one season, this may be an acceptable approach, but the usual pattern is a progression of symptoms to involve additional seasons as time goes on. Few patients are willing to limit outdoor activities to the degree necessary for such control.

Some degree of compromise is possible while still living a relatively normal life. Pollens are most prevalent in the air in the morning, as the sun rises and the air warms. Staying indoors at this time reduces pollen exposure at the most critical period of the day. Checking regional pollen counts published in major newspapers and provided by television weather forecasters in the area will indicate the days on which pollen levels in the air are exceptionally high. During these times, the pollen-allergic patient should plan on spending more time indoors. Furthermore, high winds promote widespread distribution of pollen, so that a shift from the prevailing wind direction may bring in pollens to which exposure is not expected.

Consideration of shrubs and plants that are frequently used in landscaping may be of value. Many of these shrubs are frequently planted in close proximity to the house. A privet hedge beneath the bedroom windows is a good example. In areas of the country where the windows are opened when the outside air becomes pleasant, a heavy dose of pollen may be deposited into the bedroom with the morning breezes and rising sun. Many people have little or no idea of the nature of the growing things that have been used in landscaping their home, or of their allergic potential. Even if they have been provided with a list of the pollinating plants to which they are allergic, they frequently fail to identify these with the landscaped plants growing around their home.

A visit to a good local nursery with a list of the plants to which the patient is allergic, and some clippings from the plants close to the house, can be an enlightening experience. Many commercial nurseries have on their staff one or more certified master gardeners, who are very knowledgeable and can be extremely helpful to allergic patients in planning landscaping that does not worsen their symptoms. If help from a such a person is not available, the necessary information may be obtained by visiting a botanical garden, the botany department of a local college or university, or a local branch of the Department of Agriculture. Most botanists are more than happy to have a lay person show interest in their field and are glad to cooperate in measures that have a direct clinical application.

For those unwilling or unable to base their lifestyles on the avoidance of pollinating plants to which they are allergic, methods other than environmental control are in order. If symptoms are present only for a period of a few weeks, medication may provide all the additional relief needed. If the symptoms proliferate and occupy many months, other approaches may need to be considered. Many allergic patients have to have the limitations of environmental control of pollen allergy pointed out to them. First, the physical appearance of the actual plants to which they are allergic should be made clear to them. This includes plants other than those used in landscaping the patient's home. The majority of patients have no clear idea of the appearance of the major allergenic offenders, and blame any pollen that they can see, such as slash pine pollen, on symptom production. When they know what an allergenic plant looks like, they are better able to determine how much is present in their area and how closely adjacent to their home it is.

Second, allergic patients must realize that allergenic pollen is wind-borne and will travel. Removing major allergens directly adjacent to the house may help, but it is not practical to attempt to remove large stands of allergenic plants, such as established oak trees, unless they completely envelop the house. Even then, if the allergen producer is popular in the area, patients will still have to contend with pollen blown into their area from neighboring vicinities. There have been too many instances of allergic patients embarking enthusiastically on a mission to remove all local allergenic plants, only to discover that they are the ones who have the problem, not the neighborhood. Reasonable control immediately around the home, a rational acceptance of other exposures in the area, and medical control of symptoms as necessary comprise the only practical environmental approach for the pollen-sensitive patient.

Mold Control

Unlike pollen, mold is present year round, indoors and outdoors. In addition, mold spores show a much greater size range than do pollen grains, making their removal by filtration a more difficult problem. Some of the same approaches to environmental control as are used in controlling pollen exposure also apply to molds, but others are quite different.

Unlike pollens, outdoor molds usually reach their peak level in the air in the evening hours, when the temperature drops with the setting sun. This is a good time for the mold-sensitive patient to remain indoors. Molds also show a strong affinity for dampness. Watering lawns in the evening encourages the growth of molds, which then become airborne and affect the mold-sensitive patient. The presence of bodies of water, even as small as fish ponds, enhances mold growth. Unfortunately, in many instances these are placed close to the house of the allergy sufferer. Swamps, wetlands, and low-lying areas with poor drainage are heavy producers of mold, and such areas are obviously not a good location for the home of the mold-allergic patient.

Decaying vegetation also promotes heavy mold growth. When plantings are heavy and set close to the house, allergic problems may well be caused by the presence of mold beneath and behind the plants. Such areas receive little sun and retain moisture, and removal of the decaying portion can be difficult. Like the pollen already described, the mold spores are easily carried into the home through open windows. Removing heavy plant growth from areas against the house can significantly reduce the mold problem. For the same reason, it is inadvisable for the mold-allergic patient to engage in extensive lawn work. Cuttings from trees and bushes rapidly decay and produce quantities of mold. If such work is necessary, the mold-allergic patient should at the very least wear a face mask to reduce the quantity of mold inhaled. In addition, clothes worn during this activity should go directly into the wash, and patients should immediately shower and shampoo their hair.

A word should be said here about the typical lawn. Many patients complain of severe episodes of allergic symptoms when mowing the lawn, and so suspect a grass allergy. Actually, lawn grasses do not pollinate significantly when kept closely mowed. Molds and smuts, however, are prevalent among grass roots and are thrown upward into the air when the grass is mowed.

This type of sensitivity is much more likely to be of importance than is grass pollen sensitivity under typical lawn conditions.

Indoor mold growth will appear anywhere that moisture collects. Favorite places are beneath and around drains in basements and garages, under sinks, in condensate drip pans beneath refrigerators and freezers, and around the condensers of area air conditioners. Visible mold and mildew should be cleaned with a dilute solution of bleach (one part bleach to 10 parts of water), or with a commercially available mildew remover.

Indoor green plants are also a copious source of mold growth. Indoor plants rarely pollinate, but mold will grow heavily in the planting material. Bird cages are also good mold sources. Many patients who feel that they may be sensitive to feathers actually turn out to be allergic to the bird droppings in the cage, which carry mold in quantity.

Degenerating paper, like degenerating leaves, is a prolific source of mold growth. The paper may be piled newspapers, or pages of old books in book-cases. Firewood also allows for extensive mold growth. If not kept well ventilated, stored seasonal clothing, especially shoes, may grow mold. All these may be removed from the house or protected from mold growth by various commercially available mold preventatives. A simple measure to prevent mold growth in closets is to keep a light burning in them at all times.

A special form of mold allergy commonly seen is "Christmas tree allergy." A Christmas tree does release some pine terpine and oleoresins into the air, providing the typical fragrance that is so popular, and may release a small amount of pollen. However, the primary offender affecting the victim of Christmas tree allergy is usually mold. The trees are often cut and packed in the presence of snow and frost, which subsequently melt and allow prolific mold growth. Many mold-sensitive patients find it advisable to select an artificial tree in deference to their problem.

The mold-sensitive farmer presents an essentially impossible problem in environmental control. Grain contains huge quantities of smuts and molds, all of which are airborne. Stables and barns grow copious amounts of mold, produced by animal droppings and litter as well as hay and feed. The most heroic attempts at cleanliness cannot hope to overcome this load of allergens. Medication may offer help, but the farmer with extensive mold allergy is probably doomed to a most uncomfortable life. This is one situation in which a change of occupation may deserve serious consideration.

Dust and Epidermal Allergen Control

If a group of experienced allergists were told that in the future only one antigen would be available for patient treatment, almost all would opt to select housedust. This in itself is an anachronism, as housedust does not actually represent a single allergen, but rather a combination of antigens that together act essentially in the manner of a single allergen. This lack of chemical uniformity is what has led the Food and Drug Administration to order the removal of housedust extract from the allergist's armamentarium. To date, this mandated removal has not been carried out.

The National Institute of Allergy and Infectious Diseases (NIAID) has reported that housedust contains 28 identified or suspected allergens.[1] All these balance in such a way that the overall pattern acts essentially like a single allergen. The most active allergenic ingredients of housedust appear to be degenerating lysine sugars. The potency of the allergen depends largely on the age of the dust, older dust being more allergenic. Potency is influenced to a lesser degree by the season of the year, with the fall producing the most allergenic dust. The worst allergy season for the housedust-sensitive individual is usually the winter, when low temperatures result in tightly closed houses. The dust allergy season may conveniently be thought of as the converse of the baseball season (late fall to early spring).

Housedust is generated in any living environment. It is not dirt that has been tracked into the house and dried, but rather the degenerating residue of upholstery, carpets, mattresses, bedding, and any other organic substances present in a home or workplace. Added to this substrate are an assortment of pollens, molds, insect parts, and food particles accompanied by a variety of hairs from pets and vermin. With a constant renewal of the dust supply from the sources generating it, total removal is practically impossible.

The most publicized component of housedust is the dust mite, a microscopic creature present in all dust worldwide. The prevalence of dust mites is negatively affected by altitude; the higher the altitude the fewer the mites. This is not a hard and fast rule, however, as some mites have adapted to high altitudes. Humidity also increases the mite population, as does a warm environment. Several types of mites are present in the United States, and antigens for all are becoming available. There is some, but not complete, allergenic cross-reactivity between the mites.

The dust mite is the component of housedust whose antigen pattern most closely resembles that of housedust itself. The potency of mite extract, however, is considerably less than that of housedust extract. In the future, if housedust extract per se is withdrawn from the market, it will be necessary to substitute dust mite extract, supplemented by various epidermals, to approximate the housedust pattern traditionally available for testing and therapy.

The allergenic load produced by housedust can be lowered by assiduous efforts at control, but never truly eliminated. Standard vacuum cleaners remove only a fraction of the ambient dust, and only a minimum of the dust mite population. The allergenic portion of the dust mite is contained in its fecal material. This material attaches firmly to fibers, including carpet, upholstery, and bedding, and is extremely difficult to remove. Even a commercial, high-powered vacuum cleaner can be expected to remove only a small portion of the dust mite allergens. Superfiltering vacuum cleaners are now available; these remove additional amounts of dust and prevent its dispersement back into the air during vacuuming. Although the HEPA filter vacuum (Fig. 7–4)

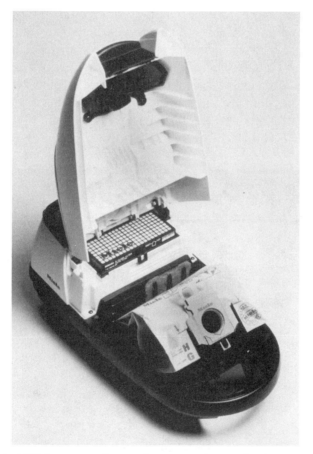

FIGURE 7–4. HEPA vacuum cleaner. A vacuum cleaner that incorporates a HEPA filter is an extremely efficient method of removing even very small allergenic particles from carpets. A less efficient alternative is the use of a high-efficiency regular vacuum cleaner with a double bag, which prevents gathered particles from escaping back into the atmosphere. (Courtesy of Allergy Control Products, Inc, 96 Danbury Rd, Ridgefield, CT 06877.)

is especially recommended in this regard, some (but by no means all) commercial vacuum cleaners have been found to be highly effective in removing dust without recirculating it. The best source of information is this regard is a publication such as *Consumer Reports*.

Some commercially available compounds (such as X-Mite) containing tannic acid act to denature dust mite allergens, but do not kill mites.[2] Other preparations contain benzyl benzoate and are effective in killing dust mites, but do not denature their antigenic protein.[3] The most commonly available such acaricide is Acarosan. Before the use of these materials, a test material (such as Acarex) may be applied to dust vacuumed from the carpets in various rooms. This indicates the level of mite fecal material present. If the level is high enough to present a potential problem, the acaricide is applied to the carpet and then vacuumed up. Acarosan is available as a powder for application to carpets. Although a foam preparation for use on upholstery is available in Europe, it has not been marketed in the United States. Typical acaricide and mite-removal products are illustrated in Figure 7–5.

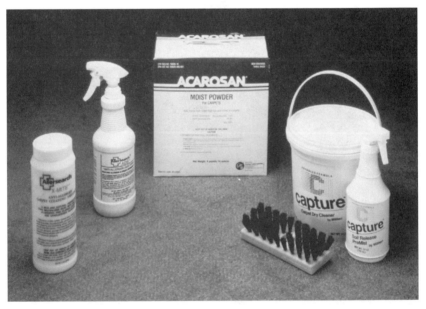

FIGURE 7–5. Acaricides and carpet cleaners. Multiple preparations are available for this purpose. Those that contain benzyl benzoate are acaricidal, whereas those utilizing tannic acid denature the mite protein. At present, no single compound appears to do both. (Courtesy of Allergy Control Products, Inc, 96 Danbury Rd, Ridgefield, CT 06877.)

Treatments with an acaricide require repetition every few months, as the mite population is soon replenished. The expense and disruption entailed in performing regular treatments of this type have limited its acceptance. In addition, some question exists as to the long-term effectiveness of acaricides in this regard. An alternative is regular vacuuming of the carpets, draperies, and upholstered surfaces in the home with an HEPA vacuum.

Dust mites are intolerant of high temperatures. Although they are unaffected by laundry detergents, regular washing of bedding in water above 140 F will destroy the mite population. Tumbling Dacron or similar pillows for 15 minutes in a dryer set to "high" substantially reduces the mite population. Pillow covers and mattress covers that are impermeable to dust mites are available from commercial allergy supply houses. These significantly reduce dust mite exposure during sleep. However, these covers must be cleaned regularly by washing in hot water. A typical mattress cover and pillow cover are shown in Figure 7–6.

The ideal home for the dust-sensitive individual is rather spartan. A significant degree of relief for the dust-allergic patient can be provided by the removal of "dust catchers" from the living area. Such items, generally those that are difficult to clean and tend to retain dust, include easily breakable items that are rarely dusted with care, and silk flowers or mounted animals, which act as reservoirs for large amounts of dust. Books in open shelves tend to accumulate large amounts of dust and mold. Ideally, dust-sensitive patients will avoid wall-to-wall carpeting in their homes and elect instead to have hardwood or tile floors with throw rugs that can be laundered. Removal of draperies and curtains is also beneficial. Closet shelves (and their contents) should be cleaned regularly, preferably with a damp sponge or cloth. The tops of window frames and door frames are typically major accumulators of dust, as are any other surfaces above eye level. Ceiling fans not only stir up dust from the room, but tend to collect large amounts of dust on the fan blades unless cleaned frequently.

Some special notes are indicated about the dust-sensitive child. The infant rarely has significant inhalant allergies, but as the child with allergic potential grows older, dust is usually the first sensitivity to appear. This development is probably a consequence of both the perennial presence of dust in the home and the exceptionally heavy dust exposure of the child crawling on the floor. Through the years, the allergy community has made a major effort to dust-proof children's rooms. This approach includes removing carpets and draperies, covering mattresses with dustproof material, replacing stuffed animals that have artificial fur with toys made of washable foam and terry cloth, and generally developing the same spartan atmosphere that is desirable for the

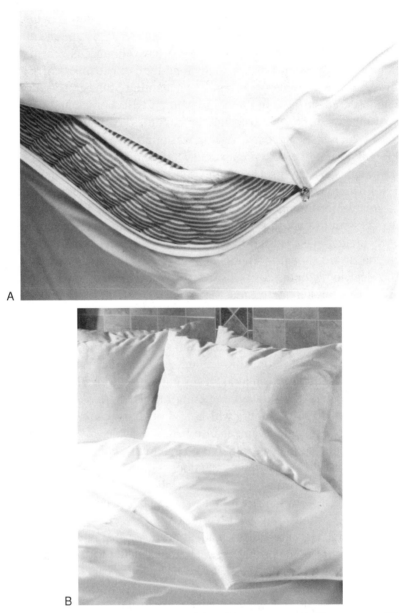

FIGURE 7–6. Barrier coverings for bedding. Newer types of pillow covers (A) and mattress covers (B) are impermeable to dust mites, yet are as comfortable as conventional covers. The use of such barrier coverings, in conjunction with hot water washing of bedding and the use of a nonallergenic pillow, is strongly recommended for patients with demonstrated sensitivity to dust mite. (Courtesy of Allergy Control Products, Inc, 96 Danbury Rd, Ridgefield, CT 06877.)

entire home of the dust-sensitive patient. The reduction of the allergenic load is certainly to be commended. It should be recognized, however, that such restrictions of comfort, if carried to an extreme, may have an adverse emotional effect on children and that unless the entire house is altered to conform to the demands of dust elimination, the benefits will accrue only when children are in the particular room that has been dustproofed. As in most aspects of environmental control, the operative word is compromise. Reduction of the overall load is to be encouraged. Altering the entire living pattern, especially with the knowledge that only a partial degree of success can be anticipated, is probably going to prove unrewarding.

SUMMARY

Environmental control of inhalant allergens is a theoretically ideal solution to the problem of inhalant allergy, but rarely effective as a single approach. Inhalant allergy problems are induced by multiple allergenic exposures, emanating from a wide variety of sources. The total adverse effects of allergy represent a sum of all the exposures encountered by the patient. Any reduction of such exposures may be expected to reduce the overall symptom level and make any additional treatment methodology more effective. Environmental control, therefore, is desirable to an extent that does not compromise normal living. It is rare for an allergic patient to be sensitive to a single class of allergens and retain only limited sensitivity indefinitely. With this in mind, it is advisable to consider as many aspects of environmental control as appear practical and institute whatever measures appear reasonable. These will vary with location and living conditions. Such precautions should not only reduce the current allergic load, but also aid in preventing future sensitization to other allergens by reducing the level of potential exposure. Environmental control serves as a baseline in the plan of overall allergy treatment. Other forms of therapy will usually be needed, but the success of these may be increased by proper environmental control.

REFERENCES

1. NIAID. Dust Allergy. Bethesda, MD: National Institutes of Health; Publication No. 83-490 (revised Nov. 1982).
2. Green WF. Abolition of allergens by tannic acid. Lancet 1984;88:77–82.
3. Lau-Schadendorf S, Rusche AF, Weber AK, Buttner-Goetz P, Wahn U. Short-term efficacy of benzyl benzoate on mite allergen concentration in house dust. J Allergy Clin Immunol 1989;83:263(abst).

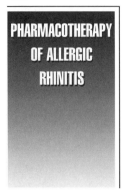

8

PHARMACOTHERAPY OF ALLERGIC RHINITIS

The best treatment of inhalant allergy is avoidance, whenever possible. Unfortunately, this treatment is often the least likely to succeed (or even occur), generally because of patients' disinclination to give up their cat, golf, gardening, or other activities that produce allergenic exposure.

The most definitive treatment of inhalant allergy is immunotherapy, properly administered over a sufficient length of time to affect the patient's immune response to triggering antigens. Although the exact mechanism by which this occurs remains a source of conjecture, there is no doubt that immunotherapy presents the only hope for a "cure" for the allergic patient.

Between these two poles lies the linchpin of treatment, which is pharmacotherapy. The patient practicing avoidance will, at some time, invariably come in contact with an allergen and require the use of one or more pharmacotherapeutic agents to provide symptom relief. Furthermore, patients receiving immunotherapy will not necessarily become totally "immune" to their triggering allergens, and an overwhelming or prolonged exposure will generally produce symptoms, which must be relieved by the use of these agents. Therefore, it is of prime importance for those dealing with upper respiratory allergy to understand the available pharmacotherapeutic tools and their appropriate use.

OVERVIEW OF AVAILABLE TOOLS

To understand the proper use of the drugs available to treat the symptoms of allergic rhinitis, it is necessary to have a clear understanding of the allergic reaction. This is detailed elsewhere in this text. In general, the medications available work in one or more of several areas.

Classic antihistamines act primarily by competing with histamine for H1-binding sites on the target organ. If an antihistamine is occupying that site, histamine cannot occupy the same site, so that the antihistamine blocks the histamine-cellular interaction, which would otherwise produce consequences including sneezing, itching membranes, and rhinorrhea. Newer antihistamines also may have direct actions on inflammatory mediators, diminishing their production and/or negating their effects. For this reason, some of these preparations may be more effective than older compounds in relieving the symptoms of a reaction already in progress. It is important to note that antihistamines exert their effect primarily on the ''wet'' symptoms of allergy, but do not decongest nasal passages.

Decongestants, whether topically or systematically administered, cause contraction of the large vascular channels in the nasal turbinates, reducing the size of this tissue. This alpha-adrenergic stimulation and the resultant diminution in pooled volume within the turbinates is the mechanism by which they produce relief of nasal congestion.

Nonsteroidal anti-inflammatory agents, often called *mast cell stabilizers* (e.g., cromolyn), were originally thought to act by preventing the degranulation reaction that occurs when an antigen bridges two adjacent allergen-specific immunoglobulin E (IgE) molecules bound to a mast cell (or basophil). This was found to be true in laboratory animals, but in humans, it is possible that these preparations also have specific mediator effects. This is certainly the case with nedocromil, and possibly some of the other new compounds in this class. In any case, these agents definitely prevent an allergic reaction when used before an anticipated antigen exposure, and it is this effect that gives them their greatest utility in the management of allergic rhinitis. They have a less beneficial effect in treating reactions already in progress.

Corticosteroids exert a nonspecific anti-inflammatory action in rhinitis of many types. In allergy, their effect is primarily on the late-phase reaction. Topical nasal steroids can inhibit the acute-phase reaction if administered regularly for 4 to 7 days. It is important to realize that corticosteroids do not prevent allergic reactions, but merely counter the symptoms produced by the release of inflammatory mediators.

Anticholinergics act to inhibit mucous production in nasal mucosa. Systemic preparations are rarely used because of undesirable side effects such as dry mouth, dry eyes, and urinary retention. However, topical anticholinergics are available that are specific in their actions. These drugs inhibit rhinorrhea without producing systemic effects or affecting other symptoms of the allergic reaction.

GENERAL TREATMENT STRATEGY

The management of the symptoms of allergic rhinitis through the use of drugs can be visualized as proceeding in a stepwise fashion. Simple measures will often relieve mild symptoms. Progressively more complex treatment schemes, using drugs with more potential for side effects or adverse interactions, may be necessary to treat severe problems. The first principle to keep in mind is to use the simplest, safest (and least expensive) drug that will get the job done.

In a survey of patients suffering from allergic rhinitis (R. L. Mabry, *unpublished data*), the attributes of drug treatment were ranked in this order of importance: efficacy, side effects, cost, and dosing regimen. A similar survey of physicians treating these patients provided a strikingly similar ranking: efficacy, side effects, dosing regimen, and cost. What is clear from this information is that both patient and physician want the medication to work, preferably without side effects that impair productivity or quality of life. After that, patients are more worried about cost than convenience, whereas the reverse is true of physicians.

OVER-THE-COUNTER MEDICATIONS

Most patients will come to the specialist already having taken one or more nonprescription medications. It is important to determine if this is the case, as the patient's response will influence the physician's choice of further drug therapy. If over-the-counter antihistamines provided good symptom relief but caused undesirable side effects, such as sedation, the substitution of a nonsedating preparation may be a valid first step. If an over-the-counter antihistamine-decongestant combination caused undesirable stimulation, this will be even more pronounced if the decongestant is combined with a nonsedating antihistamine. If there was absolutely no response to these over-the-counter remedies, it is unlikely that prescription antihistamines and decongestants will be entirely effective in controlling symptoms.

Patients with allergy often seek relief of nasal congestion from over-the-counter decongestants administered either orally or as nose drops or sprays. The systemic decongestant present in most over-the-counter combinations is pseudoephedrine, which is also used in most prescription antihistamine-decongestant combinations. Less commonly used, and less effective, is phenylephrine. Ephedrine is still encountered, although rarely, in either over-the-counter or prescription preparations. Phenylpropanolamine, which is a common prescription decongestant, is not a component of over-the-counter medications.

Because of the chronic and often severe nature of their disease, patients with allergic rhinitis often use topical nasal vasoconstrictors regularly for prolonged periods, resulting in the problem of rebound rhinitis. This should be a consideration for the physician when taking an allergy history, as the

NURSE'S NOTE

The allergy care provider, who sees patients on a frequent basis to administer immunotherapy injections, must continually remind patients about the proper (and sometimes regular) use of their medications. Some key points to remember are the following:

1. Every patient with allergic rhinitis who is receiving immunotherapy should have available basic medications for symptom prevention and relief: cromolyn, antihistamines, and decongestants. Forms of all these may be obtained over the counter, although the nonsedating antihistamines require a prescription. Patients must also be continually re-educated about what symptoms each type of medication relieves.

   For patients using over-the-counter antihistamines, it may be necessary to suggest that they take them primarily at bedtime, to avoid daytime sedation. On the other hand, decongestants are best taken in the morning, to avoid the side effect of insomnia.

2. Patients must be reminded that cromolyn and antihistamines work best when used before an anticipated allergy exposure, and encouraged to use them in this way. Some patients feel that immunotherapy gives them free reign to be exposed to their allergens without ever suffering symptoms. Unfortunately, this is not always the case, especially early in a course of treatment. Pharmacotherapy always remains a necessary tool in treating patients with allergic rhinitis.

3. Patients who have been placed on nasal steroid sprays must be reminded (or initially educated) of the proper way of administering them (as outlined later in this chapter). Furthermore, it is necessary to emphasize that these sprays are not like decongesting nasal sprays, which can be used on an as-needed basis. Rather, steroid nasal sprays should be used regularly, in the dosage prescribed, for a specific duration (usually a particular season or time of expected allergen exposure). If patients experience local side effects, such as nasal bleeding and crusting, they should discontinue the sprays and see the physician to be evaluated for septal damage.

4. If patients are placed on antibiotics for complicating infections, they must be reminded to complete the full course. Likewise, when infections produce thick secretions, patients should not depend on their antihistamines. In this situation, most patients receive from the physician a combination decongestant-mucolytic (e.g., Entex, Deconsal II, Guaifed) to be used during the infection.

first step in diagnosing (and treating) a complicating medicamentous rhinitis is asking the patient about the use of decongesting nasal sprays or drops.

A major breakthrough in over-the-counter allergy pharmacotherapy occurred in 1997 when nasal cromolyn became available without a prescription. As already noted, cromolyn is the prototypical mast cell stabilizer, and although the exact mechanism of its action remains a matter of conjecture, there is little doubt that it does prevent an allergic reaction when used before an antigen exposure.[1] Of course, it is necessary that cromolyn (or any intranasally administered drug) adequately reach the nasal mucosa to be effective. This means that it may not be feasible for use by patients with severe septal deviation and/or marked turbinate hypertrophy. Not only will polyps prevent cromolyn from achieving adequate contact with nasal mucosa, but the cromolyn also has no effect on the polyps. Rather, it prevents the allergic event when applied beforehand, and to a much lesser degree may ameliorate symptoms of an allergic event in progress. It must be reapplied every 4 to 6 hours to remain effective. Despite these shortcomings, cromolyn is especially effective for patients with allergy to well-defined inhalants that are unavoidable and are not encountered on a continuous basis. Also, cromolyn is exceptionally safe, and is probably one of the best methods of providing relief for pregnant women with mild to moderate symptoms of allergic rhinitis.

PRESCRIPTION ANTIHISTAMINES

These compounds typically exert their antiallergic action by occupying H_1-receptor sites on respiratory mucosa, preventing histamine released during the allergic reaction from producing the typical symptoms of sneezing and rhinorrhea. Newer antihistamines may have additional actions on other allergic mediators.

In 1937, Bovet and Staub noted the antihistaminic effects of certain phenolic ethers. By 1945, the first antihistamines for human use, diphenhydramine (Benadryl) and tripelennamine (PBZ), were introduced. By 1997, more than 20 different antihistamines and more than 100 different antihistamine-containing products were available in the United States. This proliferation of drugs continues, with each new preparation claiming its own advantages. However, it is necessary also to be aware of the disadvantages of each, as well as the properties that are unique for each drug or class.

Antihistamines may be classified by their chemical structure, depending on the attachment of nitrogen, oxygen, or carbon to a substituted ethylamine

TABLE 8–1. First-generation antihistamines

Classification	Generic name	Trade name (example)
Ethanolamines	diphenhydramine	Benadryl
	clemastine	Tavist
Ethylenediamines	tripelennamine	PBZ
Alkylamines	chlorpheniramine	Chlor-Trimeton
	brompheniramine	Dimetane
Piperazines	hydroxyzine	Atarax
Phenothiazines	promethazine	Phenergan
Piperadines	cyproheptadine	Periactin

moiety. Classes and examples are listed in Table 8–1 and properties are summarized in Table 8–2. These drugs are effective in reducing sneezing and rhinorrhea during episodes of allergic rhinitis. However, most are marked by side effects of drowsiness and sedation as well as anticholinergic effects, which may cause bladder neck obstruction and increased intraocular pressure in susceptible individuals. For this reason, they carry a warning against use during the operation of machinery or other tasks that require alertness. They should also be used with caution in patients with prostatic hypertrophy and narrow-angle glaucoma.

Another potential adverse effect of first-generation antihistamines is interaction with other drugs. For example, they may increase the sedative effects of tranquilizers, sedatives, and alcohol. In turn, monoamine oxidase (MAO) inhibitors may potentiate the sedative effects of antihistamines.

A lesser-known side effect of ethylenediamine compounds is the produc-

TABLE 8–2. Summary of properties of antihistamines

Action:
Relief of sneezing, itching, rhinorrhea
Mode of action:
First-generation: by competitive inhibition, occupying H_1-receptor sites
Second- and third-generation: by above action plus multiple direct actions on mediators and inflammatory processes
Side effects:
Conventional: sedation, anticholinergic effects (dry mouth, bladder neck obstruction, elevated intraocular pressure)
Second- and third-generation: arrhythmias (see below), weight gain, hair loss, urinary retention, sedation in high doses (some preparations)
Drug interactions:
Conventional: CNS depressants, anticholinergics, MAO inhibitors
Second-generation: Cardiac arrhythmias may result from coadministration of terfenadine or astemizole with systemic antifungals, erythromycin, clarithromycin, troleandomycin, nefazodone (Serzone), grapefruit juice, quinine.

tion of gastrointestinal symptoms (e.g., nausea, constipation, abdominal pain). Paradoxical stimulation by antihistamines may be seen in infants and older patients.

Because of problems with first-generation antihistamines, a new generation of antihistamines was developed. This began with the introduction in 1985 of terfenadine, followed in 1989 by the commercial availability of astemizole. Because these compounds are relatively lipid-insoluble, they do not cross the blood-brain barrier and thus do not produce sedation. In addition, they were found not to cause excessive anticholinergic stimulation, and so could be used in patients with prostatic hypertrophy and narrow-angle glaucoma. Finally, they did not demonstrate the phenomenon of antihistamine tolerance, or "tachyphylaxis," which had been observed with first-generation compounds.

Because they did not cause unwanted side effects, and because they were new, most clinicians expected these drugs to be more effective than first-generation antihistamines in controlling allergy symptoms. However, terfenadine and astemizole were determined to be equipotent with (but not better than) first-generation antihistamines such as chlorpheniramine.[2]

Like the preparations they replaced, terfenadine and astemizole were found to have side effects and potential drug interactions of their own. Both were noted to cause problems with urinary retention,[3] but these were felt to be rare.[4] Weight gain from astemizole and hair loss from terfenadine were also reported. However, the most serious and potentially catastrophic problem with these two drugs was that of ventricular arrhythmias.[5]

It has now been determined that administration of drugs or substances that inhibit the metabolism of terfenadine or astemizole, or the ingestion of very large doses (as in suicide attempts), may result in ventricular arrhythmias. Drugs incriminated in this regard are degraded in the same hepatic metabolic pathway as are terfenadine and astemizole, namely, the P-450 CLYP3A4 cytochrome oxidase path. Preparations that should not be given in conjunction with terfenadine and astemizole include macrolide antibiotics (erythromycin, clarithromycin, troleandomycin), systemic antifungals (ketoconazole, itraconazole), the tranquilizer nefazodone, and quinine in large doses. Even grapefruit juice (in quantities as small as 8 oz twice daily) has been incriminated in this regard.[6]

Because of these adverse effects, a third generation of antihistamines has been developed, including compounds that appear to be free of cardiotoxicity. The earliest members of this class were loratadine and acrivastine. Then were added cetirizine (a relatively nonsedating congener of hydroxyzine) and fexofenadine (the acid metabolite of terfenadine, with equal activity but no cardiotoxic side effects). These preparations are generally considered to be nonsedating in normal doses, although loratadine and cetirizine in large doses apparently can cause some degree of sedation.[7]

A move toward topical preparations in the treatment of allergic rhinitis has included the development of several antihistamines delivered in this fashion. This concept is not new, as the effectiveness of chlorpheniramine administered as a nasal spray was reported in 1983.[8] The first intranasal antihistamine introduced in the United States was azelastine, which appears to be equivalent to other antihistamines in potency. Unfortunately, a high incidence of taste perversion has been noted among patients using it. Topical nasal formulations of levocabastine have been introduced in Canada and Mexico, but introduction is pending in the United States. This preparation is said to be 15,000 times more potent than chlorpheniramine, with a duration of effect of 24 hours or more and few if any side effects.[9]

As has been noted, the primary effect of antihistamines is to diminish prurutis, sneezing, and rhinorrhea. The choice of the drug employed will depend on the physician's experience, the patient's circumstances, and (often) the patient's response to samples of various antihistamines. Within these parameters, "whatever works" is generally the best drug. Representative second- and third-generation antihistamines are listed in Table 8–3.

TABLE 8–3. Second- and third-generation antihistamines

	Formulation	Adult/pediatric dose
Second-generation:		
Terfenadine (Seldane)[†]	tablets, 60 mg	60 mg BID
Astemizole (Hismanal)	tablets, 10 mg	10 mg daily
Acrivastine (Semprex D)*	tablets, 8 mg	8 mg TID
Loratadine (Claritin)	tablets, 10 mg	10 mg daily
	syrup, 1 mg/mL	2–12 yr, 5 mg daily
Ketotifen (Zaditen)	tablets, 1 mg	1 mg BID
	syrup, 1 mg/mL	>3 yr, 1 mg BID
Ebastine (Ebastel)	tablets, 10 mg	10 mg daily
Third-generation:		
Fexofenadine (Allegra)	capsules, 60 mg	60 mg BID
Cetirizine (Zyrtec)	tablets, 10 mg	10 mg daily
	syrup, 5 mg/mL	6–11 yr, 5–10 mg daily
Topical:		
Azelastine (Astelin)	solution, 0.1%	2 sprays/nostril BID
Levocabastine (Livostin)	suspension, 0.5 mg/mL	2 sprays/nostril BID

* Also contains 60 mg of pseudoephedrine.
† Seldane was removed from the US market in February 1998.

PRESCRIPTION ANTIHISTAMINE-DECONGESTANT COMBINATIONS

Antihistamines may be prescribed alone or in combination with a decongestant. In the latter situation, the alpha-adrenergic agonist drug is added to relieve nasal congestion, which is the major portion of the allergic symptom complex that is not addressed by antihistamines alone. As is the case in over-the-counter combinations, the decongestant most commonly combined with an antihistamine is pseudoephedrine, in a total daily dose of 180 to 240 mg. The next most common orally administered decongestant is phenylpropanolamine, the daily dose of which should not exceed 150 mg. Much less utilized is phenylephrine (average daily dose, 40 mg), which is useful as a topical vasoconstrictor but less effective when administered systemically. Although one of the earliest treatments for allergic rhinitis was a combination of ephedrine and amobarbitae (Amytal), ephedrine is now rarely used as a systemic decongestant. Properties of decongestants are summarized in Table 8–4.

The most common side effect of systemically administered decongestants is cardiovascular stimulation. This is generally most pronounced in the case of phenylephrine and ephedrine. In patients with labile hypertension, pseudoephedrine may produce somewhat less blood pressure elevation than phenylpropanolamine, although either preparation may be used (albeit with caution) in patients with stable, treated hypertension.[10,11] Other cardiovascular stimulatory effects of these drugs include tachycardia, palpitations, and even arrhythmias.

The central nervous system (CNS) stimulation produced by decongestants is generally manifested as anxiety and insomnia. Phenylpropanolamine may also produce anorexia and, indeed, is the active ingredient in many over-the-counter diet pills. Because convulsions may be caused by overdose of

---

TABLE 8–4. Summary of properties of decongestants

Action:
　Relief of nasal congestion
Mode of action:
　Alpha-adrenergic stimulation, producing vasoconstriction in stroma of inferior turbinates
Side effects:
　Topical: habituation (rebound rhinitis), systemic effects (see below)
　Systemic: stimulation (cardiovascular and CNS), anorexia
Drug interactions:
　Tricyclic antidepressants, MAO inhibitors, beta-adrenergic blockers, antihypertensives, CNS stimulants

this drug, careful inquiry should be made as to the use of any nonprescription drugs before phenylpropanolamine is administered.

Unfortunately, the stimulatory side effects of systemic decongestants are enhanced by tricyclic antidepressants and MAO inhibitors. The potentiation by MAO inhibitors may persist for up to 2 weeks after these drugs have been discontinued. Thus, in patients receiving these drugs, decongestants should be administered cautiously and in reduced doses.

When decongestants are combined with first-generation, sedating antihistamines, the stimulatory effects of the former are often negated by the sedative effects of the latter. However, when newer, nonsedating antihistamines are combined with decongestants, patients will frequently complain of unacceptable side effects. This is especially true in some sustained-action preparations, because the release of decongestants continues throughout the evening from a tablet or capsule taken earlier in the day. Patient response is highly variable in this regard, and other than suggesting that the second dose be taken in the early evening (and never at bedtime), a trial of several medications to determine the one best tolerated is the most appropriate approach to this problem.

CORTICOSTEROIDS

In 1855, Addison presented his classic description of a syndrome resulting from destructive disease of the adrenal glands. However, it was not until 1930 that potent adrenocortical extracts were prepared. By 1942, organic chemists had isolated five biologically active steroids from the adrenal cortex: cortisol, cortisone, corticosterone, 11-dehydrocorticosterone, and 11-desoxycorticosterone. In 1949, the remarkable anti-inflammatory properties of cortisone were shown in the treatment of rheumatoid arthritis. Subsequent research led to the development of a variety of new glucocorticoids with greater anti-inflammatory effectiveness than cortisone, yet with less mineralocorticoid activity. These included prednisone, methylprednisolone, triamcinolone, and dexamethasone. During the past half-century, corticosteroids have become a favorite pharmacologic tool of the rhinologist. The properties of corticosteroids are summarized in Table 8–5.

Systemic Corticosteroids

Corticosteroids are an important means of treating various types of rhinosinusitis. However, when administered systemically, they possess a potential

TABLE 8–5. Summary of properties of corticosteroids

Action:
Multiple anti-inflammatory effects, relieving rhinorrhea and congestion
Mode of action:
Systemic preparations affect late-phase reactions. Topical preparations, after pretreatment for several days, affect both acute and late-phase allergic reactions by decreasing capillary permeability, stabilizing lysosomal membranes, inhibiting mediator synthesis, blocking migratory inhibitory factor, and blocking arachidonic acid cascade.
Side effects:
Systemic: cataracts, hyperglycemia, menstrual irregularities, hypokalemia, edema, tachycardia and hypertension, gastrointestinal irritation or activation of ulcer, anxiety and insomnia, osteoporosis, muscle wasting, aseptic necrosis of femoral head, psychosis
Topical: local crusting, irritation, bleeding, septal perforation. Systemic effects are possible if high doses are administered for prolonged periods.
Drug interactions:
Aspirin/NSAIDs/acetaminophen, anticoagulants, digitalis, thyroid and antithyroid drugs

for producing significant adverse effects. Pharmacologic doses of systemic corticosteroids may suppress endogenous cortisol production. After the administration of 20 to 30 mg of prednisone or the equivalent for 1 week, an additional week is required for adrenal recovery; after prolonged high-dose therapy, 1 year may be required before recovery of function.[12] In addition, systemic corticosteroids present a potential for adverse effects on virtually every organ system (Table 8–6.) In one study, low-dose, long-term predni-

TABLE 8–6. Potential adverse effects of systemic corticosteroids

Posterior subcapsular cataracts
Hyperglycemia (in diabetics)
Menstrual irregularities
Hypokalemia
Edema
Tachycardia
Hypertension
Gastrointestinal irritation
Activation of peptic ulcer disease
Mental aberrations (insomnia to psychosis)
Muscle wasting
Osteoporosis
Aseptic necrosis of the femoral head
Cushing's syndrome
Adrenal suppression

sone ($\leq$ mg/d) resulted in such adverse events as fractures, serious infections, gastrointestinal bleeding and/or ulcers, and cataracts.[13] For this reason, many rhinologists now prefer to use topical rather than systemic corticosteroids when possible. If systemic preparations are necessary, they may be given either as a brief burst of an oral form or as an injection of an aqueous and repository mixture (e.g., betamethasone acetate and phosphate), which possesses less tendency for adrenal suppression than a repository form alone.

Oral corticosteroids are often prescribed in the form of a commercially prepared, tapered-dose pack. However, such preparations provide truly therapeutic doses for only 2 or 3 days, the remainder of the medication being delivered at tapered doses that are often not effective in the relief of symptoms. To provide truly effective doses for about a week, while still utilizing the tapering advocated to address any temporary adrenal suppression, Marple (Bradley F. Marple, M.D., *personal communication*) has suggested the "double Dosepak" concept. Two tapered-dose packages are dispensed. The patient takes the first day's dose from pack 1 on day 1, the first day's dose from pack 2 on day 2, and so forth. The entire day's dose should be taken all at once as a single morning dose: morning dosing both minimizes the typical steroid side effect of insomnia and is less likely to cause adrenal suppression than nocturnal administration. An acceptable alternative is for the physician simply to tailor a dosage regimen. One example is the administration of the equivalent of 30 mg of prednisolone daily for 3 days, followed by 20 mg daily for an additional 3 days, then 10 mg daily for 3 more days. If the treatment has been effective, it may be stopped at this point with little risk for adrenal suppression. If therapy must be continued longer or administered for an additional day or two at any of the steps, individual adjustment is possible.

Intramuscular injections of repository corticosteroids such as methylprednisolone acetate (Depo-Medrol) or triamcinolone acetonide (Kenalog) may produce an anti-inflammatory action for 1 to 2 months, and have been popular for the symptomatic treatment of severe allergic rhinitis during the patient's most significant allergy season. Unfortunately, they may also produce systemic side effects, including marked suppression of endogenous cortisol for a similar period after such an injection.[14] For this reason, when situations arise necessitating the parenteral administration of a corticosteroid preparation to provide sustained relief, a logical choice is a mixture of betamethasone phosphate and acetate (Celestone Soluspan), which delivers an immediate steroid dose plus a sustained effect for about 2 weeks, with somewhat less likelihood of prolonged adrenal suppression.

When systemic corticosteroids are necessary, one must keep in mind not only their possible adverse side effects, but also potential interactions with other drugs. For example, corticosteroid therapy administered concurrently with acetaminophen may cause an increase in the formation of a hepatotoxic metabolite of the latter preparation. Patients receiving both corticosteroids and aspirin or nonsteroidal anti-inflammatory agents (e.g., ibuprofen, naproxen) are at increased risk for gastrointestinal ulceration or frank hemorrhage. The effect of coumarin-type anticoagulants, such as warfarin, may be either potentiated or decreased by the concurrent administration of corticosteroids. Hypokalemia induced by corticosteroids may be detrimental in patients taking digitalis and its derivatives. Even more than with many other medications, it is important that the physician consult appropriate literature for a review of possible adverse drug interactions before prescribing corticosteroids. In addition to the usual sources of such information, the *Medical Letter on Drugs and Therapeutics* (1000 Main St, New Rochelle, NY 10801) has available an excellent computer program on drug interactions.

Intranasal Corticosteroid Injection

Published data on the intraturbinal injection of repository corticosteroids dates to the 1950s. In the mid-1970s, questions began to arise as to the safety of this very effective procedure. Sporadic reports of visual loss, either transient or permanent, following such injections sparked a spirited debate among otolaryngologists at the time. This in turn led to articles elucidating the mechanism of these complications and suggesting safe injection techniques to avoid them.[15,16]

The submucosal injection of a repository corticosteroid at the anterior tip of the inferior turbinates results in a slow uptake of the material with spreading to the adjacent nasal mucosa, offering symptomatic relief of allergic rhinitis (and other forms of rhinitis) beginning within a few hours and persisting for 4 to 6 weeks. The slow absorption of the injected steroid does not generally result in suppression of endogenous cortisol production, indicating that the effect is local rather than systemic.[17]

A review in 1981 of all published and available unpublished data on visual loss following intranasal steroid injection indicated that the mechanism involved was either retinal vasospasm or embolization of the injected material into the retinal circulation through collateral channels from the nose to the eye.[18] Suggestions for preventing such complications included preparing the nasal mucosa by the application of a topical vasoconstrictor/anesthetic solution, use of a fine needle for injection, avoidance of steroid preparations with large particle size and high viscosity, placement of the injection just beneath the mucosa in the anterior tip of the inferior turbinate (as far away from retinal collaterals as possible), and use of a very gentle technique during injection. Following these guidelines, one of the authors has performed more than 20,000 such injections during almost 30 years, with no visual complications.[19] The recommended technique that has evolved from this experience is set forth below and summarized in Table 8–7.

This procedure is extremely technique-sensitive and is not recommended for those nonotolaryngologists who are not facile in the use of the head mirror or headlight to perform intranasal manipulations. Proper patient preparation and gentle technique are mandatory, and a physician who is unprepared to observe the caveats set forth here is well advised to utilize an alternative pharmacotherapeutic approach.

It is important to advise patients of what to expect. Some patients can readily be identified as potential "fainters," and it is often best to choose another method of delivering corticosteroid in such instances. Also, it is appropriate to obtain informed consent. The most common sequelae of this injection are blood-streaked nasal mucus and facial flushing on the following day. This flushing, a result of local vasodilation, is more common in female than male patients and more often seen in fair-complected and/or red-haired persons (for reasons unknown to the author). A rare patient will demonstrate an adverse reaction to the repository vehicle, manifested by back pain after the injection. Local heat and mild analgesics suffice to control this reaction, which subsides in a few hours or less. In these case, a notation should be made on the chart and the patient should not receive the same preparation (either intranasally or intramuscularly) in the future. The incidence of visual loss after one of these injections has been estimated as about 0.006%, and physicians should make their own decision about including this in the informed consent.

Preparation of the injection site by placement of a cotton pledget with a topical anesthetic/vasoconstrictor serves two purposes. When properly performed, intraturbinal steroid injection is virtually painless, even without anesthesia. However, the anesthetic also may prevent reflex vasospasm from an inadvertently painful injection. The topical vasoconstrictor decreases the caliber of the vessels within the turbinate stroma, making intravascular deposition even less likely. As most otolaryngologists perform an initial intranasal examination, followed by another evaluation after decongestion, if a solution such as 5% cocaine or a mixture of 2% lidocaine/0.5% phenylephrine is utilized for this purpose, the patient is already prepared for the injection by the time the examination has been completed.

The utilization of a fine (usually 25-gauge, 1.5-in.) needle not only contrib-

TABLE 8–7. Recommended technique for intraturbinal corticosteroid injection

I. Explanation and reassurance
   A. Explain what is to be done.
   B. Identify possible "fainters" and either prepare them or choose another treatment method.
II. Preparing the injection site
   A. Apply 5% cocaine or a solution of 2% lidocaine with 0.5% phenylephrine on cotton pledgets to the anterior portions of the inferior turbinates for about 1 minute.
   B. If this was done when the nose was decongested for examination, it need not be repeated.
III. Preparing injectable material
   A. Fit a 25-gauge, 1.5-in. needle to a tuberculin syringe.
   B. Draw up 1 mL of triamcinolone acetonide, 40 mg/mL (Kenalog-40). Utilizing the smaller needle to draw up the steroid will minimize particle aggregation and clumping. For the same reason, the material should not be predrawn and allowed to sit, to avoid settling.
   C. Alternative preparations are triamcinolone diacetate (Aristocort Forte), dexamethasone acetate (Decadron-LA), or methylprednisolone tebutate (Hydeltra-T.B.A.).
   D. Do *not* mix a local anesthetic with the injected material. It is unnecessary, and adds to the risk for clumping.
IV. Performing the injection
   A. Remove the cotton pledget (if still in place). From a slight angle, insert the tip of the needle into the anterior tip of the inferior turbinate, just submucosally.
   B. Using very gentle pressure, inject a total of approximately 0.5 mL. The "feel" will be about the same as when injecting local anesthetic into a septum. A white blanching of the tissue around the injection site should occur.
   C. If more than gentle pressure is required, rotate the needle 90 to 180 and if possible withdraw the needle slightly. If it is still impossible to inject in this area, withdraw the needle and place a piece of dry cotton at that site. Go to the other side, and then return to this side.
   D. After each side has been injected, place a piece of dry cotton over the injection site (to avoid accumulation of blood from the needle stick site and minimize leakage of injected material).
V. Completing the procedure
   A. Discuss again with the patient your expectations for the procedure.
   B. Warn that blood-streaked nasal mucus may appear for a few minutes afterward. Occasionally, patients will experience facial flushing, and they should be reassured beforehand that this will cease in a day or less without treatment.
   C. Remove the cotton, blot any blood within the nostrils, allow the patient to blow his or her nose.

utes to the comfort of the patient but also makes injection of a bolus of clumped material less likely. A tuberculin syringe allows more control during injection than a larger-capacity syringe. The preparation chosen for injection should not have a high viscosity or large particle size, and it should not be mixed with a local anesthetic (with or without vasoconstrictor), which might contribute to clumping and/or vasospasm. If the author's recommended preparation, triamcinolone acetonide (Kenalog-40), is used, the dose is 0.5 mL per side. Preparing several of these syringes at the start of a workday might at first seem to be efficient, but it also contributes to particle settling and clumping, which are undesirable.

If the procedure is properly performed, the needle tip is inserted just beneath the mucosa, and the injection spreads the material to produce a white blanching of the surrounding area (Fig. 8–1). If resistance is encountered, the needle tip should be rotated, or even withdrawn and reinserted. After each injection, brief application of pressure with dry cotton completes the procedure.

The results of an intraturbinal corticosteroid injection are usually noted within a few hours of the injection, and if triamcinolone acetonide has been injected, they last for 4 to 6 weeks. Lesser duration of action is seen with

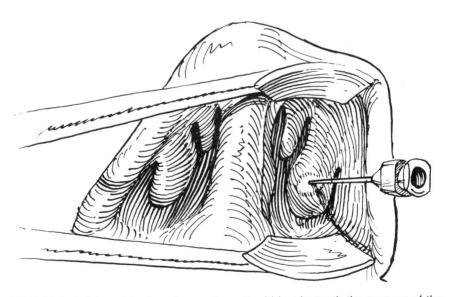

FIGURE 8–1. Direct injection of repository steroid just beneath the mucosa of the anterior head of the inferior turbinate should produce a slight, white blanching. (Reprinted with permission from Mabry RL. Intraturbinal steroid injection: indications, results and complications. South Med J 1978;71:789.)

the alternative steroids listed. The injection should never be repeated until the initial beneficial effects have worn off.

This procedure is extremely helpful for symptom relief in patients with severe nasal allergic symptoms limited to a single season. If several injections per year are necessary, the patient is probably a candidate for maintenance therapy with topical steroids. Of course, such patients are also best treated with immunotherapy, making the regular use of steroids unnecessary.

Topical Nasal Corticosteroids

In the treatment of nasal disorders, the topical application of medications seems quite appropriate, both to concentrate the therapeutic effect on the target organ and avoid undesirable systemic effects. The first commercially available topical nasal aerosol, a propellant-driven form of dexamethasone, became available in the 1970s. However, little attention was given to this form of therapy until the introduction in 1981 of topical nasal beclomethasone, followed soon thereafter by flunisolide in topical nasal form. Since then, numerous other preparations have been developed and introduced. Each new drug is purported to have advantages over its predecessors, generally in the form of less frequent dosing and a lessened potential for systemic absorption. The search for the "perfect" nasal steroid continues, and until that is found, the list will continue to grow. Topical nasal corticosteroids currently available and on the horizon are listed in Table 8–8.

TABLE 8–8. Topical nasal corticosteroids (in chronologic order of introduction of parent compound)

Generic name	Trade name	Delivery	Dosage	Margin of safety*
Dexamethasone	Dexacort	MDI	TID	1+
Beclomethasone	Vancenase	MDI	BID–QID	5
	Beconase	MDI	BID–QID	5
	Vancenase AQ DS	Pump	Daily	5
	Beconase AQ	Pump	BID	5
Flunisolide	Nasalide	Pump	BID	3.5
	Nasarel	Pump	BID	3.5
Triamcinolone	Nasacort	MDI	Daily	16
	Nasacort AQ	Pump	Daily	16
Budesonide	Rhinocort	MDI	Daily	4
Fluticasone	Flonase	Pump	Daily	8
Mometasone	Nasonex	Pump	Daily	20

MDI, metered-dose inhaler.
* Multiple of recommended initial dose to produce hypothalamic-pituitary-adrenal axis suppression.

Because their anti-inflammatory action is nonspecific, nasal steroids may be useful in the treatment of both allergic and nonallergic rhinitis. Unlike systemic corticosteroids, which almost exclusively affect the late-phase allergic reaction, pretreatment with topical nasal corticosteroids for up to a week has a beneficial effect on both acute- and late-phase allergic reactions. However, it is worth emphasizing that these compounds do not prevent the allergic reaction, but simply blunt the effects of the mediators thus released.

The effective use of nasal steroids (as with any nasal preparation) begins with the drug being able to penetrate the nasal cavity and come in contact with the target mucosa. For this reason, patients with severe septal deviation and/or markedly hypertrophic inferior turbinates will benefit to a considerably lesser degree from the use of nasal corticosteroids than will patients without such obstruction. A systemic decongestant, or a brief course of a topical decongestant, may be necessary in conjunction with nasal steroids (especially at the initiation of therapy) to ensure adequate penetration past congested areas. Although steroid nasal sprays are effective in the treatment of small nasal polyps and the prevention of polyp regrowth after nasal and sinus surgery, large polyp masses that essentially block the nasal passage will not generally yield to topical therapy. An exception is the application of topical steroids as drops, administered in the Moffatt (kneeling, head down) position. Such treatment, using budesonide drops during a period of months, has been reported to be effective by some investigators.[20] Unfortunately, nasal steroid drops are not available in the United States, and although the enterprising physician might devise a way to deliver steroids in this fashion, other, equally effective methods are more readily available.

Patients with nasal problems are accustomed to utilizing decongestant nose drops and sprays on an as-needed basis. This same approach is not appropriate in the use of nasal steroids, and the lack of efficacy of such an approach has been well documented.[21] Rather, patients requiring topical nasal corticosteroids for the relief of allergic rhinitis should begin these drugs at the onset of their anticipated season of exposure, maintaining an initial dosage level until symptom relief is obtained, then decreasing their use to the lowest effective maintenance dose throughout the remainder of that season.

In an effort to increase compliance, the current trend in nasal steroid therapy is toward once- or twice-daily dosing. To lessen patient discomfort, some of the newer preparations include improved delivery systems. Manufacturers have omitted preservatives such as phenylethyl alcohol (which has an unpleasant taste and odor), changed the vehicle from propylene glycol (which causes stinging) to polyethylene glycol and altered the propellant-delivered systems to provide a "gentler" puff into the nostrils.

Local side effects may occur with any nasal steroid preparation. In addition to local discomfort caused by preservatives and vehicles, side effects frequently involve nasal crusting and dryness, epistaxis, headache, and sore throat. Excoriation or ulceration of the nasal septum may follow nasal steroid therapy, sometimes leading to frank septal perforation. In addition to irritation from propellants and a thinning of the nasal mucosa from the steroid, the most likely contributory factor is trauma to the septum. This can be avoided by careful instruction to patients to direct the tip of nasal steroid sprays away from the septum (pointing it toward the corner of the eye), thereby avoiding contact with the septum. Nasal candidiasis may occur in patients using nasal steroids, as does oral candidiasis in patients using inhaled steroids for pulmonary disease; this responds well to the application of nystatin cream to the nasal vestibule twice daily for about a week.

Local side effects are bothersome, but much more serious are the potential systemic effects that may be associated with systemic absorption of topically administered nasal steroids. About 20% of corticosteroid administered intranasally is absorbed directly from the nasal mucosa. In addition, more than half the material is swallowed and absorbed from the gastrointestinal tract. This latter portion gains entry to the portal circulation and undergoes a significant amount of first-pass hepatic metabolism, which may vary from 80 to 99%. However, the portion that is absorbed from the nasal mucosa does not immediately undergo degradation and may result in systemic corticosteroid effects.[22]

It is often thought that administration of topical nasal steroids, even for prolonged periods, presents no potential for systemic effects. However, conflicting data are now available about systemic bioavailability after topical administration of such supposedly safe preparations as budesonide or fluticasone at normal doses.[23-26] The message from all this is that although it has been assumed for years that topical nasal steroids do not have the potential to produce systemic effects, the final answer is not yet known. Although clinicians should not be hesitant to prescribe these drugs when needed, it is incumbent on them to reduce the dosage to the lowest effective maintenance level once improvement has occurred, and to monitor patients for any adverse effects and to ensure that use of the drug continues to be necessary.

The potential adverse systemic consequences of intranasally administered corticosteroids include posterior subcapsular cataracts, menstrual irregularities, hyperglycemia in diabetics, aseptic necrosis of the femoral head, decreased growth of long bones in children, and suppression of endogenous cortisol production. Realistically, these are most likely to occur in patients taking higher than recommended doses for prolonged periods of time, also utilizing inhaled steroids for pulmonary disease, and being treated with nasal steroids that have a very low margin of safety.

The term *margin of safety* refers to the multiple of the recommended initial dose of a topical nasal corticosteroid (depending on the preparation in question) necessary to produce a systemic effect, as evidenced by suppression of endogenous cortisol production.[27] The generally accepted margins of safety for commonly available nasal steroids, taken from published data, are shown in Table 8–8. Dose-related systemic absorption of nasally administered dexamethasone is well documented, and although it remains an excellent choice to achieve rapid relief in a short period of time, it is not suitable for treatment for a period exceeding 3 weeks. Probably the greatest clinical experience with nasal steroids involves beclomethasone and flunisolide. Triamcinolone, budesonide, and fluticasone present the advantages of once-daily dosing and a greater margin of safety than the early nasal steroids. This margin of safety between topical therapeutic doses and potential systemic effect is even greater with mometasone, and undoubtedly future research efforts will attempt to provide more safety and convenience for the patient. Potency is not a major consideration, as all currently available topical nasal steroids are adequately potent.

ANTICHOLINERGIC DRUGS

At one time, it was popular to add systemic anticholinergic drugs, such as derivatives of atropine and scopolamine, to antihistamine and decongestant combinations. This "shotgun" approach was aimed at alleviating all the symptoms that could possibly be experienced by the allergic rhinitis sufferer. These combinations produced such adverse effects as overdrying, producing nasal crusting and thick nasal mucus. Other, less common side effects of systemic anticholinergics are tachycardia, hypertension, delayed gastric emptying, increased intraocular pressure, blurred vision, and urinary retention. Because of this, most such combinations have been withdrawn from the market. Instead, topical anticholinergics are now popular for the relief of rhinorrhea.

Atropine sulfate, 0.050 to 0.075% in saline solution, has been recommended as a topical anticholinergic. As no commercially available preparation currently exists, it must be prepared individually. The duration of action is about 3 hours, and no notable side effects have been reported.[28] Fortunately, it is seldom necessary to compound atropine solution, as the anticholinergic ipratropium bromide is now available in 0.03% and 0.06% strengths in a metered-dose pump spray for intranasal use. The 0.06% strength is primarily used to alleviate the initial rhinorrhea of the common cold, whereas the 0.03% concentration is utilized to control rhinorrhea caused by vasomotor or allergic rhinitis.

Although patients with allergy rarely complain of rhinorrhea without other symptoms, such as itching and nasal congestion, there are times when control of rhinorrhea is difficult with the drugs already described. In these situations, intranasal ipratropium (Atrovent nasal spray) may be added to the regimen. It appears from early work that the most important factor is a sufficient dose early in the day to control symptoms, with additional dosing as necessary.[29] The recommended dosing regimen is two sprays in each nostril in the morning on arising, with subsequent doses of two sprays in midafternoon and in the evening if needed. Often, the morning dose alone suffices. In these circumstances, the use of the topical anticholinergic is not curative but will often control symptoms that are extremely bothersome to the patient. Side effects from topical nasal ipratropium are minimal, and its long-term use does not appear thus far to present a problem.

COMBINATION REGIMENS

The patient with allergic rhinitis does not typically achieve relief of all symptoms with the use of a single medication. Antihistamines relieve the itching, sneezing, and rhinorrhea that typify this disorder. Decongestants are necessary to relieve nasal stuffiness. Often, these are combined, and although the use of individual antihistamines and decongestants allows the patient more leeway in treating individual symptoms as they occur, the use of a single tablet or capsule once or twice daily is appealing to many patients as a matter of convenience (and requires no clinical judgments on their part).

Nasal corticosteroids have become the mainstay of the treatment of patients with more severe or chronic nasal allergic symptoms. In comparisons of the effectiveness of antihistamines versus nasal steroids versus both drugs in combination, nasal steroids were more effective in relieving the majority of allergy symptoms, and combined therapy was even more effective.[30] Although the effectiveness of nasal steroids in alleviating the symptoms of allergic rhinitis is generally accepted, placing patients on them for virtually unlimited periods of time with little or no supervision presents a risk for complications that is not matched by the use of antihistamines.

Patients with mild symptoms may require little more than the use of a mast cell stabilizer, such as cromolyn, before an anticipated allergen exposure. A second- or third-generation antihistamine may be given prophylactically or to relieve symptoms as needed. When patients have severe and/or chronic

TABLE 8–9. Costs of some drugs for allergic rhinitis

Drug name	Cost for 30 days' treatment*
Antihistamines	
Azelastine (Astelin)	$51.12
Astemizole (Hismanal)	$59.91
Loratadine (Claritin)	$62.49
Cetirizine (Zyrtec)	$44.59
Fexofenadine (Allegra)	$51.56
Mast cell stabilizers	
Cromolyn (Nasalcrom) (available over the counter)	$12.52
Nasal steroids	
Beclomethasone (Vancenase, Beconase)	$20.46–$24.37
Beclomethasone (Beconase AQ)	$22.08
Beclomethasone (Vancenase AQ DS)	$22.08
Flunisolide (Nasalide)	$33.11
Triamcinolone (Nasacort)	$46.93
Triamcinolone (Nasacort AQ)	$33.15
Budesonide (Rhinocort)	$39.37
Fluticasone (Flonase)	$44.17

* Cost to patient for 30 days' treatment at the lowest initial dosage for adults, according to wholesale price (AWP) listings in Drug Topics Red Book Update, April 1997. From Med Lett Drugs Ther 1997 May; 9:46 (vol 39).

symptoms that necessitate medication on a daily basis, it is appropriate to switch to the use of a nasal steroid. This should then be used daily throughout the expected season of allergen exposure, and may be augmented by antihistamines and/or decongestants on an "as-needed" basis. Once a patient has been on topical nasal steroids for a week or more, the effect on the acute-phase allergic reaction is sufficient to make the additional use of nasal cromolyn redundant.

In situations in which rhinorrhea does not respond to either nasal steroids or topical ipratropium, a combination of the two may be effective. The patient should be maintained on a nasal corticosteroid in the usual dosage, adding ipratropium daily with the usual morning dose and supplemental doses of ipratropium once or twice later in the day as needed. This same approach may be used in patients whose rhinorrhea is only partially relieved with antihistamines, and who (for whatever reason) are not candidates for nasal steroid therapy.

It is increasingly true that along with safety, effectiveness, and convenience, the factor of cost must be considered when a treatment regimen. Some comparative costs of a number of common medications used in the treatment of allergy are presented in Table 8–9.

NEW DIRECTIONS IN PHARMACOTHERAPY OF ALLERGIC RHINITIS

Research is continuing to focus on alleviating the symptoms of nasal allergy through multiple mechanisms. Newer antihistamines are more than just "histamine blockers"; they also affect multiple mediators of inflammation released during the allergic reaction.

Leukotriene inhibitors show promise in the treatment of asthma. Their action is primarily on the late-phase allergic reaction, and it is unlikely that they will become a mainstay of treatment of the acute phase. However, all this could change with further research.

Peptides, such as pentigetide, have been shown to inhibit cutaneous and systemic IgE-mediated allergic reactions in humans. Preliminary studies show that these substances, administered as intranasal sprays, produce a significant reduction in the symptoms of itching, sneezing, rhinorrhea, and nasal congestion. The biochemical mechanism by which these compounds exert their antiallergy activity is unknown, but research is proceeding in this area.

It is impossible to predict where the next breakthrough in the pharmacotherapy of allergic rhinitis will occur. Informed health care professionals will closely monitor presentations at scientific meetings and articles in reputable journals, constantly updating their armamentarium to provide symptom relief to the allergy sufferer.

REFERENCES

1. Mabry RL. Intranasal corticosteroids and cromolyn. Am J Otolaryngol 1993;14:295–300.
2. Choice of antihistamines for allergic rhinitis. Med Lett Drugs Ther 1987;29:105.
3. Lin AY, Zahtz G, Myssiorek D. Astemizole-associated urinary retention. Otolaryngol Head Neck Surg 1991;105:893–894.
4. Spaulding HS, Sutherland RS, Sklarew PR, et al. Effect of terfenadine on urination. Ann Allergy 1994;72:441–445.
5. Monahan BP, Ferguson CL, Killeavy ES, et al. Torsades de pointes occurring in association with terfenadine use. JAMA 1990;264:2788–2790.
6. Honig P, Baraniuk JN. Adverse effects of H_2-receptor antagonists in the cardiovascular system. In: Simons FER, ed. Histamine and H_1-Receptor Antagonists in Allergic Disease. New York: Marcel Dekker; 1996:383–412.
7. Meltzer EO, Welch MJ. Adverse effects of H_1-receptor antagonists in the central nervous system. In: Simons FER, ed. Histamine and H_1-Receptor Antagonists in Allergic Disease. New York: Marcel Dekker; 1996:357–381.
8. Kirkegaard J, Secher C, Borum P, et al. Inhibition of histamine-induced nasal symptoms by the H_1 antihistamine chlorpheniramine maleate: demonstration of topical effect. Br J Dis Chest 1983;77:113–122.
9. Mabry RL. Topical pharmacotherapy for allergic rhinitis: new agents. South Med J 1992; 85:149–154.

10. Beck RA, Mercano DL, Seguin SM, et al. Cardiovascular effects of pseudoephedrine in medically controlled hypertensive patients. Arch Intern Med 1992;152:1242–1245.
11. Kroenke K, Omori DM, Simmons JO, et al. The safety of phenylpropanolamine in patients with stable hypertension. Ann Intern Med 1989;111:1043–1044.
12. USP Drug Information for the Health Care Professional. 17th ed. Rockville, MD: US Pharmacopoeial Convention; 1997;958–983.
13. Saag K, Koehnke R, Caldwell JR, et al. Low-dose long-term corticosteroid therapy in rheumatoid arthritis: an analysis of serious adverse events. Am J Med 1994;96:115–123.
14. Mikhail GR, Livingood CS, Mellinger RC, et al. Effect of long-acting parenteral corticosteroids on adrenal function. Arch Dermatol 1969;100:263–268.
15. McCleve DE, Goldstein JC, Silver S. Corticosteroid injections of the nasal turbinates: past experience and precautions. Trans Am Acad Ophthalmol Otolaryngol 1978;86:851–857.
16. Mabry RL. Intraturbinal steroid injection: indications, results and complications. South Med J 1978;71:789–791.
17. Mabry RL. Evaluation of systemic absorption of intraturbinally injected triamcinolone. Otolaryngol Head Neck Surg 1981;89:268–270.
18. Mabry RL. Visual loss after intranasal corticosteroid injection. Arch Otolaryngol 1981; 107:484–486.
19. Mabry RL. Intranasal steroids in rhinology: the changing role of intraturbinal injection. Ear Nose Throat J 1994;73:242–246.
20. Lildholdt T, Fogstrup J, Gammelgaard N, et al. Management of nasal polyps by steroid nose drops. Am J Rhinol 1991;5:25–27.
21. Juniper EE, Guyat GH, O'Bryne PM, et al. Aqueous beclomethasone dipropionate nasal spray: regular versus as required use in the treatment of seasonal allergic rhinitis. J Allergy Clin Immunol 1990;86:380–386.
22. Lipworth BJ. New perspectives on inhaled drug delivery and systemic bioactivity. Thorax 1995;50:105–110.
23. Edsbacker S, Anderson KE, Ryrfeldt A. Nasal bioavailability and systemic effects of the glucocorticoid budesonide in man. Eur J Clin Pharmacol 1985;29:477–481.
24. Knutson U, Stierna P, Marcus C, Carlstedt-Duke J, et al. Effects of intranasal glucocorticoids on endogenous glucocorticoid peripheral and central function. J Endocrinol 1996; 144:301–310.
25. Day J, Alexander M, Drouin M, Frankish C, et al. Budesonide aqueous nasal spray and pressurized metered-dose inhaler in the treatment of adult patients with seasonal allergic rhinitis. Am J Rhinol 1997;11:77–83.
26. Banov CH, Woehler TR, LaForce CF, et al. Once daily intranasal fluticasone propionate is effective for perennial rhinitis. Ann Allergy 1994;73:240–246.
27. Mabry RL. Corticosteroids in the management of upper respiratory allergy: the emerging role of steroid nasal sprays. Otolaryngol Head Neck Surg 1992;107:856–860.
28. Georgitis JW, Shilstone J. Atropine sulfate nasal solution: efficacy and safety of 0.05% and 0.075% for severe rhinorrhea. Ann Allergy 1993;70:81(abst).
29. Mygind N, Borum P. Anticholinergic treatment of watery rhinorrhea. Am J Rhinol 1990; 4:1–5.
30. Brooks CD, Francom SF, Peel BG, Chene BL, Klott KA. Spectrum of seasonal allergic rhinitis symptom relief with topical corticoid and oral antihistamine given singly or in combination. Am J Rhinol 1996;10:192–199.

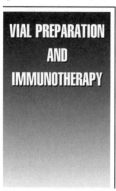

9

RATIONALE AND BACKGROUND OF IMMUNOTHERAPY

In the mind of the public, specialty allergy care is equated with immunotherapy. Patients of all ages are familiar with immunotherapy. This treatment approach, which has been in use since about 1910 and has proved effective in a large percentage of cases, is available only from a specialist. Other approaches to allergy management are available but have drawbacks. Environmental control has always been difficult, and before the use of air conditioning, both in homes and public buildings, became widespread, environmental control represented an essentially impossible approach for the patient faced with avoiding more than a few isolated offenders. The limitations of geographic relocation have already been discussed. Although it is true that various medications have been used to treat allergic problems for the better part of a century, drugs that are truly effective in controlling allergy symptoms while relatively free of side effects have been available only for slightly more than a decade. Even today, as noted in the discussion of pharmacotherapy, the effects of long-term use of many of the newer medications are unclear. Like environmental control, pharmacotherapy, although greatly improved in today's medical climate, has its limitations.

The current generation is also more likely to choose immunotherapy because it has been taught to emphasize maintaining fitness and wellness, limit costs of drugs, and inquire about the availability of other approaches. Patients have been advised by the media to take charge of managing their medical problems to the greatest degree possible. Many patients are reluctant to take medicines, which they consider foreign substances, regularly for prolonged or indefinite periods. This attitude is by no means universal, but every practitioner has heard patients voice concern about the possible risks and side effects of drugs. Although immunotherapy may be perceived as an inconvenience, it is potentially "curative," and therefore many patients are willing to "put up with all those shots" rather than depend on medications for a lifetime.

Furthermore, patients are presented daily, through many sources, with treatment options for allergy that are outside the mainstream of standard medical practice. Although some of these approaches may eventually be validated, others remain merely ineffective nostrums that may delay appropriate treatment. Knowledgeable patients, and those educated by the physician, are generally willing to avoid such uncertain methods of management, opting instead for immunotherapy, which has been proved effective by many decades of experience.

From a more pragmatic standpoint, numerous medications for allergy control are now available over the counter, and most allergic patients have tried a number of these before electing to engage the services of a physician. Probably, the referring physician has utilized one or more prescription preparations in an attempt to control the patient's symptoms. The physician offering more medications of a similar nature without at least discussing immunotherapy is likely to encounter little enthusiasm on the part of the patient. This is especially true in the present era of managed care, when referral to a specialist may be difficult to obtain. Once this referral has been obtained and consultation accomplished, something more definitive in the way of care is usually expected. In most cases, the patient who has proceeded this far is prepared for immunotherapy.

BENEFITS OF IMMUNOTHERAPY

Immunotherapy offers one benefit not currently provided by any other form of therapy. It is the only approach that offers the probability of providing long-term, permanent relief from most or all of the patient's allergic problems by a direct action on the immune system. Many patients are not aware of the fact that immunotherapy today is not expected to be continued for a lifetime, and that about 80 to 90% of patients, properly treated, will be able to discontinue immunotherapy after 3 to 5 years and remain comfortable. Some medical supplementation may be required when allergen exposure is especially heavy, but this will usually be on an as-necessary, temporary basis rather than a regular one. This makes immunotherapy the only currently available definitive approach to allergy care.

The limited and defined duration of treatment needed under an immunotherapy program has several benefits. First, albeit on a somewhat nebulous basis, it tends to reassure the somatically focused patient. Because a specific, limited treatment time is projected, the patient feels that the body is being cured rather than symptoms simply being masked. To many patients, this factor is of major importance.

Some patients are concerned about the mechanism of immunotherapy. The patient may be advised that the allergens used for treatment are essentially merely the substances that are causing the allergic reactions, and not foreign material. The offenders are being presented to the patient's immune system repeatedly in such a way that the immune system is able to adjust to the exposure and build up protection rather than experience an adverse reaction.

Patients also question why continual exposure to an allergen during the blooming season does not build up resistance. The answer is the need for higher antigen levels to accomplish this. The amount presented in a single injection of ragweed, for instance, generally exceeds the normal body exposure to ragweed during a single season. This is, of course, an oversimplification, but many patients are able to relate to it.

Clarification of another benefit of a defined and limited course of immunotherapy may require some education of both the patient and the third-party payer involved in reimbursing for care. The initial negative reaction to immunotherapy, in addition to discomfort, involves cost. Immunotherapy, including both testing and treatment, is perceived as quite expensive. It usually surprises both patient and payer to find that immunotherapy is not only the most definitive form of allergy care, but allows significant savings over a lifetime of pharmacotherapy. This cost balancing requires a little explanation. There can be no question that when all costs are considered, properly administered immunotherapy on properly selected patients is the most cost-effective form of allergy care. The operative words, however, are "properly selected" and "properly administered." In addition to a savings on medications, other benefits that accrue to the patient treated by immunotherapy are fewer sick days, improved quality of life, and increased productivity.[1]

PRINCIPLES OF PATIENT SELECTION FOR IMMUNOTHERAPY

Treatment Choices

A variety of formats for providing immunotherapy are in common use. In this text, the format that will be primarily discussed is the one practiced almost exclusively by otolaryngologists, as well as many other physicians from other disciplines. This format is derived from skin endpoint titration (SET), and such immunotherapy based on quantitative testing provides the same safety and efficiency found in the SET testing methodology. Before presenting the details of immunotherapy, we should first consider the results that can be expected from it, as well as details about patient selection.

Age

It is rare to find significant inhalant allergy in a patient less than 2 years of age. There simply has not been enough time for exposure to potential allergens to have resulted in sensitization. If no significant inhalant allergy is present, it is axiomatic that no immunotherapy is indicated, as immunotherapy functions by building specific blocking mechanisms against specific allergens. If these have not yet become a part of the patient's makeup, even if the genetic propensity is there, immunotherapy will not prevent the development of allergy. Unless there is a very strong history of inhalant allergy symptoms under very specific exposure conditions, testing with a view to immunotherapy in a child under the age of 2 would be rare. It is advisable to explain this to the parents, who may well be anticipating a recommendation for immunotherapy. The physician does not want to generate the impression that such a response represents a wish to avoid treating small children, which the parents may easily feel to be the case. After all, small children tend to be noisy, time-consuming, and frequently messy. They can disrupt the smooth function of a busy office. Children of any age, however, tend to respond extremely well to appropriate allergy care and frequently provide some of the best advertising obtainable for the new allergist.

Allergy care for the very young child should be approached initially by history and dietary regulation, as foods are a more frequent offender than inhalants in the first 2 years of life. This approach is more likely to be successful than immunotherapy, is easier for the parents to provide, and instills in the parents a feeling that the physician is sincerely motivated to provide the best care for the child. If it is necessary to demonstrate the presence or absence of inhalant sensitivity, a very limited number of allergens may be tested by radioallergosorbent testing (RAST). These should include perennials: the dust group, pets in the home, and a representative mold. If these produce no significant responses, the test will have convincingly demonstrated that immunotherapy need not be considered. If positive responses are obtained, as avoidance and environmental control are possible for all these antigens, such measures should be instituted before any consideration of immunotherapy.

For the child of roughly 2 to 5 years who is genetically predisposed to become allergic, inhalant allergy may be developing if the allergen exposure is heavy. Usually, the first sensitivity to be seen is to perennial allergens. If the child has definite symptoms of inhalant allergy at this stage of development, limited testing by either skin testing or RAST methods may reveal an allergic response strong enough to warrant immunotherapy. If such a response is demonstrated, it may be wise to inform the parents that spontaneous resolution of the condition is unlikely, as there is still a popular opinion among the laity that most such children will "outgrow their allergies." This impression may be the result of seeing food-allergic children improve symptomatically as the lining of the gastrointestinal tract matures, limiting the absorption of macromolecules of food that previously stimulated the immune system to produce reactions indistinguishable from those of inhalant allergy. This response to foods, known as the "leaky gut" syndrome, is not uncommon in small children and is not in any way related to the mechanism of inhalant allergy. When inhalant allergy becomes manifest, the tendency is for the sensitivity to the established allergens to increase, and for new allergies to appear as exposure to new potential allergens continues.

Immunotherapy at an early age will probably be successful, but it is necessary to realize that it is effective only for the allergens that have already produced a hypersensitivity reaction. If new allergies develop, the apparent success of the immunotherapy already under way will gradually be diminished, as only a limited number of the total offenders are being treated. The physician treating an allergic child must be prepared to test for new allergens according to the emerging symptom pattern, and to add these to the treatment regimen when they have been identified. This may require a second treatment vial and an additional injection for a short period of time, as a maintenance level of vaccine concentration may have been reached for the allergens already under treatment, whereas a dosage escalation schedule will be necessary for the new offenders. The antigens may be combined into one vial when a maintenance level has been reached for all.

Pollen sensitivity rarely appears before the age of 5 years. When a seasonal pattern emerges, it may be time to consider an inhalant allergy screen. This may not be necessary if only a single season of short duration is involved, but the probability is that the single season will expand into additional seasons and may eventually become a perennial problem. Certainly if more than one season produces allergic symptoms of significant severity, the course of the allergic disease is becoming evident and demands attention. If results of the initial screening tests (described in Chapter 5) are positive, they may be expanded to include all the likely offenders. This should be done before instituting immunotherapy, as the addition of more allergens to a treatment regimen entails additional injections. It has already been mentioned that new allergies may be expected to develop from time to time as new prolonged exposure occurs, but at some point a decision must be made about the benefits of delaying definitive care to allow for the possibility of the eventual appearance of new sensitivities.

The decision as to whether or not to start immunotherapy at the earliest sign of active sensitization must be an individual consideration. If the child is not responding to dietary manipulation and environmental control, if the symptoms are severe and not controlled easily by medication, or if the patient reacts poorly to medical therapy, immunotherapy may be indicated. If this is not the case, it may be advisable to defer immunotherapy until the patient is a little older.

Although new problems may develop with time, there is an additional benefit to instituting immunotherapy in children as soon as a significant pattern of allergic disease has been identified. This is the reduction of the "total allergic load," a condition related to the "priming effect." The more uncontrolled allergy that is present, the greater the symptoms that are produced by the same allergen exposure. *Priming* is the phenomenon whereby at the start of an allergy season, high degrees of allergen exposure may be needed to produce symptoms, whereas toward the end of the season, a minor exposure will produce severe symptoms. Priming may also cause exposure to minor allergens to result in marked symptoms, although such exposure produced no symptoms at the start of the season. The patient's immune system has become "primed." By the same token, in the patient whose allergic problems have been brought under control, severe symptomatology is much less prone to develop after new exposures because the allergic load has been reduced.

Avoiding priming and minimizing the total allergic load allows the allergist to treat for a more limited number of key antigens, concentrating on the more severe offenders and still obtaining good results. It should be evident that it may be impossible (and certainly impractical) to treat routinely for every major and minor allergen to which a patient has any degree of sensitivity. For example, antigenic extract is not available for some of the more minor substances, and other allergens may not be evident to the investigator. Cross-reactivity, significantly further reduces the total number of allergens needed for treatment, so that immunotherapy with a reasonable number of antigens is effective.

The above discussion has been directed primarily at considerations of immunotherapy for the developing child, but many of the same considerations are equally applicable to the allergic adult. Allergy may appear at any time in life, and when the criteria described are met, immunotherapy is one of the treatment modalities deserving consideration.

Season and Circumstances

Immunotherapy is a valid means of therapy for inhalant allergy, but it may not always be the best choice. Not every patient demonstrates the same progression of disease; the rapidity of the progression is highly variable. For the patient who has symptoms only on specific exposure to avoidable antigens, such as the cat-sensitive patient, careful avoidance and environmental control may be all that is needed. The patient with symptoms only during the relatively short tree-blooming season, for example, may find medical treatment to be entirely adequate. The exception is the patient who responds poorly to medication and resists taking any such medication, either because of side effects or merely personal preference. These patients may request immunotherapy, and there is no reason to deny their requests, as the immunotherapy should be as effective as that given to patients with multiple-season symptoms. The ideal candidate for immunotherapy, of course, is the patient whose symptoms have progressed to last 6 months or more of the year and who is young enough to anticipate many decades of problems requiring treatment of some type.

Patient Cooperation

For the full benefits of immunotherapy to be achieved, the patient must be prepared to cooperate in the program. Achieving this cooperation requires a significant degree of discussion with the patient before such a course is undertaken, usually augmented by some printed material that may be reviewed by the patient at regular intervals. It is best to identify potential "dropouts" before treatment is begun. Immunotherapy may be the most cost-effective form of allergy care, but this is true only if a full course of treatment is carried out.

One of the major benefits of immunotherapy, and also one of the factors most subject to misunderstanding on the part of the patient, is the early response to treatment usually seen in patients treated by SET-based immunotherapy. Because treatment for each antigen is started at the highest concentration found to be safe by testing, beneficial results are frequently seen within a matter of several weeks. This response may represent a double-edged sword. The benefits are evident: prompt improvement, even during a major allergy season, with little potential risk for reactions. The drawback is the tendency of the patient to feel that because improvement has occurred, further treatment may safely be neglected. Stopping treatment too early is not dangerous to the patient's health, but it definitely negates the potential long-term benefits of this form of treatment. Likewise, the allergist must not be lulled into a false sense of security by early favorable results from immunotherapy, holding the dosage at a symptom-relieving level. As will be pointed out later, escalation must continue past this early stage.

A decade or more ago, before the current degree of understanding of the immune system was reached (it is still far from complete), it was recommended that allergy patients undergoing immunotherapy continue their injections throughout life. Allergy was known to be a genetically determined condition, and it was assumed that such a problem would be irreversible. Within the past decade, it has been determined that providing immunotherapy at high dosage levels during a period of about 5 years will, in the vast majority of patients, produce an immunologic response that makes further immunotherapy unnecessary. The exact nature of this response is still unclear. It appears to involve not only changes in the ratio of immunoglobulin E (IgE) to immunoglobulin G (IgG), which tend to reverse after treatment is discontinued, but also some effect on the lymphocyte population that further prevents the allergic reaction. Currently, a maximum of about 5 years of immunotherapy, most of which is at maintenance level, is still recommended. It is possible that as a result of ongoing research in this area, in the future treatment may be advised for only about 3 years. It is not yet known with total certainty how long immunotherapy must be administered without a risk for regression when it is discontinued. However, all indications are that as our knowledge increases in this regard, the recommended duration of treatment will shorten rather than lengthen.

Time Requirements

If a patient does not continue treatment as long as is necessary for a more permanent reversal of the allergic process to develop, immunotherapy must be resumed when the initial beneficial effects disappear. If the process of prematurely discontinuing therapy is repeated, the same result may be expected. This sequence does not harm the patient, but it reinforces the earlier, erroneous concept of lifetime dependence on immunotherapy. When inadequate or repeatedly interrupted immunotherapy is administered, the cost benefits are lost. In our modern climate of managed care, it is often necessary to emphasize to a third-party payer the benefits of covering immunotherapy care on the basis of the limited and finite time needed for such care. The coverage for immunotherapy must be weighed by the third-party payer against a lifetime of symptom-relieving medication, which is not inexpensive. If this long-term benefit of immunotherapy provided for 3 to 5 years is not evident, it is not surprising to see a denial of all coverage for immunotherapy.

The selection of patients for immunotherapy, as for all other forms of therapy, depends heavily on patient commitment and is strongly influenced by information supplied by the physician. Immunotherapy is an excellent form of treatment, and probably the best choice currently available for the management of inhalant allergy. Its greatest benefit, however, is the potential for long-term success after a well-defined period of treatment. The time and dedication that the patient is prepared to commit to immunotherapy directly affect the degree of success that may be expected. A patient in transit, for example, who cannot or is not willing to follow through on regular injections, is a poor immunotherapy candidate. Improvement will often occur, but it will rarely be maintained. A patient with a history of starting allergy injections but discontinuing them after a few months will not often benefit from immuno- therapy to the degree expected. The unfortunate part of this situation is that the patient usually blames the failure either on the physician directing the treatment or on the treatment modality itself. After a few failures, it is difficult to persuade the patient to accept responsibility for the poor result and again commit to a trial of therapy of the same basic type. Even if the patient listens closely to the new information provided and takes more printed material home to study at leisure, the commitment professed often weakens over a period of time. This is not to say that no successful responses to immunother- apy ever occur in such patients, but the physician should be alerted to the likelihood of another failure through no fault on the part of the clinician. Failures breed guilt, and the new allergist is especially susceptible to such situations. For some reason, patients who have failed in the past to respond to competent therapy because of poor compliance tend to converge on the new allergist. This may be a consequence of rejection by those who have previously initiated proper therapy, only to see minimal compliance produce failure, or of an eternal search on the part of such patients for a quicker, simpler form of treatment that will entail no need for cooperation on their part. Regardless of the reason, the physician just starting to offer good, comprehensive allergy care may expect to see an abnormally high number of poor-risk patients congregate to the practice in its early stages. This may, but should not, discourage the properly trained clinician utilizing appropriate techniques from pursuing this new aspect of practice.

SPECIFIC INDICATIONS AND CONTRAINDICATIONS FOR IMMUNOTHERAPY

The administration of immunotherapy is predicated on the patient's meeting the criteria for an acceptable candidate for such treatment. Such patients should have proven atopy (mediated by IgE) to one or more antigens that are not readily avoidable. They should have symptoms that are inadequately relieved by pharmacotherapy, or should be intolerant to pharmacotherapy

---

NURSE'S NOTE

Testing has been done. Results indicate that the patient is allergic, and the patient has symptoms that correspond with the test results. Furthermore, the patient is willing to follow through a course of immunotherapy that will last 3 to 5 years. It is time to prepare for treatment. However, at this point, the allergy care provider should again go over the anticipated benefits of immunotherapy, remind the patient (and the family, if the patient is a child) of the commitment of time and effort necessary, explain the usual time course of 3 to 5 years involved, and be certain that the patient's expectations of the results of immunotherapy are realistic. It is always better to do this at the time immunotherapy is begun than to deal with problems that arise later from unrealistic expectations or lack of understanding.

(because of side effects or other considerations). Their symptoms should be multiseasonal, spanning more than one allergy season, or if present during only a single season, the symptoms should be severe. The patients should be motivated and likely to be compliant with a program of allergy immunotherapy.

Indications

Although the best treatment of inhalant allergy is avoidance, there are many circumstances in which complete (or even effective partial) avoidance of an inciting allergen is impossible or impractical. Each case must be considered on its own merits, and patients should not be denied immunotherapy simply because the allergist feels that they ''should'' be able to avoid their antigenic triggers.

The admonition to treat only multiseasonal allergies with immunotherapy is firmly entrenched in tradition. However, given the track record of safety and effectiveness of the methods for testing and immunotherapy described in this text, patients with single-season allergies (especially if severe) should be considered for definitive treatment by allergy immunotherapy.

Some patients are content to utilize various pharmacotherapeutic measures to relieve their allergic symptoms, and if such treatment is not disruptive of their lifestyle and they experience no adverse effects, there is no need to press the matter of immunotherapy. As a practical matter, most patients ''don't like to take pills'' or use nasal sprays on a regular basis, and are happy to consider a therapeutic program that may eventually allow them to use their medications less frequently. Although great strides in the pharmacotherapy of inhalant allergy have been taken in the past 50 years, none of the medications currently used is free of potential side effects, drug interactions, or other adverse effects.

It is important for the physician, nurse, or some other member of the allergy team to counsel patients before immunotherapy, frankly detailing the expenditure of time, effort, and money involved. A great deal of needless frustration can be avoided if immunotherapy is begun only after a joint commitment on the part of both patient and health care provider.

Contraindications

The only absolute contraindication to allergy immunotherapy is the absence of allergy. In addition, patients who test positive for human immunodeficiency virus (HIV) should not receive immunotherapy, as its efficacy in these patients is uncertain and it could conceivably accelerate the progress of the disease. Relative contraindications to the initiation of immunotherapy include beta-blocker therapy, pregnancy, and immune dysregulation.[2]

It is unusual, but not impossible, to encounter HIV-positive patients with severe nasal allergic symptoms. When such instances occur, symptomatic control should be sought through appropriate pharmacotherapy. Only if prolonged systemic corticosteroid therapy is required for the management of allergic symptoms in such patients is consideration of immunotherapy justified.[3]

It appears that patients receiving beta-adrenergic blocking drugs may be more prone to severe allergic reactions (from any cause) than other patients.[4] Beta blockade may be "proallergic" through blocking smooth-muscle relaxation (contributing to possible bronchospasm) and amplifying production of various mediators of inflammation produced in an allergic reaction. Although some question exists as to the exact degree of increased risk, it is probably even more important to realize that noncardioselective beta blockers significantly affect the possible treatment of an anaphylactic reaction, should one occur during testing and treatment.[5] If epinephrine is given to a patient in the presence of a beta-adrenergic blocker, unopposed alpha-adrenergic stimulation may occur, resulting in a hypertensive crisis. This is discussed in detail in Chapter 12, Allergic Emergencies. It is prudent to discuss with the patient's primary care physician a possible change to another agent, such as a calcium channel blocker, before skin testing and initiation of immunotherapy. If this is not possible, a switch to a cardioselective beta blocker may reduce the risk for potentiating bronchospasm, but it does not alleviate the possibility of an enhanced hypertensive response to epinephrine.

It is generally accepted that immunotherapy that has been initiated before pregnancy may be continued during pregnancy.[6] However, it is unwise to begin immunotherapy in a pregnant patient for a number of reasons. First, it is likely that the degree of sensitivity of the patient will vary with the immunologic changes that occur during pregnancy. Thus, levels of reactivity determined during pregnancy may be inaccurate after delivery. More importantly, there is a very real risk for hypoxia and fetal damage if the mother experiences anaphylaxis. Because most reactions to immunotherapy occur during initiation and dose advancement, subjecting a pregnant patient to this risk is ill-advised. On the other hand, patients who are receiving immunotherapy and become pregnant may continue to receive their injections (with the approval of the obstetrician). It is best not to attempt to increase the dose of antigen administered during this period, but maintenance therapy is generally considered to be safe.

The question of immunotherapy in patients with autoimmune disorders remains controversial.[7] Although immunotherapy has not been definitely shown to cause or worsen autoimmune disorders, sufficient questions have been raised in this regard to require a thorough consideration by such patients and their physician of the risk-to-benefit ratio of immunotherapy for inhalant allergy.

PREPARING THE TREATMENT EXTRACT

The decision has now been made to treat the inhalant allergic patient by immunotherapy. Before the treatment is started, a vial of treatment extract must be prepared specifically for the patient to be treated. This should be done in advance of the first treatment visit, with the same care and freedom from interruptions required for proper preparation of testing dilutions. This vial will serve to initiate treatment, and to allow early progression of immunotherapy toward a point of symptomatic relief. It would be rare to have this first treatment vial represent a final level of maintenance, but unless problems arise, the preparation of successive treatment vials of increasing strength will be based on the formula used in the initial vial.

For the beginning allergist, treatment vials may be made directly from the testing board. Later on, as the patient volume increases, it may become desirable to make a separate board for treatment, using larger vials or extract with the same fivefold dilutions prepared in the testing board but with all successive dilutions containing 10% glycerine as a preservative. This will not be necessary at the start, and many allergists prefer always to make their treatment vials from the testing board, adding glycerine to the vial after preparation to bring the glycerine concentration to 10% or above. This concept will be clarified shortly. Initially, let us concentrate on the procedure for making the initial treatment vial.

The treatment format is based on SET, taking advantage of the relative quantification of sensitivity to the various allergens and highest safe initial dose provided by this testing procedure. It has been established that the endpoint identified by this form of testing is a safe level at which to initiate immunotherapy for any specific allergen.

Treating for a Single Allergen

Strictly speaking, treatment of a single allergen need not be discussed under preparation of vials for therapy. There is really no need to prepare a vial to treat a single allergen. Such patients may receive treatment from the stock antigen vial on the board. For teaching purposes, however, we begin by considering treatment with one antigen.

It has been established that the endpoint is a safe level at which to initiate treatment. In establishing this endpoint, several negative wheals have been produced, all containing minute amounts of antigen insufficient to initiate an immunologic reaction. In addition, the endpoint wheal has been produced. This wheal contains 0.01 mL of extract, the amount necessary to produce a 4-mm wheal. A confirmatory wheal has also been produced from the next stronger dilution. This wheal contains the same 0.01 mL of extract, but it is five times more concentrated, making it the equivalent of 0.05 mL of the extract producing the endpoint. Thus, during testing the patient has received 0.06 mL of the endpoint extract, plus an additional small amount from the negative wheals. If no adverse reaction has occurred during testing, it may be assumed that it is safe to administer 0.05 mL of the endpoint dilution as an initial treatment dose. The first treatment dose will therefore be 0.05 mL of the endpoint strength.

To treat for a single antigen, this dose may be drawn from the vial producing the endpoint and administered subcutaneously. Such treatment injections are given subcutaneously for slower absorption, using (if available) special treatment syringes rather than those used for skin testing. Successive doses may be drawn directly from the testing vial and given as described above. There is no need to prepare a treatment vial unless the patient is to take it elsewhere for therapy. Should the patient need to take the vial elsewhere for treatment, the same procedure used in preparing a multiple-antigen, multiple-dose vial is followed.

NURSE'S NOTE

Two reminders are necessary. The first is that the larger the number, the more times the antigen has been diluted. The second is that the larger the number of the patient's endpoint, the higher the patient's sensitivity (and the greater the need for caution). For this reason, antigens at #4, #5, and #6 strengths are frequently placed in a vial separate from the #3, #2, and #1 strengths. This allows greater flexibility in adjusting doses.

Preparing the Multiple-Antigen, Multiple-Dose Vial

The vast majority of patients requiring immunotherapy are sensitive to a number of allergens. Theoretically, treatment for any number of allergens could be performed exactly as described for single-allergen treatment, starting each allergen treatment with a 0.05-mL dose of the extract producing the endpoint. Practically, this would involve multiple injections of different allergens at each visit, which would make the patient quite unhappy. The simplest solution to this problem would be to place 0.05 mL of each antigen in the same syringe and give it all as a single dose. This approach, however, is also impractical, as the total quantity of extract used in adding 0.05 mL of the endpoint of 10 or 15 different antigens quickly produces a larger amount of fluid than is comfortably tolerated in a single injection. Furthermore, the amount would increase even more with each successive injection while the treatment dose is escalated. What is needed is a means of reducing the volume of extract while preserving the potency needed to equal that of the endpoint of each antigen, allowing escalation without an undue increase in volume. Each injection should also contain all the antigens to be treated for in a single dose. Although this may seem like a monumental project, it is actually quite simple to carry out once the principle is understood.

The principles used in both testing and treatment by SET are based on certain human limitations, specifically the ability to measure wheals accurately and to measure minute quantities of extract contained in a syringe. Whenever the logistics of vial preparation are described, the question always seems to arise of why the calculations cannot be shortened, with certain steps skipped. Decades of experience have shown that any such shortcuts invariably produce a poor understanding of the process, resulting in problems in vial preparation. Adhering to the proven format gives a uniform, reproducible system that experience has shown to be effective.

Testing requires that extracts be diluted in such a way that wheals of a uniform size, which can be produced repeatedly, will respond uniformly. Treatment requires concentration of the same extracts in such a way as to allow for easy, reliable measuring for vial preparation and injections. The fivefold dilutions made for testing are basically reversed to provide the material needed in treatment.

Step 1. Calculations and Procedure to Make the Initial Treatment Vial

The results of SET are recorded on a testing sheet indicating the endpoints identified for each allergen (Fig. 9–1). At the right side of the sheet, immediately after the numbered columns, is a column in which the endpoints identified by testing are recorded. From these endpoints, the calculations are made to determine the contents of the treatment vial.

The definition of endpoint for SET has been covered in Chapter 6, Testing Methods for Inhalant Allergy. Briefly, the endpoint of titration represents the antigen strength that produces the first positive (reacting) wheal followed by progressively larger positive wheals—that is, the endpoint concentration is the dilution that initiates progressive positive whealing.

Even if the initial testing has been done by RAST, the principles involved in vial preparation are based on SET. In the past, it has been popular to utilize different methods to calculate vial composition when testing has been done by in vitro methods such as RAST. This is unnecessary. One of the major advantages of the Fadal-Nalebuff modified RAST (F/N mRAST) is that the increments of that scoring system match the fivefold dilutions determined by Rinkel in his modified titration system to yield the most accurate and reproducible results. Experience has shown that F/N mRAST classes parallel the endpoint classes in SET, although the results of SET generally indicate a sensitivity about one class greater than is found by F/N mRAST. In other words, an endpoint by SET of #5 would correspond to an F/N mRAST class IV. For further explanation of this relationship, the reader is referred to Chapter 11. This correlation may also exist with other in vitro methodologies, but the practitioner will have to ascertain whether such is the case before utilizing those results in preparing vials by this method. Because of this relationship, if vials are to be prepared from RAST results instead of SET, one may substitute in the endpoint column a number equal to the RAST class score plus one. Because a higher number indicates a more dilute solution, this has been called a *RAST minus one* level, but actually it represents the *addition* of one to the RAST score. This has been a source

SKIN ENDPOINT TITRATION

NAME PATIENT #4   CLINICAL DX. PNA, Bronchitis   DATE

ANTIGEN	6	5	4	3	2	1	EP	Use-Vol	Use Diln.
RAGWEED	5	5	⑦	9					
PIGWEED	5	5	5	5	⑦	9			
BERMUDA GR.	5	6	⑧	10					
TIMOTHY	5	⑦	9						
ELM	5	5	7	⑦	9				
COTTONWOOD	5	5	5	6	⑦	9			
OAK	5	5	⑦	9					
A.P. DUST	5	5	5	6	⑨	11			
H.D. MITE	5	5	5	5	⑦	9			
DOG HAIR	5	5	5	5	5	6			
CAT HAIR	5	5	5	5	5	5			
ALTERNARIA	5	5	5	5	⑦	9			
HORMODEND.	5	5	5	5	6	7			
CEPHALOSP.	5	5	5	5	6	8			

Total Vol. _____

Diluent   _____

Final Vol. _____

FIGURE 9–1. Completed titration sheet for skin testing.

of confusion to many novices. For a RAST class IV response, the "endpoint" 5 would be entered. Vials may then be prepared in the usual fashion.

The mathematical calculations needed to determine the volume and specific dilution of each antigen that must be placed in the treatment vial are simple and very basic. However, it is important to understand the principles behind these calculations, as at some time it may be necessary to make a change in the procedure. This may occur, for instance, as a result of the developing standardization of extracts. Alterations in the set formula are required should the physician wish to make a smaller or larger treatment vial to accommodate the needs of particular patients. The format presented has been developed to require the smallest number of calculations practical, and to correlate the calculations with the established fivefold dilution format to avoid confusion. Repeated studies have shown that the new allergist or the technician preparing the treatment vials is able to follow this format with a minimal risk for error. This simplicity is of special benefit during training of a new allergy assistant. It is not the most economical method of preparing a treatment vial (because the examples involve 5-mL vials), but the minor waste of antigen in the early stages of practice is more than compensated for by the simplicity of the preparation and reliability of the result.

The principles involved in preparing the vial are as follows:

A. The extract should be concentrated as much as possible to reduce the volume of fluid in the injection while maintaining the amount of antigen to match the endpoint concentration.

B. It would not be productive to prepare a new antigen mixture each time the patient is due to receive an injection. A reasonable number of escalating injections should be planned and prepared at the same time in the same vial.

C. To treat properly with immunotherapy, during escalation each injection should normally contain a greater amount of antigen than was contained in the previous injection. This escalation schedule, which may vary, is discussed below in the section on escalating the treatment dose. How many injections are actually contained in a single vial will vary, but an arbitrary number must be selected to prepare the vial. For ease of understanding the calculations, the number of injections selected for calculation purposes is 10.

D. When a dose of 0.50 mL is delivered from the first vial, it will correspond to a dose of 0.10 mL from the next stronger vial because the contents of the new vial are five times stronger than the contents of the first. This means that instead of raising the injection volume from the first vial above 0.50 mL, one may (and should) proceed to the next stronger vial, which will further reduce the fluid volume without altering the amount of antigen present. This will become clearer when escalation of doses is discussed. For the present calculations, what is necessary is understanding that the maximum dose normally delivered from a vial will not exceed 0.50 mL. Doses above this level will be delivered from a new vial, five times stronger than the first.

Now for the calculations: We would like to reduce the volume of each antigen put into the master vial as much as possible without altering the amount of antigen present, so that we can add all the positive antigens together in a convenient volume and bring the total volume up to the desired amount. This can be done by removing diluent from the injected material. If we prepare a vial from bottles that contain five times less diluent per milliliter than the endpoint vial, we end up with an extract that contains more antigen per milliliter, so that 0.1 mL of the new vial contains the antigenic equivalent of 0.5 mL from the endpoint vial. Using as a stock vial one that is two fivefold dilutions stronger than the vial producing the endpoint provides another reduction of five times the amount of diluent. This concentration is 25 times greater than the endpoint dilution (with the same antigenicity) and represents about as much concentration as is practical while still allowing accurate measurements to be performed. The mathematical calculations would be (for example) as follows: 0.50 mL of a #6 (1 : 312,500) dilution equals 0.10 mL of a #5 (1 : 62,500) dilution equals 0.02 mL of a #4 (1 : 12,500) dilution. The amount of antigen in each successively reduced amount of extract is exactly the same (Fig. 9–2).

The patient will receive increasing doses, up to a maximum of 0.5 mL, from the initial treatment vial. The second calculation determines the amount of each antigen needed to provide what has been estimated to be a reasonable number of doses, to be included in the initial treatment vial. To illustrate this calculation, we will assume the amount to be 10 doses of 0.5 mL. This amount of extract in the vial will probably not actually be used, but placing such an amount in the vial will provide more than enough properly mixed extract to allow for all the injections necessary from this vial before it reaches its expiration date.

We need to calculate the amount of extract from each vial of antigen, at a concentration two dilutions stronger than the vial producing the endpoint dilution, to provide 10 doses of 0.5 mL each. This simply requires multiplying the amount needed for a single maximum injection of 0.50 mL by 10. We have already determined that 0.02 mL of extract from the vial two dilutions stronger than the vial producing the endpoint is equivalent to 0.50 mL of the endpoint vial. Then, 0.2 mL (0.02 × 10) from the vial two dilutions stronger will supply the amount of antigen needed for 10 doses of 0.50 mL of the endpoint dilution. All that has been removed is diluent. The calculation

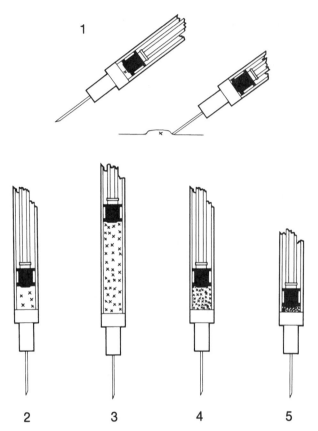

FIGURE 9–2. Concentrating an antigen dose: 0.01 cc cannot be measured in the syringe, but produces a 4 mm wheal in the skin: (1) A 0.05 cc represents a usual starting dose for immunotherapy, and contains 5 of 0.01 cc "units" present in the endpoint dose; (2) 0.05 cc contains 50 of these "units," and at this level the dose will have reached the strength of the next stronger dilution; (3) if diluent only is removed from this dose, an amount containing only one-fifth the total volume but the same amount of antigen (50 "units") will result. This is the same as 0.01 cc of the next stronger concentration; (4) if the same procedure is repeated, the same 50 "units" will be contained in 0.02 cc of the dilution 2 stronger than the endpoint. Diluent has been removed by reversing the titration preparation process, but the amount of antigen present has been preserved. (From Cowen DE, Dixon BJ, revised by Ward WA. Skin endpoint titration technique. American Academy Otolaryngic Allergy (manual). Washington, D.C., p 4; with permission.)

If a treatment set of 10 doses is made to simplify measurement, multiple antigens are included, as in the following example:

		Antigenic equivalents of a 50X of each of ten doses
Pollen	Endpoint #6	0.02 of #4 × 10 = 0.20 ml. of #4
Pollen	Endpoint #3	0.02 of #4 × 10 = 0.20 ml. of #1
Pollen	Endpoint #6	0.02 of #4 × 10 = 0.20 ml. of #4
Pollen	Endpoint #5	0.02 of #4 × 10 = 0.20 ml. of #3
Pollen	Endpoint #6	0.02 of #4 × 10 = 0.20 ml. of #4
Pollen	Endpoint #4	0.02 of #4 × 10 = 0.20 ml. of #2
		= 1.20 ml.

FIGURE 9–3. Summary of the actual calculations necessary to make a multiple-dose, multiple antigen treatment set. (From Cowen DE, Dixon BJ, revised by Ward WA. Skin endpoint titration technique. American Academy Otolaryngolic Allergy (manual). Washington, D.C., p 4; with permission.)

simply involves determining the strength of the endpoint dilution of each antigen, increasing that strength by two concentrations, taking 0.20 mL of extract from this vial, and placing it in a treatment vial (Fig. 9–3). The same calculations are valid for all antigens, although in some instances (such as with standardized antigens or antigens that do not come in $1:20$ weight/volume [w/v] stock concentrations), correction factors must be applied.

An added advantage of the system described is the ease of measuring small volumes of extract. Although 0.02 mL is essentially impossible to measure accurately, 0.20 mL may be measured with considerable accuracy by any diligent nurse or technician.

After 0.20 mL of each antigen for treatment has been placed in the treatment vial, an appropriate amount of diluent must be added to the vial. The above calculations have been described for preparing a 5-mL vial. To the vial must be added enough diluent to bring the total contents of the vial to 5 mL. This merely requires adding the volume of antigen (in milliliters) already placed in the vial, subtracting that from 5 mL, and adding that amount of diluent.

It has been found by experience in numerous courses and teaching situations that making a 5-mL vial in this manner presents few problems for the novice. When the calculations of students during teaching situations have been examined, a consistent tendency to err has appeared when additional calculations have been introduced. Most of these errors involved a failure to carry out consistent mathematical calculations through the entire process.

Whatever the reason, the problem has appeared frequently enough to result in the development of the format presented. It is simple, easy to teach to a new physician, nurse, or technician, and easy for any colleague employing SET to understand if a patient must be transferred to another physician. The beginning allergist is strongly advised to follow the procedure described scrupulously, at least in the earlier stages of the practice; it also has many benefits when continued indefinitely. When necessary, it is quite possible for the experienced technician to use the same methods to produce larger or smaller vials.

Step 2. Preparing the Actual Vials and Calculating Diluent

Dividing the Vials

The preceding section has explained the concept and described the steps involved in preparing a single treatment vial. These must be understood before the steps outlined below for making vials to treat sensitivity to multiple antigens can be understood. In most cases, the allergic patient will demonstrate a variety of sensitivities to multiple antigens of different strengths on testing, all of which require treatment. Often, a wide range of sensitivities will be present: SET endpoints at #6 and #2 or RAST responses ranging from class VI to class II. It should be noted here that SET endpoints on #1 or RAST class O/I sensitivities are not always considered indications for immunotherapy unless the symptom pattern strongly indicates a relationship between the weak responses and the patient's symptoms.[8] With SET, it is also necessary that the response exceed the wheal diameter for the 10% glycerine control (because this is the glycerine concentration in a #1 dilution), indicating that the reaction is immunologic, not irritative. It is quite possible to place many or all of the individual antigens usually needed for treatment at varying concentrations in the same treatment vial. However, this is not an ideal solution.

Although SET indicates a safe starting point for initiating therapy for each antigen, it does not establish the treatment level needed for maintenance. This is established clinically. Allergens with higher endpoints (e.g., SET #6, RAST class V) generally represent a higher level of sensitivity, and these require therapy to be started at considerably more dilute doses than allergens with endpoints indicating less sensitivity (e.g., SET #2, RAST class I). In addition, the allergens to which the patient is most sensitive are more likely to precipitate an adverse reaction during immunotherapy, and therefore must be treated with more caution. Because treatment for the allergens with high endpoints must be started at a more dilute level, more injections will generally be necessary for these allergens before maintenance doses are reached. For all these reasons, it is more efficient to start treatment with two vials rather than one: one vial containing the allergens with high endpoints (SET #4, #5, #6 or RAST class III, IV, V) and the other vial containing allergens with low endpoints (SET #2 and #3 or RAST class I, II). Injection doses from the two vials may then be increased individually until maintenance levels of therapy are reached, as discussed later. If a single vial containing all the antigens is used initially, it will often be necessary to divide the vial at some point early in treatment because of local reactions. Starting initially with vials for high and low sensitivity avoids this problem.

Number of Antigens per Vial

The question always arises as to how many antigens should be, or can be, placed in a single treatment vial. Simple mathematics will give the answer to the second part of this question. Adding 0.2 mL of each antigen to a vial will allow a total of 25 antigens to be placed in a 5-mL vial, with no room for diluent. Such a situation will rarely, if ever, arise. If such a high number of antigens are placed in one vial, one immediate problem must be considered. Stock vials of antigens are normally purchased in a 50% glycerine solution. Glycerine is an excellent preservative, but it is also quite irritating. This is the reason why a glycerine control is needed during testing. You will recall that this consists of 2% and 10% glycerine solutions, representing the amount of glycerine contained in the #2 and #1 SET testing dilutions, respectively. If a treatment vial contains a large number of antigens taken from concentrate or the #1 dilution, the total glycerine level may easily exceed 10%. Injections containing this much glycerine are almost guaranteed to produce a local irritation. This is not harmful, but a local reaction is normally the earliest indication that a maximum tolerated dose has been reached. If such a reaction were the result of glycerine irritation, dose escalation would be halted on the assumption that the injected antigens were producing the local reaction, and treatment would not be carried to an appropriate maintenance level. If a quick mathematical calculation shows that a vial will contain more than 10% glycerine, it is well to divide the vial. In some instances, when a large number of antigens are treated using concentrates for preparation, it may even be advisable to divide the antigens among three vials.

Diluents

This brings up the question of the amount and type of diluent appropriate for a treatment vial during initial treatment and dose escalation. In this respect, more than one approach is possible. Several diluents are available for both testing and treatment mixes. By far the most widely used is buffered phenolated saline solution.

Human serum albumin (HSA) has previously enjoyed some popularity for the preparation of testing vials, but it is more expensive than saline solution. Contrary to popular belief, HSA does not act as a preservative. HSA provides only one advantage, the reduction of "walling," which is the tendency of small amounts of extract to adhere to the walls of a glass vial. This is of no real importance in therapy, and of little consequence in testing. In addition, much of the public has become concerned about the use of blood products, fearing the possibility of transferring viruses such as hepatitis virus or HIV. In point of fact, commercially prepared HSA is heated above the temperature at which pathogenic viruses can survive. Nevertheless, HSA has little to recommend it for routine use as a diluent.

Buffered saline solution contains 0.4% phenol to prevent any viral or bacterial growth, and is buffered to match the pH level of human blood. It does not contain a preservative, and antigens mixed with saline solution alone may be expected to maintain full potency for only about 6 weeks if kept refrigerated when not in use. This is the reason why all testing boards should be remade every 6 weeks, replacing all dilutions starting with #1. No glycerine is ever added to a testing vial, as the glycerine alone will usually produce a skin reaction, obscuring any allergic response. In preparing treatment vials, however, another option exists.

In the initial stages of treatment and while escalating doses, there may be an advantage to not adding glycerine to the treatment vials. One of the indications that the maximum tolerated dose is being approached is the presence of a local reaction at the site of an injection. If no glycerine has been added to the vial, such a reaction may be assumed to be a consequence of immunologic activity, and the level of the vial producing the local reaction can be maintained for the time being. Proceeding in this manner provides a simple indicator of progress and a clear point at which to evaluate treatment results. This may be a real benefit to the treating physician, especially the novice. The limitation of this approach is that the vial being used in treatment maintains its potency for only a little more than 6 weeks, even when refrigerated, and therefore if the escalation is still proceeding after 6 or 7 weeks, the vial must be discarded. If the patient is on a schedule of two injections a week, this is usually not a problem. However, if the injections are given at weekly intervals, the potency of the extract may become significantly reduced by the time it is necessary to advance to the next stronger vial.

When preparing treatment vials, it is often helpful to be certain that the vial contains a glycerine level of about 10%. In this way, the potency of the vial will be maintained for at least 3 months, sometimes longer. In some instances, this may involve using 10% glycerine as a diluent. A simple way to prepare a large bottle containing 10% glycerine is by diluting a stock bottle of 50% glycerine (which may be purchased separately from the allergy supplier) in the proportion of 1 mL of 50% glycerine to 4 mL of buffered saline solution (i.e., a 1:5 dilution), just as is done in making a glycerine control. (In the future, the 10% glycerine control may be taken from this stock bottle, and a 2% glycerine control may be made by a further 1:5 dilution with buffered saline solution.) When all antigens have been placed in an empty treatment vial, a quick calculation will show about how much glycerine is already in the vial, based on the strength and number of antigens that have been placed in the vial.

The glycerine content of the vial can be calculated easily if one considers that antigens added at concentrate level contain 50% glycerine. Because 0.2 mL of each antigen is added to a vial that will ultimately contain a volume of 5 mL, if five antigens at concentrate level are added, 5 times 0.2 equals 1 mL of 50% glycerine. Adding 4 mL of diluent (or other antigens containing less glycerine) will leave a final concentration of 10% glycerine in the vial. Therefore, if five or more antigens at concentrate level are contained in a 5-mL vial, no additional glycerine need be added. If more than one but fewer than five antigens at concentrate level are present, the difference between the volume from these antigens and a total of 1 mL may be made up by adding 50% glycerine. In other words, if two antigens at concentrate are present, they provide 0.4 mL of 50% glycerine. Add 0.6 mL of 50% glycerine from a stock bottle, then add other antigens and diluent to a total volume of 5 mL. If no antigens at concentrate level are present, using 1.0 mL of 50% glycerine as diluent for a 5 mL vial will bring the glycerine concentration to at least 10%.

Some local reactions may be expected from injections from vials with a glycerine content of 10% or greater, but they will generally be minor. A marked increase in local reactions will indicate a treatment level close to a maximum tolerated dose. If a large number of antigens at concentrate level have been placed in the treatment vial, the amount of glycerine in the vial may already be high. In this case, only saline solution need be added. All vials to be used for maintenance therapy may be prepared in this manner to maintain potency for at least 3 months, which will usually allow the vial contents to be exhausted before the expiration date.

NURSE'S NOTE

It is imperative that the person preparing treatment vials thoroughly understand the concepts just presented. This review will allow the process to be seen from a second viewpoint, although the principles are exactly the same.

For ease in calculations, a 5-mL vial will be prepared containing 10 doses. To allow several antigens to be mixed in the same vial, providing a dose in a quantity that the patient can easily tolerate, the antigen strength is concentrated 25-fold. The antigens (in concentrated form) are then mixed, and diluent is added to reconstitute them. This is the beauty of a fivefold dilution system: 5 mL of #4 (1:12,500) equals 1 mL of #3 (1:2500) equals 0.2 mL of #2 (1:500).

Each antigen is added to the vial in the strength (determined by the SET or RAST endpoint) that indicates a safe starting point. Suppose we wish to make this vial:

Timothy grass #4 (1:12,500)
Ragweed #3 (1:2500)
Oak tree #2 (1:500)
Dust mite #2 (standardized extract; see below)

Each antigen would be taken at two concentrations stronger, so that we would use the following:

Timothy grass #2 (1:500)
Ragweed #1 (1:100)
Oak tree concentrate (1:20)
Dust mite concentrate (standardized extract; see below)

For standardized extracts, a rule of thumb is that a strength of 30,000 allergenic units (AU) or Biologic Allergy Units (BAU) may be used as concentrate, whereas a strength of 10,000 AU or BAU is integrated into mixing as though it were a #1 (1:100) concentration.

To match strengths with RAST results, use a dilution weaker by one than is indicated by the RAST score (the RAST minus one level), so that a RAST I level would be treated as a #2 (1:500) level.

Remember that in making vials, a level stronger than concentrate cannot be used. So, for either a #2 or #1 endpoint, the vial would be made from concentrate.

Each antigen is prepared from a stock vial 25 times more concentrated than the desired eventual strength, so to make a 5-mL vial (10 doses of 0.5 mL each) would require 0.2 mL (5 mL ÷ 25) of each antigen. Using the example above,

NURSE'S NOTE *(continued)*

Timothy grass	0.2 mL of #2
Ragweed	0.2 mL of #1
Oak tree	0.2 mL of concentrate (1:20)
Dust mite	0.2 mL of concentrate (30,000 AU/mL)
Total volume of extract	0.8 mL
Diluent to be added	4.2 mL
Total vial size	5.0 mL (10 doses of 0.5 mL)

If this vial were to be used for treatment only, not for testing, we would try to prepare it in such a way as to contain 10% glycerine. Looking at the above calculations,

Timothy grass	0.2 mL of #2
Ragweed	0.2 mL of #1
Oak tree	0.2 mL of concentrate - in 50% glycerine
Dust mite	0.2 mL of concentrate - in 50% glycerine
Total volume of extract	0.8 mL, of which 0.4 mL is 50% glycerine

To make the total vial contain 10% glycerine would require that 10% of the vial size (10% of 5 mL = 1 mL) be glycerine. So, 0.6 ml of 50% glycerine is added   0.6 mL

Regular diluent is added to bring the total to 5 mL.

Diluent	3.6 mL
Total volume	5.0 mL (10 doses of 0.5 mL, which will maintain potency for 3 months)

If the vial contains less than 10% glycerine, it must be remade in 6 weeks (if kept refrigerated when not in use). If it contains 10% glycerine, it will retain its potency for 3 months. If it contains 25% glycerine, it will retain its potency for 6 months. If it contains 50% glycerine (as is the case with stock antigens), its potency will be retained for 2 to 3 years.

After the treatment vial is made, a typical dosing regimen might be as follows: 0.05 mL, 0.10 mL, 0.15 mL, 0.20 mL, 0.25 mL, 0.30 mL, 0.35 mL, 0.40 mL, 0.45 mL, 0.50 mL. You will note from this that if the injections are given weekly, the vial will expire before 10 doses can be given, unless glycerine is added to bring the concentration to 10%, as already noted.

STARTING IMMUNOTHERAPY

The Vial Test

After the initial vial for treatment has been made, it is time to prepare for administering the first treatment dose of allergenic extract. As would be expected, the first injection is critical, as it is the one most likely to precipitate an adverse reaction. Such a reaction is most unlikely if proper precautions have been taken in preparing the treatment vials, but not impossible. If the testing has been done by RAST, the extracts used in testing are not those that will be used in treatment, as is explained on Chapter 11. Even if the testing has been done by SET, combining the extracts in a single vial may on rare occasions allow a reaction to occur. Usually, this is caused by unrecognized cross-reactivity between some of the antigens included in the vial, most often several cross-reacting grasses, resulting in the administration of a larger effective dose of allergen than anticipated. Therefore, it is imperative to "test the water before jumping in." This involves a bioassay of the extract in the treatment vial, performed by intradermally injecting the patient with a small amount to form a skin wheal before administering a full therapeutic dose. The concept of the vial test is described in Chapter 11, but it is summarized briefly at this point.

In performing a vial test, the vial to be used in the initial treatment is treated as if it were a testing vial. Positive (histamine) and negative (diluent) controls should be placed, as described already, to ensure proper skin reactivity. If the initial testing was by SET and the result of a saline solution control was negative (ruling out dermatographia), this procedure probably need not be repeated. If initial testing was by RAST, both controls are advisable. A small amount (about 0.05 mL) of extract is withdrawn from the treatment vial and a 4-mm wheal is made by intradermal injection, as described in Chapter 6. The wheal is observed for 10 minutes. If the wheal has grown to 13 mm in diameter by this time, the vial is considered safe to be used in treatment; however, enough antigen has been delivered in the skin test to equal the amount contained in an initial injection, so no more extract is given at this time. If the wheal diameter is 11 mm or less, it is safe to give an initial injection of 0.05 mL subcutaneously at this time. If the wheal measures more than 13 mm, the vial should be titrated, as described below.

Titrating the Vial

In titrating the vial, the initial treatment vial is treated like a vial of antigen concentrate being serially diluted for testing. Initially, 1 mL of the mixed extract is withdrawn from the vial and introduced into a vial containing 4 mL of buffered saline solution. This procedure is repeated serially several times, just as in making serial dilutions for testing. An idea of the number of serial dilutions required may be obtained by measuring the size of the original large test wheal, then estimating the number of serial dilutions that will probably be necessary based on a 2-mm reduction in size for each successive dilution. A new test wheal is then made using the lowest-strength dilution that has been made. Testing may then be continued with stronger concentrations until a clear progression is demonstrated, ending with a wheal measuring 7 to 11 mm. When this point has been reached, an initial injection of 0.05 mL from this diluted vial may be given at the following visit. This dilution represents the initial safe concentration for immunotherapy. As a practical matter, the first fivefold dilution of the original treatment vial will often provide an acceptable vial test reaction.

The question often arises as to why an endpoint wheal in SET is 7 mm in diameter, whereas a wheal of 11 to 13 mm is acceptable for vial testing. The answer is that SET is performed with a single antigen, and the vial test with several antigens at different concentrations. Experience has shown that the figures quoted represent a safe level for initiating immunotherapy.[9]

In performing SET, each antigen is bioassayed and a safe dose determined. However, the possibility of errors in compounding always exist, and for this and other reasons, a vial test is recommended even if initial testing was done by SET. The experienced clinician may eventually choose to omit this step, but it is mandatory for the novice. It has been emphasized that if testing is carried out by in vitro means, a vial test is mandatory before immunotherapy is begun.

The Initial Injection

Immunotherapy should be considered from the most conservative position possible. In many cases, it would be quite safe to begin treatment at a slightly higher level than is recommended in this text, and also to progress more rapidly than described. However, it is the goal of the authors to provide the new allergist with an approach to immunotherapy that is both effective and safe. An adverse reaction during treatment, like one during testing, not only represents an impediment to good patient care, but reflects exceptionally badly on the physician who has recently added allergy to the practice. The confidence of patients in physicians in general is currently at an all-time low, and no physician is more vulnerable than one with limited experience in a new aspect of practice. Good patient care always dictates that good results with minimal chances for side effects should be a primary consideration on the choice of a method of treatment.

The initial immunotherapy injection should consist of 0.05 mL of extract from the initial treatment vial, given after the vial testing described has been completed. A dose of 0.05 mL has already been proved safe because the antigenic material administered in forming the 7-mm wheal during testing, which established the endpoint, plus the 9-mm confirmatory wheal have already provided the equivalent of 0.06 mL of each antigen. The injection is normally given subcutaneously in the posterior area of the upper arm. This is an area where local reactions may be easily observed and where subsequent local trauma, such as contact with clothing, is likely to be at a minimum. Also, a tourniquet may be placed above this site in the unlikely event that a systemic reaction occurs. According to current standards, the patient should be instructed not to leave the office for 20 to 30 minutes after receiving the injection.[10,11] In some countries, a wait of 1 hour has been suggested, but studies have shown that the chance of a serious systemic reaction occurring after 20 minutes is minimal.[12] In this era in which adverse reactions often result in litigation, it is advised that the allergy practice prominently display in the injection area a sign advising all patients to remain in the office for at least 20 minutes after receiving a therapeutic injection. Although testing and treating using the SET format is extremely safe, reactions remain a definite, albeit unlikely, possibility. If a patient elects to leave immediately after receiving an injection, and subsequently sustains a systemic reaction, the physician has made a demonstrable, reasonable effort to keep the patient under observation for the suggested time frame.

After the initial allergy injection, it is wise to have the patient rechecked by the person administering the injection after 20 minutes to record and evaluate any possible local reaction. This may lead to a change in dose or even vial composition before the next injection. Even if no reaction occurs, the patient has seen evidence of the importance in therapeutic decisions of even a minor local reaction. After the first injection, the patient is encouraged to report any significant local reaction from the preceding injection before that day's shot is given. However, the allergy care giver should always inquire if the patient makes no such report. All too often, when this question is omitted, it is only after an advancing dose has been administered that the patient remembers to report a large local reaction after the previous injection.

ESCALATING THE TREATMENT DOSE

For the developing allergist, *caution* should be the watchword. The first immunotherapy injection is at a dose of 0.05 mL, for the reasons described above. Subsequent injections are given at weekly or semiweekly intervals. If the patient is able to receive injections twice a week, maintenance and the accompanying symptom relief may be achieved much more rapidly. After the first injection, each successive dose is increased by 0.05 mL, establishing a pattern of 0.05 mL, 0.10 mL, 0.15 mL, 0.20 mL, 0.25 mL, 0.30 mL, 0.35 mL, 0.40 mL, 0.45 mL, 0.50 mL. With experience, especially with a nonbrittle patient (not asthmatic, no high degrees of sensitivity, not in season for most reactive antigens), this progression may be made in larger increments (i.e., 0.1 mL, 0.2 mL, 0.3 mL, and so forth), but in the beginning the more conservative approach is advisable. Safety is more important than speed, and the only disadvantage to the more conservative approach is a minor delay in reaching maintenance levels and an increase in the number of injections necessary to achieve this status. The maintenance dose is not affected by the progression used in reaching it. The injections from the initial vial are escalated in the manner described to a dose of 0.50 mL. If a maintenance dose has not been reached at this point, and it rarely will have been, it is time to progress to the vial of the next strength.

One of the benefits of SET is that immunotherapy may be started when an offending pollen is in season. In the immunotherapeutic approach for seasonal allergens (i.e., pollens) used by most general allergists, treatment is not normally started when the offending allergen is in season, because of the risk for systemic reactions. If testing is not done in a quantitative fashion, such as with SET or RAST, a safe starting dose has not been accurately determined, so that dosing must begin with an arbitrarily selected, extremely small dose to avoid risking an early overdose response. In this approach, initiation of immunotherapy for seasonal offenders is normally deferred until the offender is no longer in bloom, with a standard dose escalation program started when the season is over, so that some defense will have been achieved before the next blooming season. Under these circumstances, pharmacotherapy is the patient's sole line of defense until the season is over. This would be less of a problem if patients typically sought help via immunotherapy at the end of a season, but such is practically never the case. Patients resist visiting the doctor until they are truly miserable, and then they wish for immediate relief. Immunotherapy based on SET or RAST will not provide immediate relief, but a significant degree of symptom reduction may be expected within a few weeks of the initiation of injection therapy. If this is augmented by appropriate pharmacotherapy, even the most miserable of patients may be made comfortable in a fairly short period.

SET testing will indicate a safe dose at which to start immunotherapy, no matter whether testing is done "in season" or not. Retesting at the end of the season is generally not necessary because by then immunologic changes generated by immunotherapy have occurred, and some degree of symptom relief is noted. However, if in a patient in the early stages of immunotherapy increased symptoms and/or unacceptable local reactions suddenly develop following allergy injections, retesting might be a consideration. Most often, the change will be caused by one or more common scenarios. These include an increased exposure to the antigen as the season progresses, the "priming effect" already described, a complicating infection, exposure to other allergens not included in the initial treatment mix, or the concomitant ingestion of foods that cross-react with one or more of the inhalants for which the patient is being treated. Usually, it will be necessary to lower the immunotherapy dose during the blooming season of antigens to which the patient is significantly sensitive, and to raise it again when the season ends. Sometimes, all that is needed is to halve the dose at the beginning of the season and to continue careful escalation, but if the symptoms have been severe, it is safer to retest for the pollens in season and begin escalation at the new level. Because the maintenance level will be determined by skin and systemic reactions, the only disadvantage in retesting is a minor delay in reaching a maintenance dose.

Preparing Vial #2, of the Next Strength

Because this text is being presented in the same sequence that the physician and/or person administering allergy care would be expected to follow in the evaluation and treatment of a typical patient, some of the arrangement of material may seem incongruous. The preparation of the initial treatment vial has been described, followed by the first stages in treatment. When the maximum dose appropriate to this first vial has been reached, it is time to prepare the next stronger vial. It seems more practical to discuss the preparation of this vial at the stage of treatment at which it will be needed rather than before that point. If two vials, a high- and a low-sensitivity vial, have been prepared and used, the maximum dose of 0.50 mL of each may not have been reached at the same time. This does not present a problem. When the treatment dose from either vial has reached 0.50 mL, it is time to move the treatment to the next stronger treatment vial for that mixture of antigens.

Preparation of the next stronger treatment vial does not involve any major new calculations. All the initial calculations for preparing the initial vial have been completed, including the means of concentrating the antigen to deliver the endpoint dose in a much smaller volume of fluid. Because the serial dilutions are prepared on a 1:5 basis, the next stronger concentration will be five times as strong as the initial one, or one endpoint higher (i.e., from SET #5 to SET #4). In making the next stronger concentration, all that is necessary is to change the endpoint from the one used in making the initial dilution to an endpoint that is one concentration stronger, and place 0.20

mL of that extract in the second treatment vial. In other words, if the endpoint of one antigen is at a #5 concentration, the initial vial would be made from 0.20 mL of extract from dilution #3, two endpoints stronger. The second vial would be made from 0.20 mL of extract from vial #2, one endpoint (or five times) stronger than that in the first vial. The same procedure of increasing the strength of each antigen extract by one (fivefold) degree of concentration is used for each antigen, and the vial contents are brought to a total volume of 5 mL with an appropriate diluent, as described in preparation of the initial vial. It should be noted that less glycerine may be needed for this vial because the stronger concentrations used may have a higher glycerine content.

An exception to the rule of raising each antigen by one dilution may apply at this point if a concentrate of any antigen has been used in making the initial vial. The concentrate contains antigens at the strongest concentration that can be used in treatment, so if a level of mixing from concentrate has been reached, the strength of this antigen cannot be increased. When the next stronger vial is made, if the initial treatment vial called for concentrate for any antigen, concentrate is used again in the preparation of the next stronger vial. In considering the level of antigen used in reaching a maintenance level, it should be borne in mind that employing antigen at a concentrate level in making treatment vials actually produces a treatment vial in which the level of antigen is two dilutions weaker. Thus, if concentrate (1:20 w/v) is used in preparing the mixture, 0.5 mL from that vial delivers the antigenic equivalent of 0.5 mL of the #2 (1:500) dilution. If this is not obvious, it would be wise to review the earlier material on vial mixing.

Continuing Dose Escalation

The antigens in treatment vial #2 are at a concentration five times stronger than the concentration of those in vial #1, the initial treatment vial. Therefore, 0.10 mL of mixed extract from vial #2 contains the same amount of each antigen as 0.50 mL of mixed extract from vial #1, simply held in five times less diluent (which, of course, has no immunologic activity). If the patient has tolerated a dose of 0.50 mL from vial #1, it should be safe to go immediately from this dose to 0.10 mL of extract from vial #2. Vial #2, however, is a new vial, freshly prepared, which could be (and probably is) slightly more potent antigenically. Furthermore, it presents the possibility of some variation from vial #1 even though it has been prepared from the same stock antigens. The recommended approach is to start treatment from vial #2 at a slightly reduced dose, 0.05 mL, just as was done with vial #1, and to progress

NURSE'S NOTE

If dose advancement is desired, the next vial will be as follows:

Timothy grass	0.2 mL of #1
Ragweed	0.2 mL of concentrate
Oak tree	0.2 mL of concentrate
Dust mite	0.2 mL of concentrate
Total extract	0.8 mL (0.6 mL containing 50% glycerine)
50% glycerine	0.4 mL
Diluent	3.8 mL
Total volume	5.0 mL

An injection of 0.1 mL from this vial should antigenically be equal to 0.5 mL from the previous (five-fold weaker) vial. However, because the contents of this vial are fresher and thus theoretically antigenically more potent, the first injection from this vial is generally 0.05 mL, followed by 0.1 mL, 0.15 mL, and so forth (Fig. 9–4).

In advancing to the next stronger treatment vial, it is assumed that the patient has shown symptomatic improvement, with no local reactions exceeding 25 mm in diameter. If the patient tolerates this advancement, with continued symptom relief, it continues until repeated local reactions of greater than 25 mm occur, or until all antigens are being mixed from concentrate.

With the same formula, a five-dose or even a two-dose vial may be made.

	10 doses	*5 doses*	*2 + doses*
Vial size	5 mL	2.5 mL	1.25 mL
Amount of each antigen	0.2 mL	0.1 mL	0.05 mL
Total 50% glycerine (if added)	1 mL	0.5 mL	0.25 mL

upward in the same manner to a level of 0.50 mL (Fig. 9–5). If at this point a maintenance dose has not been attained, vial #3 is prepared in the same manner as vial #2, with the endpoint used in preparing vial #2 raised by one strength, and any concentrates kept at the level already in use. Injection escalation will then proceed in the same manner as in treating from vial #2. A vial #4 can be made following the same format if needed.

One question always arises concerning the use of successively stronger treatment vials. Initial treatment vials require a vial test to determine the safe starting dose, for the reasons described. In theory, a vial test should be performed with any new vial before it is used for treatment. However, when vial #2 is made, it is five times stronger than vial #1. Because insufficient

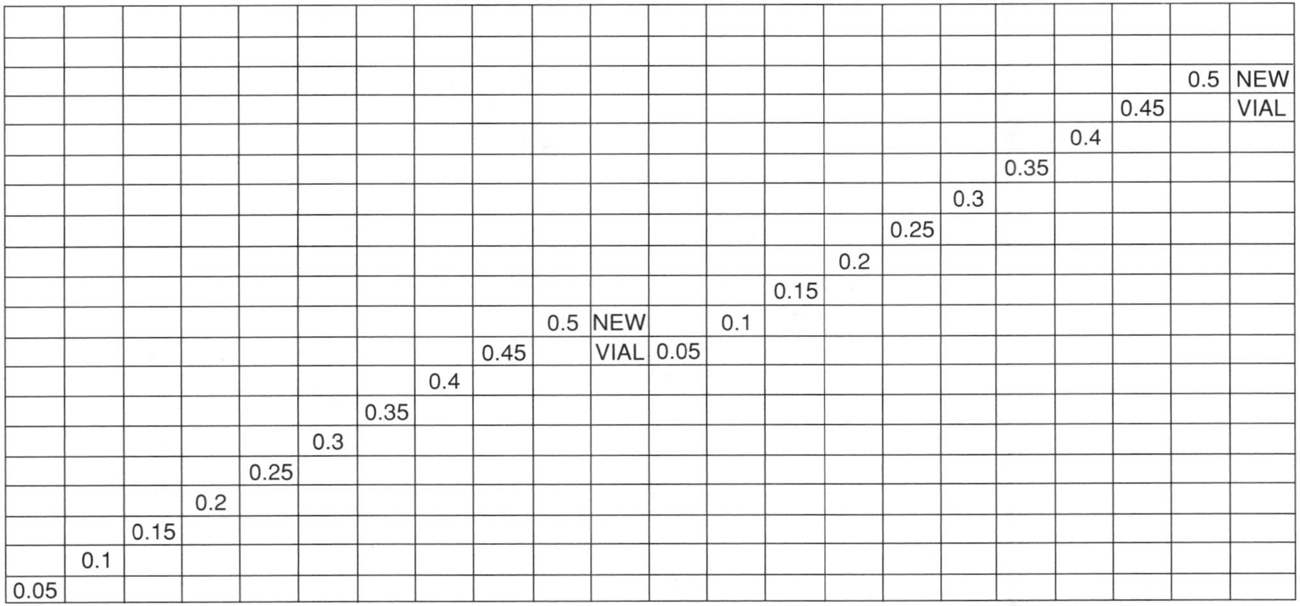

FIGURE 9–4. Dosing proceeds stepwise through the first treatment vial. If no indication to stop appears, a new vial is prepared containing antigens at a fivefold stronger concentration. A slight decrease in equivalent dosing is made to compensate for any increased potency in the fresher vial. Escalation then continues through this vial, and vials prepared at even stronger concentrations if necessary. The important point is that dose escalation continues to a point determined by the clinical response, not to an arbitrary amount.

Vial #1

Vial #2

Vial #3

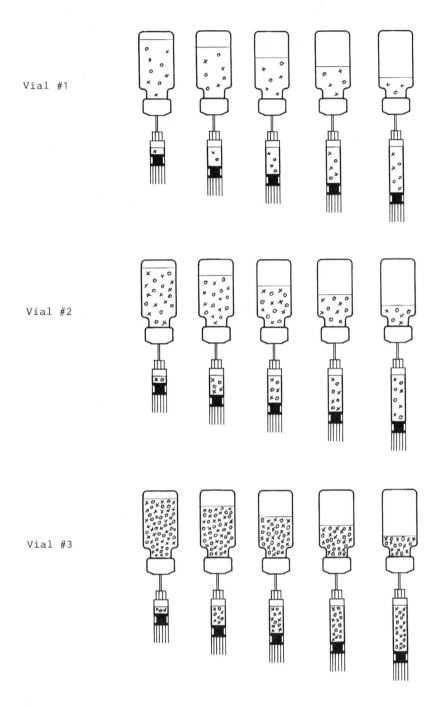

immunotherapy has been administered to affect skin reactivity at this point, a vial test would be expected to produce a significant skin reaction, just as the next stronger dilution above the endpoint in SET produces a reaction. If the rules of vial testing for the initial vial were followed, treatment would never progress beyond the level of the first vial, as the vial test would require reducing the dose to the initial starting level. This situation, unfortunately, has frequently occurred, preventing the process of dose escalation and rendering the administration of immunotherapy ineffective. As a practical matter, reducing the dose initially given from vial #2 by 50%, by starting at 0.05 mL as already described, compensates satisfactorily for the problem and is the generally accepted approach. If stronger vials are required and prepared as described, the same dose progression from the vial should provide a safe approach.

ESTABLISHING A MAINTENANCE DOSE

The initial goal of immunotherapy is to reach a dose of antigen extract that will relieve the patient's symptoms. The second goal is to reach a dose that, if administered for a period of time, will eliminate or reduce the patient's allergic symptoms. Such improvement may be only partial or temporary, but in ideal situations it will be permanent except when the patient is subjected to severe allergen challenges. To reach this point, indefinite dose escalation is neither possible nor desirable, and a lifetime of closely spaced injections is certainly not pleasant for the patient. The prospect of a specific, limited period of time during which frequent injections are necessary should be clearly understood by both physician and patient, as in the not-too-distant past it was taught that successful immunotherapy did require a lifetime of regular injections. Even today, it is not unusual to find a physician unaware of the fact that in the vast majority of cases, immunotherapy may eventually

◄────────────────────────────

FIGURE 9–5. Graphic representation of dose escalation and preparation of subsequent vials. Only every other dose is shown because of space limitations. In actuality, 10 doses would be withdrawn from vial #1, the patient's initial multiantigen vial, and administered starting with a dose of 0.05 mL. Doses would increase by increments of 0.05 mL to a final dose of 0.5 mL. At this point, if further dose escalation is necessary, the patient is treated from vial #2, prepared at a concentration five times stronger than that of vial #1. Because this vial is fresher and theoretically more potent, the initial dose would be 0.05 mL, although a dose of 0.1 mL would constitute the antigenic equivalent of the 0.5 mL dose last administered from vial #1. Thereafter, dose escalation proceeds as before, with preparation and administration of a vial #3 if indicated after the patient tolerates a dose of 0.5 mL from vial #2.

be discontinued without sacrificing its benefits, provided a proper maintenance dose has been reached and administered for a sufficient time period
(generally a total of 3 to 5 years).

The Symptom-Relieving Dose

When antigen doses are escalated, at some point the injection of extract will
produce a significant local reaction. This skin response, which may vary in
size, consists of subcutaneous induration, generally associated with redness.
It usually itches and is warm to the touch. The reaction should disappear
within 24 hours. It will be noticeably larger than reactions to previous escalated doses, even if the mix contains 10% glycerine. If high-sensitivity and
low-sensitivity vials are being used in treatment, such a local reaction will
generally not occur simultaneously at both injection sites. The physician or
allergy care provider generally depends on the patient to report this reaction,
as it may develop after the patient leaves the office. If educated and encouraged to do so, the patient can normally be trusted to describe and measure
this reaction satisfactorily, as there will have been enough previous injections
not producing such a reaction for the patient to recognize the change. This
local reaction indicates an approaching maintenance level of immunotherapy.

The size of the local reaction may vary from the diameter of a nickel (20
mm) to that of a quarter (25 mm) or a half-dollar (30 mm). The nickel-sized
area of redness and induration generally indicates that escalation may be
continued, but with caution. A local reaction with the diameter of a quarter
suggests that the same dose should be repeated on the next visit. If a reaction
of the same size results, the dose should be kept constant or decreased by
a small amount (probably 0.05 mL). The development of a local reaction
with the diameter of a half-dollar is a warning that some overdosing may
be occurring, and the subsequent dose should be one-half the dose that produced the large local reaction. Cautious advancement may then be carried
out if this decreased dose produces no local reaction; the point at which
an ''acceptable'' (quarter-sized or smaller) reaction is produced should be
sought.

If a single vial is being employed containing all the antigens being used in
treatment, the first appearance of a local reaction may coincide with symptom
relief, and at times symptom relief may be noted before a dose is achieved
that causes a noticeable local reaction. When such symptom relief occurs
and is maintained for at least a week, the dose producing the relief is referred
to as the *symptom-relieving dose*. In the past, this dose served as a maintenance dose, and further dose advancement was discouraged. If symptoms

recurred on this regimen, the symptom-relieving dose was adjusted up or down through a small range to compensate for seasonal change and exposures. Such a treatment format would usually successfully control a patient's symptoms, and it is still being employed in some quarters, but it never achieves the second goal of immunotherapy, which is making it possible to discontinue injections without recurrence of symptoms. This long-term response requires a higher dose.

If two or more treatment vials are being used simultaneously in the administration of immunotherapy, it is usual to see a local reaction appear following an escalated injection from one of the vials before symptom relief has been achieved. This is to be expected because a symptom-relieving dose may have been reached for some of the antigens being used in treatment but not for others, contained in another vial. Symptom relief is a generalized response, and a majority of the antigens producing the symptoms must often be administered to an adequate level before the patient feels significantly better. In this situation, the first development of a significant local reaction may serve as a useful guide. The reaction tends to indicate that injections from the vial producing it have been escalated to a currently satisfactory level, and that further escalation should be deferred for the present. This does not mean that injections from this vial should be stopped, but only that they should be continued at the level producing the local reaction, or at the level of the dose immediately below the one producing the first local reaction if that reaction was substantial. Injection doses from the other vial or vials should continue to be escalated until either a similar local reaction is seen or symptoms are relieved.

The Maximally Tolerated Dose

As understanding of the immune system has improved through the years, it has been recognized that although it may be successful in relieving symptoms for a period of time, usually a week or 10 days, treatment at the symptom-relieving dose is rarely adequate to produce long-term relief and allow eventual discontinuance of injections. Altering the body's immune response in such a way as to provide this prolonged response requires a higher dose of antigen than is provided by the symptom-relieving dose. Much of the understanding of this situation has come from studies of stinging-insect allergy, which is a type I, IgE-mediated reaction. Although not a perfect immunologic model, immunotherapy of stinging-insect allergy has provided a great deal of insight into immunotherapy for other IgE-mediated conditions and has confirmed the benefits of high-dose immunotherapy for long-term relief.

If immunotherapy has been advanced properly, it is extremely rare to see a significant general reaction during escalation from symptom-relieving to maximally tolerated doses. Enough immunologic changes seem to have occurred during careful dose escalation to protect the patient from a major reaction. Of course, as at any stage in testing and treatment, *caution* is the watchword.

The symptom-relieving dose is generally considered a temporary stage in advancement of immunotherapy. To establish the next level, dose escalation (of each vial) is continued to a point at which the local reaction produced signals that further advancement would be imprudent, while symptom relief is still being provided. This has historically been designated the *maximally tolerated dose*. As already noted, the local reaction at which dose advancement is stopped has approximately the diameter of a half-dollar (30 mm). Mild symptoms may accompany the reaction. At this point, one should halve the dose producing the reaction and gradually advance again to the amount that produces a local reaction no larger than the diameter of a quarter (25 mm) without causing adverse symptoms. Such "fine tuning" establishes the maximally tolerated dose for this vial.

As already noted, the patient's sensitivity may be affected when a new allergen comes into bloom early in the treatment program. This may require an adjustment in dose, or may even signal the need to maintain the same treatment level until allergen exposure diminishes or some degree of tolerance is achieved from the injections. On the same basis, when the physician is attempting to ascertain a maintenance dose for immunotherapy, if the allergen is not in the air, by definition the patient cannot receive a symptom-relieving dose for that allergen. There are no symptoms to relieve. Attempting to raise the dose to a maximally tolerated level at this point may result in reaching a level so high that when the pollen comes into bloom, that dose will produce a local (or systemic) reaction.

The Maximum Dose

A third term, the *maximum dose*, must be considered during immunotherapy. The maximum dose is not the same as the maximally tolerated dose. There is a maximum amount of antigen that most patients can tolerate at any given time. In such situations, when this antigen is in season, local reactions may occur during immunotherapy without concomitant symptom relief. In the majority of cases, this antigen will probably be a single pollen to which the patient is quite sensitive. It is always wise to treat for any seasonal antigen to which the patient is highly sensitive using a separate vial during the

If a local reaction occurs, these are the things to check:

1. Is evidence of an infection developing? Viral infections frequently begin with a prodrome that mimics allergic symptoms, and infections can result in large local reactions after an allergy injection at a dose that was previously well tolerated.

2. Has there been an increased exposure to any antigen? Dust-sensitive patients frequently note increased symptoms when moving or cleaning. Has the season changed? Cool nights and warm days increase the release of pollen, and windy conditions aid in pollen dispersal.

3. Has the patient been exposed to large amounts of irritants, such as cigarette smoke, air pollution, or chemicals?

4. Has the patient's stress level increased? For example, students often complain of nasal congestion and/or rhinorrhea at exam time.

It might be noted here that some patients may either demonstrate no local reactions or produce large local reactions (i.e., 30 mm or greater in diameter), with no smaller reactions between. It is important to remember that the occurrence of a local reaction is not a stopping point; it is just a point at which to maintain therapy until the body can adjust to the dose increase. This may occur after a few weeks, or the dose may have to be kept constant until the end of that particular season. Typically, trees pollinate in the spring, grasses from late spring to fall, and weeds in the late summer to fall. If the dose cannot be advanced after a season change, advancement may be attempted again after the first freeze of the season.

blooming season of this antigen, allowing advancement of other antigen doses in the usual fashion while the dose for this allergen is held stable or advanced very cautiously as dictated by local reactions. The doses of allergens being treated for at a maximum dose may be adjusted to a maximally tolerated level after the blooming season has passed, in the same fashion as already described.

It should be noted that although there is no such thing as an arbitrary maximum dose for therapy, certain guidelines have been determined through years of experience with immunotherapy. As early as 1956,[13] it was found that a dose of raw antigen of less than 40 μg was rarely effective in controlling allergy symptoms and that doses above 1000 μg rarely were required; higher doses added little in the way of benefits and at times appeared to be even less effective. Forty micrograms of raw antigen corresponds roughly to 0.50 mL of an SET #4 dilution, and 1000 μg of raw antigen corresponds roughly to 0.10 mL of an SET #1 (or 0.50 mL of #2) dilution. This range serves only as a rough guide, but if relief is achieved at a level significantly below the 40-μg level, it is well to advise the patient that the relief will probably be temporary and that further advancement will probably be necessary in the future. On the other hand, if the 1000-μg level is reached with no relief, it may be well for the allergist to consider other factors, including antigens not investigated for which the patient is not under treatment.

TECHNIQUE OF ALLERGY INJECTIONS

The injection begins with both the person administering the injection and the patient identifying the proper treatment vial (Fig. 9–6). The appropriate amount of antigen is carefully drawn up into an allergy syringe. The site generally chosen for the injection is the subcutaneous tissue on the back of the upper arm, below the insertion of the deltoid muscle. This site affords less chance for an inadvertent injection into muscle, which often results not only in discomfort but a significant local reaction afterward. The site is cleansed with an alcohol wipe. The person administering the injection holds the syringe like a dart in the dominant hand, and with the opposite hand grasps the tissue above the injection site and bunches it to pull the subcutane-

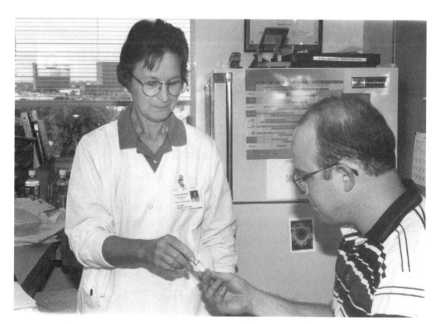

FIGURE 9–6. Both the person giving the shot and the patient should ascertain that the correct treatment vial has been chosen before an injection is given.

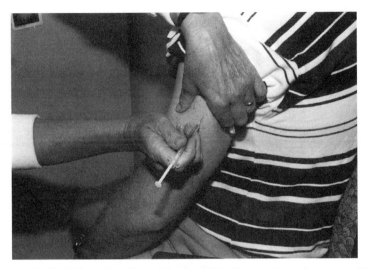

FIGURE 9–7. Technique for allergy injection. Note the location chosen, and that the injection is given subcutaneously, not intramuscularly.

ous tissue into prominence (Fig. 9–7). The needle is inserted quickly and the forefinger of the hand holding the syringe exerts pressure on the undersurface of the plunger to aspirate and ensure that no intravenous injection occurs. The forefinger then presses the plunger to inject the contents of the syringe fully. A brief wipe of the injection site with an alcohol wipe after the needle is withdrawn completes the process. Massaging the injection site should be avoided, as that can produce erythema and may force injected material into the superficial tissues, where it can produce induration in the same manner as in a skin test. Patients rarely bleed at the site of a properly administered injection, but a spot bandage may be applied to avoid staining clothing with the drop of blood that sometimes results.

CONTINUING IMMUNOTHERAPY

Once the maximally tolerated dose has been reached for all the allergens for which the patient is under treatment, they usually may be combined into a single treatment vial if this has not already been done. Most patients will request this to reduce the number of injections required, and it should be done by the time advancement has reached this stage so that practically all antigens are being treated at a #3 or #2 level (taking antigens from the #1 vial or from concentrate). Immunologically, such a combination rarely presents a problem. On a very few occasions, the combination will initially result in a pronounced local reaction (not seen when the antigens were given separately) and the antigens will have to be separated again, but this is rare. More often, the difficulty encountered is a result of unsuccessful attempts to recalculate the contents of the vials to provide a single vial and proper doses. This situation provides fertile ground for error, but if the basics of calculation are understood, it should present little problem. When the new vial is made, doses may be begun at a low level (generally 0.05 or 0.1 mL) and advanced to the point of a maximally tolerated dose, as before.

Providing different doses from two treatment vials by combining them into one injection in a single syringe is not recommended for a number of reasons, one of which is that vial cross-contamination is quite possible in this maneuver.

When vials are prepared for maintenance therapy, the glycerine content must be considered. These vials usually contain several antigens in concentrate form, and the glycerine content from these is likely to make the total glycerine level of the treatment vial high. It will be unnecessary to add more glycerine to the vial to keep the level above 10% if at least one fifth of the vial volume consists of antigen at concentrate. If more than this amount of glycerine is present, because of the presence of even more antigens at concentrate, injections may result in significant local reactions. A glycerine level above 10% is not dangerous, but it is wise to try to avoid the discomfort produced by such injections. The best means of doing this is to draw up an equal amount of diluent into the syringe before drawing up the maintenance dose from the treatment vial. This results in an injection of increased volume but renders it less painful. Note that the diluent should be drawn into the syringe first to avoid contaminating the diluent bottle with antigens by inserting a needle that has first been inserted into a treatment vial.

Although throughout this text we have warned that glycerine may produce local reactions, it should be noted that the currently available product is much more purified that the glycerine used years ago, and a true ''glycerine reaction'' is noted only occasionally.

ADMINISTERING INJECTIONS IN OR OUT OF THE OFFICE

A constant debate flourishes as to whether or not to send antigens for injection out of the office. It would be safe to state that, given the option, any allergist would prefer to have all patients receive every injection in the office under supervision. Treating under office conditions provides as near an approach to complete safety as can be obtained, as the properly equipped office has equipment at hand for treating emergencies immediately and the staff has been (or should have been) fully trained in coping with such emergencies. It is quite possible to go through an entire career of allergy care without seeing more than one or two emergency problems, but preparation is essential, and the patient receiving injections in the office should be well protected.

An additional benefit to having patients receive injections in the office is the enhanced level of communication provided by regular contact between the patient and the allergist or trained surrogate. This contact aids greatly in adjusting proper escalation and adjustment of immunotherapy doses. Immunotherapy, when carried out using the format described in this text, produces results much earlier than when administered according to some of the traditional formats, but such results do not appear immediately when therapy is started, nor does each escalated injection necessarily alter the course of the following injection. There are times when changes in the escalation sequence are indicated, such as at the onset of a blooming season of major allergens or in the presence of a respiratory infection, but these conditions should be interpreted by the allergist or surrogate, not the patient. This is averred despite the current medical climate in which patients are urged (generally by family, friends, and the media) to "take charge" of their health care. Faster, better, and safer results will be obtained if all injections are received in the office. This is particularly true during the escalation process, before maintenance doses have been reached.

Like most ideals in the world in general, this one is frequently impossible to achieve. Patients who reside at a distance will present themselves for allergy management. These patients are unable to come to the allergist's office at the frequent intervals necessary to receive immunotherapy in the office. Others will have jobs or other responsibilities from which they are unable to be absent long enough to receive their injections. Mothers may be unable to obtain child care for the period needed for an injection. All these situations present problems that the allergist cannot afford to ignore if the practice is to flourish and (more importantly) they are to deliver adequate care to patients seeking it from them. No solution to these dilemmas is as satisfactory as administering the injection in the office, but some adjustments allow for a reasonable approximation of the ideal therapy format. Many approaches are in widespread use today, and the following discussion presents some of the good and bad aspects of each.

Administering All Injections in the Office

This section is included simply as a reminder that this approach is the best one, against which all the others must be weighed. It is highly recommended that it be used as much as possible in the escalation stage of therapy, and it should be considered essential for the first treatment dose from each vial, which carries the highest risk for adverse reactions. The procedure for making a multiantigen, multidose vial has already been presented; it is the initial step in any format of immunotherapy. This vial, individually tailored for the particular patient, should be kept under refrigeration as an added means of preserving potency. After vial testing, the first injection is given from the vial, after which, if all is well, escalation proceeds according to the schedule described.

Escalating Injections to Be Given by Another Physician

For medicolegal reasons, this approach is probably the second best available. However, as will be pointed out later, it also presents potentials for error. Many patients who have come from a distance have a personal family physician in their area willing to give allergy injections if proper instructions and assistance are provided. If this approach must be chosen, it is essential that the allergist or allergy care provider discuss the immunotherapy procedure personally with the person who will be administering the injections. It is possible to send full instructions with the treatment extract, and this should be done, but communicating in writing to the person who will be administering the injections a list of all the errors possible in performing this service is likely to either discourage the person from providing the care at all or result in having the instructions ignored. However, even at the risk of discouraging the distant physician and staff from administering immunotherapy, it should be made clear to them that they will be expected to be able to recognize and treat appropriately reactions to these injections, including full-blown anaphylaxis. Written instructions on how to accomplish this should be made available if necessary. Failure to do so subjects the patient to a significant risk in the unlikely (but not impossible) event that a systemic reaction follows such an allergy injection. Likewise, it is even more important than when injections are administered in the allergist's office that patients be encouraged to remain in the nonallergist's office for 20 minutes after allergy injections.

Practice guidelines have addressed the situation in which the antigen mix is administered in an outside office. The primary area of potential liability for the allergist is in the preparation of the antigen or in the dose schedule provided. In addition, the allergist also must make the administering physician aware of the possibility of local and/or systemic reactions, and provide instructions for dose adjustment when local reactions occur. Finally, the allergist providing the extract must make the administering physician aware of the possibility of anaphylaxis, the need to be able to treat it rapidly, and the need for the patient to wait in the office for at least 20 minutes after the injection. If these requirements are fulfilled, it is the posture of the Joint Council on Allergy, Asthma and Immunology that the allergist is not liable for negligence of the administering physician or staff.[14]

For the allergy office, the procedure of immunotherapy is simple and straightforward. For the inexperienced person, a multitude of questions may be expected to arise, all of which may affect the expected response to therapy. The issues raised below, and their solutions, are based on decades of experience in treating allergy.

The first consideration is in what form the allergy treatment extract will be provided to the nonallergist physician. Two options are available. The first of these is the multiple-antigen, multiple-dose vial, such as has been prepared for administration of immunotherapy in the allergist's office. This is the method most commonly chosen, but it is fraught with opportunities for confusion and error. The second option is the provision of unit-dose vials, each containing the exact amount of antigen required for a single injection. Preparation of these individual treatment vials requires more time and effort on the part of the allergy nurse or technician, but the end result is a significant reduction in the opportunity for error, leading to greater safety and greater acceptance by the individual charged with administering the injections.

Multiple-Antigen, Multiple-Dose Vials

No matter what procedure is used for subsequent doses, the vial test and first treatment dose from every new vial should be administered in the allergist's office. This should be made clear in the instructions that accompany the multidose vial to the secondary physician's office. Detailed instructions should accompany the vial, outlining the escalation sequence and how to adjust for any local or general reactions. Instructions should also strongly urge that the person administering the injections communicate with the allergist should any questions arise. Finally, the instructions should advise this person when to contact the allergist's office to arrange for preparation of the next vial. At that time, a report of responses to injections from the first vial will need to be reviewed. For this purpose, a reporting sheet is beneficial.

Potential Problems With Multiple-Dose Vial Therapy

The usual procedure when a physician unfamiliar with allergy is given a vial of allergy treatment extract and asked to supervise injections of its contents is for the physician to pass the vial on to an assistant. The only advice generally given at that point by the physician is an admonition to follow the instructions supplied by the allergy office. Rather than the secondary physician, the person in the secondary physician's office who will actually be administering the injections is the person with whom the allergy care provider must stay touch. Maintaining contact solely through the secondary physician leads to an exchange of third-hand information and provides an increasing opportunity for mistakes to be made. Should more than one person be charged with administering the injections, it is advisable that the allergy office communicate with all of them. However, if at all possible, it is beneficial to ask that one person in the secondary physician's office be designated the "contact" for allergy injections.

In the early steps of dose escalation, the amount of extract used in each injection is quite tiny. This presents two possible sources of error. First, 0.05 mL is difficult to measure unless the person making the measurement is supplied with an allergist's syringes. This problem may be avoided by sending the appropriate number of 0.5-mL or 1-mL allergist's syringes along with the vial, and instructing the person administering the injections to use these syringes.

The second risk is related to the first, and it may also be reduced by providing the appropriate syringes with the vial, along with specific instructions about dose measurement. This second error is the most common one seen when injections are given by someone inexperienced in allergy. The scenario proceeds as follows: The patient's personal physician, trying to be cooperative, receives the treatment extract and passes it on to an employee who skims the instructions and attempts to comply. If no allergist's syringes have been provided, a larger syringe (often a tuberculin syringe) will be used. When the tiny amount of solution represented by a dose of 0.05 mL is withdrawn, the person administering the injection assumes that an error has been made and moves the decimal point to the right, resulting in 10 times the prescribed dose being given (e.g., 0.5 mL). It is a testimonial to the safety of SET that the most severe reaction reported from this error has generally been a massive local reaction and minor allergic symptoms. There is no guarantee, however, that such will always be the case.

One other potential problem may arise when dosing from a multiple-dose vial. This will not occur during the period of dose escalation but may be seen when maintenance doses are to be given. The maintenance treatment vial is prepared to administer 10 identical doses of extract. If an allergist's syringe is used, the quantity in the vial will provide this number of doses because of the hubless construction of the unit. Should a tuberculin syringe with an added needle be substituted, however, about 0.05 mL of fluid is left in the barrel of the syringe and the hub of the needle. This means that the patient will not be able to receive all the doses expected, as after 10 doses a total of about 0.50 mL will have been left in the syringes and needles and discarded. The patient will be deprived of a dose for which payment has been made, resulting in an unhappy patient. A similar, but more minor, complaint in this scenario is the difficulty of withdrawing the last few drops of extract from the multidose treatment vial. The amount of antigen contained in these few drops is of little significance, but coupled with the missing dose, it serves to compound the patient's annoyance.

Individual-Dose Treatment Vials

Individual-dose treatment vials have been in use for several decades and have almost always been the choice of general allergists as well as many otolaryngic allergists. They greatly simplify the administration of treatment, reduce the opportunity for error, and avoid most of the problems already described that may result from the use of multidose vials.

Preparation of Unit-Dose Treatment Vials

Unit-dose vials are prepared simply and directly, using as a source the multiple-antigen, multiple-dose vial from which the patient would receive all injections if they were administered in the allergist's office. The procedure is simple and not terribly time-consuming. The ideal unit vial is an empty 1-mL vial with the same type of rubber and aluminum cap used on the larger testing and treatment vials. These vials are available from almost all allergy supply houses. The number of unit-dose vials prepared will depend on the individual situation (e.g., escalation vs. maintenance, interval between injections, whether glycerine has been added). As an example, consider the preparation of six such vials, without added glycerine, for weekly escalation of dose in an outside office. Additional vials, without added glycerine, would lose significant potency after the sixth week. As a first step, the vials are labeled with the patient's name and numbered 1 through 6. The date on which the injection is anticipated may be added, although it may be a source of confusion if an appointment is changed. The name or initials of the person preparing the vials are also added. The vials are lined up in order from #1 to #6. The amount of extract that would be administered to the patient for the first such injection during dose escalation is withdrawn from the patient's multiple-dose vial and inserted into vial #1. The second anticipated dose is placed into vial #2 and so on, until the antigen mix has been added to all vials. To each vial is then added an amount of diluent to reach a volume that allows a convenient injection. A total of about 0.5 mL is adequate, although the volume may be up to 1 mL. The exact amount added is not critical, as the entire contents of the vial will be administered. A simple and rapid means of estimating the amount of diluent to be added is to place the unit vials against a white backdrop, such as a piece of paper or cardboard. The desired total amount of diluent is measured into an empty vial, and a line is drawn on the backdrop at that level. The treatment vials are simply filled with diluent to that line after the extract needed for each injection has been placed in the vial.

Administration of Unit Doses from Unit-Dose Vials

No measurements by the person giving the injection are necessary in treating from unit-dose vials, as they are with multidose vials. On the appropriate visit, the entire contents of the sequentially numbered unit-dose vial are withdrawn using an allergist's syringe and administered as a single, subcutaneous dose. The date and number of the vial are recorded in the chart, along with any local reactions that result.

Advantages and Disadvantages of Unit-Dose Vials

Two minor disadvantages to unit dose vials are the additional cost of the vials, which is not great, and the time necessary for unit-dose preparation. This time does not represent a significant problem, as each dose would have to be measured in any case before being injected. The time factor may actually work to the advantage of the person preparing the vials, as unit-dose vials can be prepared in the patient's absence, allowing greater freedom of time allocation.

The advantages of unit-dose vials are numerous. First is the safety factor. The opportunity for error is greatly reduced when a single, premeasured dose is given in a designated order. Second is the size of the dose. The antigen is distributed through a sufficient volume that even if it is administered with a tuberculin syringe, the amount of antigen remaining in the hub is an insignificant percentage of the total quantity contained in the vial. For the same reason, a drop or two of extract that cannot be aspirated from the unit-dose vial does not represent a major loss of antigen. Although it is of psychological rather than medical importance, providing what the patient perceives to be a substantial amount of extract per injection engenders a feeling of having received an adequate dose for the cost incurred. Overall, the advantages of single-dose vials far outweigh the cost involved in purchasing the unit vials.

It should be noted that the same considerations apply to the use of unit-dose vials for maintenance therapy as for dose escalation. The maintenance vials are prepared in the same manner. Because the master vial from which these are made generally contains 10% glycerine and should be stable for up to 12 weeks, 10 unit-dose vials can be prepared. In this case, each dose will be identical. The contents of each vial are brought to the desired volume, generally from 0.5 to 1 mL, with diluent. Because each vial is the same, it is not important to number them, but the date of preparation should be marked on the label.

Taking Injections at Home

Taking immunotherapy injections at home presents a greater risk from a medicolegal standpoint than receiving injections in a physician's office. However, it may at times be the only viable option, and when the proper precautions are followed, it need not be avoided. As already discussed, it is difficult, if not impossible, for many people to be absent from work, school, or other obligations with the frequency required to come to the allergist's office for injections at weekly intervals. Although every effort should be made to administer advancement immunotherapy in the office of the treating allergist, maintenance immunotherapy administered by the patient after proper preparation and instruction on the part of the allergy staff has proved safe in the authors' hands over many years.

The American Academy of Allergy, Asthma and Immunology (AAAAI) in 1994 published a position statement advising the restriction of home administration of allergens to exceptional cases, after "very careful consideration of the potential benefits and risk."[15] This generated a firestorm of criticism from those members who had been allowing such immunotherapy for years, but the AAAAI remained adamant in its opposition to the practice.[16] On the other hand, otolaryngic allergists, practicing immunotherapy based on the quantitative methods of SET and/or RAST, have for years allowed allergy injections to be taken at home, primarily when patients are at a maintenance level, provided proper precautions are taken. The safety of this practice has been underscored by several investigations of the risk for reactions to immunotherapy given in this fashion.[11,17] In these reports, emphasis was placed on the need to train the individuals administering the injections and provide them with both the knowledge and the materials to render initial treatment of any reactions that might occur.

Many aspects of home-based immunotherapy are similar to those described for injections in another physician's office. In addition, some special aspects to home therapy require further comment.

Drawbacks of Multiple-Dose Vials for Home Immunotherapy

As already described, measurements of tiny amounts of extract are difficult, even for trained personnel. Most patients taking injections from multiple-dose vials at home must be thoroughly briefed on making these measurements, and they may indeed make them more accurately than an inexperienced allergy assistant. However, a little arthritis, poor light, a distraction, or other factors can results in a dose error. As already described, the patient may observe the small quantity used in the injection and decide that more is needed. This tendency of patients today to "play doctor" is very real and represents a significant danger when patients are allowed to receive immunotherapy at home from multiple-dose vials. No matter how strongly the patient is admonished to follow the injection schedule provided, experience has shown that a large percentage will vary the dose and treatment schedule based on their immediate symptoms or anticipated needs. The result may be either overdosing or underdosing, but in either case, significant problems may result. On one occasion, the patient may feel that symptoms have been aggravated by a previous injection and reduce the next dose, not realizing that the prior changes were related to a temporary increase in allergen exposure. On another occasion, the patient may feel that not enough progress has been made and increase the amount of extract in the next injection. Physicians, nurses, and health care personnel are familiar with patient noncompliance, as evidenced by the typical story of several antibiotic capsules left over after a full course has been prescribed. If such noncompliance occurs when a course of medicine is to be taken for only a few days, imagine the degree of noncompliance in a course of therapy that lasts for years. If injections are given from a multiple-dose vial, patients administering their own injections may note that a rather significant volume of extract remains when the expiration date of the vial arrives. This is the converse of the situation sometimes seen when injections are given in the office of the nonallergist, when enthusiasm for giving an adequate amount and/or misplacement of the decimal point results in the consumption of the entire vial during the first few shots.

Advantages of Unit-Dose Vials for Home Immunotherapy

Treating with unit-dose vials on an at-home basis presents the same advantages as treating with these vials in a nonallergist physician's office. There is appreciably less medicolegal risk than with the use of a multidose vial. The volume of each injection need not be measured, and the amount contained in the vial not only appears substantial but is easier to draw up and administer. It is, of course, still possible for the patient to "play doctor," altering the prescribed doses, but with unit-dose vials such dose alteration is not easy. Thus, although noncompliance is possible, it is difficult enough that most patients will cooperate by administering the dose prescribed.

Other Factors Affecting Injections at Home

If maintenance immunotherapy is to be provided on at at-home basis, preparation should begin with a session with the allergy nurse or assistant. During this time, the patient (or the person who will be giving the injections) is shown the proper technique for withdrawing material from a unit-dose vial and placing the injection subcutaneously in the soft tissue of the posterior aspect of the upper arm. Patients are instructed in the early signs of a systemic reaction and provided with written instructions for dealing with such reactions (Table 9–1). A prescription is given for a commercially available, premeasured epinephrine injection apparatus (EpiPen, Ana-Kit). If any question of a general reaction arises, patients are instructed to use the epinephrine, take an oral antihistamine (which they should always have on hand), place a tourniquet above the injection site, and proceed immediately to the nearest emergency room or source of urgent medical care. Finally, they are taught to watch for, record, and report any local reactions or adverse effects from the injections, and to consult the allergy office before taking the next injection if any reaction occurs. Failure to provide this education and support places patients in jeopardy and the allergy office in grave medicolegal risk.

For the patient who has difficulty or discomfort in taking injections in the subcutaneous tissue of the posterior arm, the injections may easily be taken in the layer of subcutaneous fat around the waist, usually to either side and a little below the level of the navel. This area is minimally sensitive, making the injections essentially painless, and any local reaction may easily be seen and evaluated. Another alternate site is the soft subcutaneous tissue of the thigh. These areas do not offer the advantage that a tourniquet can be placed above them, but they are much more accessible for self-injections than the upper arm.

When a patient is to take injections at home, one additional precaution should be stressed. Although adverse reactions are quite rare, the possibility always exists. The patient should never take an injection when alone.

No matter what treatment format is to be employed, it is wise to provide only the amount of extract necessary to administer a limited number of doses.

TABLE 9–1. Instructions for patients regarding reactions to allergy injections

REACTIONS TO ALLERGY SHOTS

The techniques we use for testing for the presence and degree of sensitivity to an allergen, and the way in which dosage is advanced, makes a reaction to an allergy injection unlikely. However, this information is furnished to make your treatment even safer. Please read it carefully, call us if you have questions, and *keep this sheet where it can be easily found if you need it.*

To treat a possible reaction, you will need an *antihistamine* and *epinephrine.* Any antihistamine, either prescription or over-the-counter, will do. Examples are Allegra, Zyrtec, Claritin, Chlor-Trimeton, and Benadryl. Epinephrine is available in an automatic injection form called EpiPen, EpiPen Jr., or Ana-Kit. You will receive a prescription to purchase one of these. It is unlikely that you will ever need it, but *it must be available when you receive your allergy shot.* Don't forget to check the expiration date from time to time.

The combination of an allergy shot with higher-than-usual allergen exposure may sometimes result in a *local reaction,* which is an area of firmness (not necessarily redness) at the injection site larger than a 50-cent piece persisting for at least 24 hours. Redness and/or firmness can also be caused by a complicating infection, or by a reaction to glycerine in the mixture. If a local reaction around an injection site occurs, take an antihistamine and *report this to the nurse before your next injection, for dosage adjustment if necessary.*

A true *severe reaction* must be treated immediately. It begins within 5 or 10 minutes of the injection with intense itching of the throat, nose, and chest membranes. If this occurs, take an antihistamine immediately. If the reaction progresses to any swelling of the face or throat, difficulty swallowing or breathing, and generalized itching or redness of the body accompanied by a feeling of distress, *immediately administer one dose of epinephrine,* injecting into the soft tissue of the arm opposite the site of your allergy shot. Put a tourniquet (e.g., a belt) above the place where you had the allergy shot to slow the absorption of the material into the system. *If it is necessary to administer epinephrine, go immediately to the nearest hospital emergency room or urgent care center,* where you can receive medical attention while the doctor is being notified.

For maintenance therapy, in which the antigen is contained in 10% glycerine, this may be up to 12 doses during a 12-week period. Situations in which injections are taken more frequently than once a week, or in which doses are being escalated, are generally inappropriate for treatment outside the office. When a specific number of doses are provided for a corresponding number of weekly injections, the degree of compliance is automatically determined as the patient requests more vials. If the patient or nonallergist physician does not notify the allergist's office at an appropriate time to have the next set of vials of allergy extract supplied, the allergist is immediately aware that the recommended treatment schedule has not been followed and can take appropriate steps to rectify the situation.

It is helpful to provide a record documenting injections, as well as re-

TABLE 9–2. Information for monitoring out-of-office injections

(Heading with Practice Information)

PATIENT NAME: DATE:

INSTRUCTIONS: TAKE ALL OF ONE VIAL AT _____ INTERVALS. KEEP THIS FORM WITH YOUR VIALS AND COMPLETE WHEN INJECTION IS GIVEN. RECORD ANY SYMPTOMS OR LOCAL REACTION IN SPACE NEXT TO DATE OF INJECTION.

DATE OF INJECTION   SYMPTOMS/LOCAL REACTION

_____

_____

_____

_____

_____

_____

_____

WHEN YOU HAVE TAKEN ALL VIALS, RETURN THIS FORM **IMMEDIATELY** TO THE CLINIC. YOU MAY MAIL IT TO THE ADDRESS ABOVE, OR FAX IT TO THE NUMBER ABOVE. **THIS FORM MUST BE RETURNED BEFORE YOU CAN RECEIVE MORE VIALS!!** AFTER RETURNING THE FORM, PLEASE CALL TO MAKE YOUR NEXT APPOINTMENT FOR AN INJECTION AND TO PICK UP YOUR VIALS.

sponses, to be returned to the allergy office when the supply of antigen has been exhausted and a new supply is being requested (Table 9–2).

MAINTENANCE THERAPY

Maintenance treatment levels have been reached when all antigen doses have been escalated to the maximally tolerated dose level. At a level somewhat below this, a symptom-relieving dose should have been reached at which the patient experienced a major improvement in symptoms lasting at least a week. As the level has been escalated above this to the maximally tolerated dose, there may have been a slight temporary increase in symptoms accompanying the increasing local reaction. In establishing a maintenance dose for continued use, the injection strength is reduced to the highest level that does not provoke symptoms or an unacceptable local reaction (i.e., greater than 25 mm in diameter). This will be the maintenance level of treatment. In 80%

or more of cases, treatment at this level for a period of 3 or more years successfully alters the allergic response, allowing the patient to discontinue injections without the recurrence of allergic symptoms. This relief from symptoms will most often last indefinitely (although possibly affected by situations in the future, such as massive allergen exposure or some insult to the immune system). In rarer circumstances, allergic symptoms may recur in the future, making it necessary to treat the patient again with immunotherapy. Coping with this situation is discussed elsewhere.

The final maintenance dose may be reached in stages, because as patients undergo immunologic changes with therapy or as seasons change, it may be possible to advance their dose yet further. This should be continued until the amount of antigen administered in each injection reaches the levels already described, with optimum symptomatic relief. Once the patient is receiving a maintenance level of treatment, the dose is not expected to change further unless problems arise. A brief increase in allergy symptoms should not pre-cipitate a re-evaluation of the treatment program, especially if it can be explained by a change in allergen exposure or some other temporally limited factor. Even the best immunotherapy is unable to protect from sudden allergic overloads, such as massive allergen exposure. In most cases, this overload is brief and best controlled by the temporary use of appropriate pharmaco-therapy. Unless the symptoms are associated with unacceptable local reac-tions, altering the maintenance dose under these circumstances usually repre-sents overreaction on the part of the therapist and should be avoided if possible. There will be times when the maintenance dose will require adjust-ment, but these will be rare, and adjustment should not be attempted until it is evident that the increase in symptoms represents a prolonged situation, generally more than a month.

For best results, injections at escalating and maintenance doses are contin-ued at weekly intervals for a year. This length of time normally results in adequate reprogramming of the immune system to begin extending the period between injections. If the patient's symptoms reappear before the week is up, an additional injection of the same strength may be given. This additional treatment does not alter the overall course of treatment, but if it is required repeatedly, a proper maintenance dose may not truly have been reached. In these circumstances, further increasing the dose cautiously may be beneficial.

It should be noted that respiratory infections may induce a large local reaction after an injection, coupled with an increase in nasal symptoms. A search for infection should be made before a dose schedule is altered under these circumstances.

After a year of weekly immunotherapy, including achievement of a proper maintenance dose that has been administered for at least 8 months, the interval between injections may be extended to 2 weeks. If symptoms do not reappear at these intervals after several months, it may even be possible to extend the interval further, but this is not necessarily recommended. First, immunotherapy administered on a 3-weekly schedule often results in a gradual breakdown of symptom control. Second, although it is simple to remember a weekly schedule or a fortnightly schedule, rarely is one able to comply regularly with a 3-weekly schedule that simply does not fit into the established pattern of the patient's lifestyle. If for reasons of economy or personal circumstance a lengthening of injection intervals to every 3 weeks is contemplated, it is best to defer this until the patient has completed 2 years of therapy, the first year receiving injections at least weekly and the second year at intervals of every 2 weeks. Extending the interval between injections to every 4 weeks is possible near the end of a course of immunotherapy, but injections at intervals of more than 4 weeks seem to carry an increased risk for producing an undesirable reaction.

Symptom control is not maintained in every patient when injection intervals are increased to every 2 weeks. If this situation arises, the weekly doses may be resumed. After a month or so, extending the interval between doses may again be attempted. Sooner or later, most patients will be able to extend the interval successfully. The best time to make the move to a longer period between injections is after the patient's worst allergy season has ended.

A useful approach is to administer immunotherapy at weekly or, less frequently, biweekly intervals until a true maintenance dose has been reached. Weekly injections are continued for a total of at least 1 year. If antigens are being given at adequate concentrations at a maximally tolerated dose, after a year of therapy and after the patient's worst season has passed, the interval may be increased to every 2 weeks. This is continued for a total of at least 3 years of immunotherapy. Many patients will be able to come off injections at this point, although some (especially those with very high sensitivities to grass pollens) may require therapy for 5 years. Experience will assist in judging further the appropriate schedule for most patients.

There will be occasions when a dose has been reached that produces local reactions at the highest limits of acceptability, yet the patient has not experienced adequate symptom relief. This situation does not indicate that immunotherapy has failed, but rather suggests that some elements of the allergic problem have not been brought under control. The administration of the maintenance dose established for the antigens for which the patient is currently under treatment should be continued while the allergist searches for the offending elements that are as yet untreated. Such elements may include airborne allergens that the patient is exposed to locally, either indoors or outdoors, but that are not widely present in the general area and therefore have not been included in the allergist's usual testing battery. The missing elements may also be foods or chemicals to which the patient is sensitive, requiring a different approach to diagnosis and treatment. These situations are considered elsewhere in the book. The important aspect in considering maintenance care is that even if the immunotherapy injections appear to have been unsuccessful in relieving symptoms adequately, they should not be discontinued at this time. Testing has clearly demonstrated the presence of inhalant allergy, and this has been treated by an appropriate means. The imperfect response simply indicates that the allergist's job is not yet done.

It should be noted that if symptom relief is inadequate despite immunotherapy, the patient frequently becomes discouraged. It is necessary at this point for the allergist to re-examine the patient (looking, for example, for complicating infections) and explore further the patient's history. This should be accompanied by an honest explanation of the situation and assurances that other avenues will continue to be explored as necessary to improve on the situation. Patients who simply have injections continued without further evaluation or explanation are likely to (quite properly) consider the treatment a failure and remove themselves from the care of the physician. This underscores our philosophy that regular visits with the allergist are necessary during a course of immunotherapy, as well as evaluation of patients at any time that they do not seem to be doing well. To do otherwise degrades allergy management from the practice of medicine to a technical exercise.

One alternate approach to the discouraged patient is to suggest that the injections be discontinued for a short time. Frequently, the patient will return within a few weeks, having realized that in fact the treatment had provided more improvement than had been recognized.

DISCONTINUING THERAPY

The unique advantage of immunotherapy over other forms of inhalant allergy treatment is that in at least 80% of patients, treatment may be discontinued after a finite period of a few years without a return of symptoms. The exact duration of therapy before this happens varies among individual patients, and, as has been mentioned, there may be as many as 20% of patients for whom immunotherapy will be successful but who must continue treatment indefinitely if they are to remain symptom-free. It has been estimated that about 3 to 5 years of treatment, most of which is at a maintenance dose administered every 2 to occasionally 3 or even 4 weeks, is adequate to

NURSE'S NOTE

Each treatment vial is labeled with the name of the patient and the expiration date of the vial. If the patient is being treated from more than one vial, these must be identified in some way, such as vial A, vial B; red vial, blue vial. The injections are then given in a manner that allows identification if one vial causes a local reaction. These injections may be given on separate days but are more commonly given in separate arms, with documentation of which arm received the injection from which vial.

It is important that both the person giving the injection and the patient receiving the injection identify the vial as the proper one before the shot is given (Fig. 9–6). If any symptoms are present, these should be determined and documented beforehand, along with any change in general status or medications. At the time of injection, documentation should include the date, the amount administered, which vial was the injection source (if more than one is used), the site of injection, and the person administering the injection. Any local reactions or change in symptoms following the injection should be charted.

When a patient reports symptoms, it is important to explore the possible causes. This allows measures to be taken to minimize these symptoms. Patients should be continually counseled regarding proper use of their medications. For instance, a patient reporting symptoms on mowing grass who cannot arrange for someone else to do the mowing can at least use medications (e.g., antihistamines, cromolyn) before the exposure and minimize continued exposure by using a mask, showering and shampooing after mowing, and rinsing the nose with saline solution. Unfortunately, most patients do so well on immunotherapy that they forget environmental control measures and the proper use of necessary medications.

Before each injection, the patient must be assessed to determine if the dose can be increased, should remain the same, or should be decreased. This will vary with the patient's sensitivity, the length of time on therapy, and the amount of exposure to allergens during the preceding week.

establish long-term relief for most patients. This estimate, however, is based primarily on an analogy with stinging-insect allergy therapy and has not been fully correlated with inhalant allergy care. It is known, however, that the necessary duration of treatment varies among patients, and the factors responsible for the variation have not yet been identified.

Immunotherapy may be discontinued if the following criteria are met: The patient should have received injections for a minimum of 3 years, most of that time at maintenance doses that deliver an adequate level of antigens to form blocking antibodies. This means that for practical purposes, the treatment vial should have been made with concentrate or #1 dilutions. The patient should have experienced symptom relief manifested through all four of the major seasons immediately past. Finally, in climates in which this is a consideration, it is wise to continue immunotherapy past the first freeze of the year when pollens are a significant contributor to the patient's allergic symptoms. Patients who are exquisitely sensitive to one or more antigens (especially grasses) may require longer escalation phases to reach maintenance levels, and it is often helpful at the outset of immunotherapy to advise them that they may require injections for up to 5 years. However, at some point between 3 and 5 years, discontinuing therapy should be considered. Unfortunately, although most patients welcome this news, some are unwilling to give up the "security blanket" represented by their injections. This is easily managed by reassuring them that the injections can be restarted if necessary, as outlined below.

A current recommendation is that after 3 or more years of treatment, it is reasonable to discontinue immunotherapy. If the symptoms remain under control, no more injections should be given unless problems arise. If symptoms begin to develop after 6 or 8 weeks, it is usually safe to reinstitute maintenance care, starting at a lower dose and raising the dose progressively to the previous maintenance level. How much reduction is necessary will vary with the time since the previous dose was given. If the interval has been less than 2 months, and if the patient is not exceptionally brittle, it is usually safe to try one-half the maintenance dose, given in the allergist's office. If this is tolerated, the next dose may be brought to the previous maintenance level. If a longer period has ensued, further reduction of the dose may be necessary. If the interval since the previous dose has been 3 months or longer, it is wise to introduce additional safety factors, such as a vial test, as described below.

The first consideration is that after 3 months, the previous maintenance vial will have expired, making the production of a new vial a necessity. In the interest of saving the patient as much time and money as possible, the simplest approach is to make a vial identical to the maintenance vial but use saline solution as a diluent. This vial may then be serially diluted (as already described) and titration skin testing carried out to determine a safe starting dose, as has already been described under vial testing. Treatment may then be started at this dose and escalated to the level of maintenance in the usual fashion. Most of this vial will be used up in the process of dose escalation. At this point, a new maintenance vial may be made using the necessary amount of glycerine to provide a 10% level. This approach will be successful in a large number of cases, and the patient will again have the symptoms under control. The gradual extension of the interval between injections may then proceed as before.

Some explanation of the rationale behind this approach is indicated. First, it is well established that the potential for allergy is genetically determined. If the previous immunotherapy has been successful, the major allergens in the area to which the patient is sensitive should have been identified and treated for to provide relief. Unless there have been significant ecologic changes in the area or the patient has encountered new exposures by relocating or changing activities, the same allergens that generated the previous problem will be the ones causing recurrent symptoms. For this reason, retesting as an initial step is probably not productive. All that has changed is a breakdown in the allergy-blocking mechanism, which needs to be re-established in the same way as before.

With regard to retesting under these circumstances, it is noteworthy that in most cases immunotherapy results in a reduction in skin sensitivity, even if all the symptoms have not been controlled. It is rare to see a new vial prepared for renewing treatment produce skin reactions at points more than one or two dilutions below the previous maintenance level. This circumstance allows resumption of treatment with safety at a level as close to the previous maintenance level as possible. However, such a situation is not always the case, so that titrating the new vial, even through several dilutions, may represent the safer approach.

It would be expected that because allergy is genetically determined, the above approach would be effective in all cases, regardless of the time during which the patient did not receive therapy. Clinically, however, this does not always prove to be the case. If a patient has gone more than a year without immunotherapy, it is usually necessary to retest and start over.

RETESTING

There was a time in the not-too-distant past when many allergists felt that it was necessary to retest the patient on immunotherapy at frequent intervals, often annually. Such retesting usually indicated a reduction in the patient's allergic sensitivity as manifested in the skin, thereby directing the treating physician to raise the antigen dose in compliance with the decrease in skin reaction. As has been noted, however, the change in skin reaction is not predictable, and during escalation and maintenance immunotherapy, it does not always mirror the ideal treatment dose. With increasing knowledge of the immune system, it has been established that retesting is rarely necessary and should be limited to unexplained failures in treatment, or the recommended retesting after a recurrence of symptoms a year or more after immunotherapy has been discontinued. When accurate and appropriate initial testing has been performed and escalation of doses to a symptom-relieving and then maintenance level has been completed with good results, it is not advisable to retest. For whatever reason, immunotherapy manipulation based on frequent retesting is not as effective as dose adjustment based on the initial test results and clinical judgment. To quote the old adage, "If it ain't broke, don't fix it!"

ESTABLISHING A SUPPORT SYSTEM

For various reasons, some of which have been described, most of the problems in treating allergy tend to occur early in the practice. Bearing this in mind, it will be wise for the novice allergist to seek out the guidance of a colleague with as much experience as possible in the field, who can serve as a mentor and sounding board during the early stages of practice. This support is usually not difficult to obtain. Unlike other medical conditions, most allergic problems are diagnosed and treated on the basis of history, supplemented by appropriate laboratory testing. Physical examinations are usually of limited importance after the first comprehensive examination has been performed. Under these circumstances, most problems can be discussed on the telephone once a cooperative relationship has been established between novice and mentor. If the aspiring allergist wishes to enter into such a relationship, it is well worthwhile to schedule a visit of a few days to the established practice to observe how actual care is delivered. This provides several benefits. First, the novice will be able to see patients at all stages of evaluation and treatment. He will see patients with allergic problems, many of whom are not even aware that allergy may be affecting their condition. Patients will be present in the office who are undergoing initial testing—both initial screening and, when indicated, comprehensive testing. Patients who are undergoing immunotherapy will be receiving injections, and the neophyte allergist will be able to discuss with them their reactions to treatment. Other patients will be on maintenance therapy, and the novice will be able to evaluate their responses. There is no other situation, including nationally recognized courses, that will permit the beginning allergist to observe so many aspects of allergy evaluation, testing, and treatment as a visit to an established practitioner's office. This same approach has been successfully utilized in the training of residents in many programs, either through a rotation in private offices or (in a fortunate few instances) in a private faculty otolaryngic allergy clinic.

SUMMARY

Immunotherapy has been the approach that the public associates with allergy care since the early part of the century. It is only one means of treating inhalant allergy and may not always be the most appropriate one. However, immunotherapy is currently the only form of treatment that offers the hope of long-term or permanent relief of symptoms. The preceding material has been a rather exhaustive discussion of the indications, drawbacks, and methodology of providing immunotherapy. When this form of care is initiated, as when any new technology is to be added to a practice, it is highly beneficial for the novice to attend several teaching seminars and then to visit a physician experienced in this form of practice for long enough to feel comfortable in undertaking it independently. This is not always possible, however, and even when the aspiring new allergist has undergone all this preparation for adding allergy to the practice, questions inevitably arise when patient care actually gets underway.

REFERENCES

1. Fell W, Mabry RL, Mabry CS. Quality of life analysis of immunotherapy for allergic rhinitis. Ear Nose Throat J 1997;76:528–536.
2. Gordon BR. Immunotherapy: rationale and mechanisms. Otolaryngol Head Neck Surg 1992;107:861–865.
3. Saxon A. AIDS: more common in allergy practice than once believed. Respir News 1989; 9:2.
4. Toogood JH. Risk of anaphylaxis in patients receiving beta-blocker drugs. J Allergy Clin Immunol 1988;81:1–5.
5. Gordon BR. Prevention and management of office allergy emergencies. Otolaryngol Clin North Am 1992;25:119–134.
6. Metzger WJ. Indications for allergen immunotherapy during pregnancy. Compr Ther 1990;16:17–26.
7. Phanuphak P, Kohler PF. Onset of polyarteritis nodosa during allergic hyposensitization treatment. Am J Med 1980;68:479–485.
8. Mabry RL, Mabry CS. Significance of borderline levels of specific IgE obtained by FAST-Plus assay. Otolaryngol Head Neck Surg 1992;106:250–253.
9. Mabry RL. Blending skin endpoint titration and in vitro methods in clinical practice. Otolaryngol Clin North Am 1992;25:61–70.
10. Board of Directors of the American Academy of Allergy, Asthma and Immunology. Guidelines to minimize the risk from systemic reactions caused by immunotherapy with allergenic extracts. J Allergy Clin Immunol 1994;93:811–812.
11. Cook PR, Bryant JL, Davis WE, et al. Systemic reactions to immunotherapy: the American

Academy of Otolaryngic Allery morbidity and mortality survey. Otolaryngol Head Neck Surg 1994;110:487–493.
12. Food and Drug Administration. Deaths associated with allergenic extracts. FDA Med Bull 1994;p 7.
13. Johnstone DE. Study on the role of antigen dosage in the treatment of pollinosis and pollen asthma. AMA J Dis Child 1957;94:1.
14. Joint Council of Allergy, Asthma and Immunology. Allergists' liability in providing antigens for administration by another physician. JCAAI Rep 1996;21:1–3.
15. Board of Directors of the American Academy of Allergy, Asthma and Immunology. Guidelines to minimize the risk of systemic reactions caused by immunotherapy with allergenic extracts. J Allergy Clin Immunol 1994;93:811–812.
16. Lockey RF. Reply to letters to the editor. J Allergy Clin Immunol 1995;95:1062–1063.
17. Davis WE, Cook PR, McKinsey JP, Templer JW. Anaphylaxis in immunotherapy. Otolaryngol Head Neck Surg 1992;107:78–83.

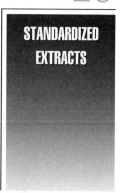

10

STANDARDIZED EXTRACTS

In attempting to find a more consistent and accurate way to measure the strength of allergy extracts, the Food and Drug Administration (FDA) has, in its quest for standardization, created a true dilemma. The definition of a dilemma is ''a situation that requires one to choose between two equally balanced alternatives.'' In the case of a change from nonstandardized to standardized extracts, however, the alternate definition seems more applicable: ''a predicament that seemingly defies a satisfactory solution.''

It has long been recognized by allergists that allergenic extracts are quite different from other forms of medication. It is unfortunate that a large percentage of nonphysicians involved in managed care, or as third-party payers, do not seem to understand the reasons why allergenic extracts do not follow the familiar pattern established for commercially prepared drugs. Equally unfortunate is the fact that many physicians not involved in allergy testing and immunotherapy also appear to be confused by this situation. It is nonetheless necessary to understand the unique nature of allergenic extracts to carry out allergy diagnosis appropriately and administer immunotherapy properly. One special area of confusion currently exists: the matter of the introduction of new formulations of allergy extracts that conform the demands of the FDA for ''standardization.''

In general, drugs from all manufacturers may be assumed to be uniform in potency, conforming to the standards set by such agencies as the FDA and the United States Pharmacopeia (USP). These drugs consist of a designated amount of clearly identified, chemically defined medication at a measured level of potency, contained in an inert vehicle. Allergenic extracts, on the other hand, are mixtures derived from active biologic material by a variety of means. The extract generally contains not only the desired allergen, but also a number of other organic substances present in varying amounts in the material from which the extract is made. The amount and potency of immunologically active material varies from one batch of extract to another, even when identical extraction methods are used, because of natural variations in the level of allergen in the particular batch of pollen or mold from which the extract is made. To date, it has not been possible to prepare such substances synthetically on a commercially feasible scale. The allergenic substances are grown by nature, and nature varies in uniformity. Extracts of the same allergen, therefore, will not be exactly uniform.

This discrepancy among various samples of a product has been recognized since the earliest days of immunotherapy. It has led to a constant search by practitioners and researchers alike for a means of accurately providing quantification, and thereby some form of standardization, for allergy extracts. This goal has never been fully achieved. Today, medicine is closer than ever before to achieving a degree of standardization for allergenic extracts, but perfect standardization for all antigens has not yet been reached. Moreover, the transition period between the use of extracts quantified by historically proven methods and of the new governmentally mandated standardized antigens has produced a level of confusion that is likely to persist for some time to come.

To understand the new methods of defining extract potency, it is necessary to know how antigens are currently quantified. In this regard, a brief historical review of the various designations of allergenic extracts may be of value.

Leonard Noon is considered by many to be the father of allergy testing and immunotherapy. As early as 1911,[1] he felt it necessary to establish some form of standardization for allergy testing to compare the degree of sensitivity to different allergens manifested by various patients. His approach resulted in the designation of what is now known as the *Noon unit*, which is defined as the amount of antigenic material that can be extracted from 0.001 mg of Phleum (Timothy grass) pollen. When this amount of antigen was placed in the conjuncitival sac of an allergic patient, the reaction could be compared on a unit basis with the amount of extract required to produce a similar reaction in another patient. Although the principle was valid for comparison purposes between patients, the procedure never become popular as a means of standardization. Nevertheless, today one may find references to a Noon unit, representing 1 μg of antigenic material.

The next approach to standardization, and the one still in the widest use today, is the weight/volume (w/v) formulation. This is simply the amount of dry allergen extracted in a given amount of diluent. As an example, 1 g of pollen extracted in 20 mL of diluent would represent a 1 : 20 w/v concentration. This designation is simple to understand. It does not always represent biologic potency in a reliable manner, but it has served for decades as a practical means of designating allergen extract strengths for testing and immunotherapy. Those practitioners familiar with the weaknesses of the system, in that equality in w/v designation does not guarantee bioequivalence, have simply allowed an appropriate margin of safety when changing to a new stock extract or to a new supplier. Today, the strength of the majority of allergenic extracts is designated by specifying the w/v value.

The other well-established designation for allergen standardization is the protein nitrogen unit (PNU). This standard was introduced in 1933 and is still in widespread use. However, it has been well demonstrated that the PNU does not indicate the allergenic potency of the extract, but rather tends to serve as a measure of the amount of all proteins present (both allergenic and nonallergenic).[2] It is also worthy of note that there is no reliable factor to convert between strength measured in w/v and PNUs.

When these limitations are considered, it is easy to see why a method of standardizing allergenic extracts would be highly desirable. The w/v extracts available from different suppliers, and even different batches of extract from the same supplier, have been shown to vary in biologic potency by a factor of up to 2000%. Despite this, the w/v designation has adequately served for defining testing and treatment antigen strengths since early in the century.

A variety of methods have been developed in recent years in an attempt to improve both qualitative and quantitative uniformity of extracts,[3] the most important of which is the standardized allergy unit (AU). As has been made manifestly clear in the past few years, the FDA is attempting to mandate that all allergenic extracts available be measured in standardized AUs as soon as possible.

Although the concept of extract standardization is certainly laudable, the FDA's attempt to proceed at top speed with its efforts has resulted in a multitude of problems. The first of these is that standardization may give a false sense of security. The fact remains that even with standardization as currently carried out, a variability in biologic activity of up to 400% between extract batches is still acceptable. Although certainly a major improvement over the 2000% variability found in the w/v extracts, such standardization still does not compare with what is found in other drugs, and treating physicians must still take reasonable precautions when changing batches of extracts or (more importantly) when changing antigen suppliers.

Antigen suppliers are also finding compliance with standardization to be a problem. AUs are not simply a different measurement scale. Antigens produced under the new mandates must meet different standards for potency assays than before. Because this may necessitate changes in the manufacturing process and quality control assays, there is generally no applicable conversion factor by which to compare the older antigen extracts supplied as w/v concentrates with the new antigen extracts supplied as concentrates measured in AUs. Initially, the FDA allowed new extracts to be labeled according to both w/v and AUs, but this convenience is being phased out. This would probably have been necessary eventually, but several problems have appeared during the period of transition, and it is not yet clear how some of these are to be resolved.

PROBLEMS WITH STANDARDIZATION

There is no disagreement with the fact that better standardization of antigenic extracts should eventually be beneficial. If immunotherapy were a new field, many of the problems of changing antigen potency measurements would not occur. Immunotherapy is not a new field, however, and millions of patients have undergone treatment in the past. A large percentage of the patients currently under treatment are receiving fairly large doses of antigen as maintenance treatment and will continue to receive these injections at intervals for the requisite number of years to achieve a degree of permanent disease control. These maintenance injections consist of antigens measured by w/v. As these antigens disappear from the market and are replaced by antigens measured in AUs, either the patient must be started anew on escalating doses of the new antigens, negating months or years of successful treatment escalation, or an attempt must be made to convert the dose currently being received to a comparable dose of the new extract. Such a conversion will be inexact at best and inevitably carries with it the risk for an adverse reaction to treatment.

At present, a relatively small number of antigens are available as extracts measured in AUs. As more appear, however, they will replace the traditional w/v extracts. The effect of this replacement of individual antigen extracts one by one would be to make it necessary to change the patient's treatment formula repeatedly as each new AU extract appeared. The old maintenance treatment vials containing antigens measured in w/v would have to be re-mixed without any antigen now available only in AUs. Retesting and dose escalation for this antigen would then be required on an individual basis, separately from the maintenance vial, until maintenance levels for it had been reached before the vials could be combined. As each new antigen became available only in AUs, the same process would need to be repeated. This approach is the one that theoretically should be employed, but the logistic nightmare of implementing such a program would be likely to discourage both physician and patient from even considering immunotherapy.

The problems with standardized extracts do not end at that point. Although no general conversion formula is available by which to equate extracts measured by w/v with those measured in AUs, it is inevitable that individual suppliers will become aware to some degree of the relative potency of each of their antigens in the new, AU-measured strengths in comparison with their older, w/v-measured material. It now appears that in very few cases are the standardized extracts at the highest available concentrations as potent as the older, nonstandardized extracts. This will often result in a patient's requiring a much larger volume of fluid in the injection to reach the same level of potency as that found in the nonstandardized extract. The size of the injection and the resulting discomfort may discourage the patient from continuing the treatment program.

NURSE'S NOTE

Limited testing may be done to compare the antigenic activity of various extracts as they are standardized. Both w/v and standardized extracts, diluted in the usual fashion, may be skin-tested side by side in selected patients and the results compared.

When a change is made from w/v to standardized extracts, a rule of thumb that is often helpful is to use the strength of 30,000 Biologic Allergy Units (BAU) or Allergy Units (AU) in the same fashion as the older 1:20 w/v concentrate, considering the strength of 10,000 BAU or AU roughly equivalent to a 1:100 (#1) concentration. This will vary from antigen to antigen but may serve as a rough guide.

When a change is made from w/v to standardized extract in treatment vials, often a new vial test may be all that is necessary.

ATTEMPTING TO COPE WITH THE PROBLEM

Let us begin by saying that there is really no good solution to the problem of conversion to standardized extracts as the situation now stands. Many consider it unfortunate that the conversion was not deferred until all, or essentially all, extracts could be made available in standardized form. This, however, is not the case, and it will probably be years before such a stage is reached. What is probably the most realistic approach to the situation follows:

1. Find an allergen extract supplier with whom you are well satisfied.
2. During the period of conversion, which will probably last for several years, do everything possible to avoid changing suppliers.
3. Purchase as much w/v concentrate as you expect to need for patients already under treatment, and as can be used before the expiration date on the concentrate arrives.

4. Ask the antigen supplier to estimate the factor for converting from w/v to AUs for each antigen manufactured. The FDA will not allow labeling of the antigen with a conversion factor, but it is currently permissible for the supplier to give this information to a physician requesting it. As new antigens become available from this supplier, the same information may be obtained for each one.

Inevitably, the conversion to all standardized extracts will become a reality. It has already been noted that there will be no exact factor to convert between nonstandard and standardized extracts, but immunotherapy by its very nature is an inexact science. When extracts are made from biologically active substances, there will be differences in each batch—less with standardization, but still present. It has already been found that moving from in vitro testing to in vivo treatment requires only the basic precautions of vial testing to minimize the possibility of adverse reactions. The same consideration applies in general to converting to standardized extracts. For some, piecemeal conversion extract by extract as each becomes available, checking for approximate equality in potency with the supplier, may prove acceptable. For others, especially when treating established patients on maintenance, delaying the conversion as long as possible may offer the best benefits. Many of these established patients may have completed their maintenance course and be able to discontinue therapy before the older extracts have expired, thus saving any conversion problems and minimizing any risk for reactions. For new patients, it will of course be advisable to start with the available standardized extracts, as eventually all extracts will be in this category.

As would be expected, preparing serial dilutions of standardized extracts presents an additional problem. Conversion tables must be developed to cope with the period of conversion, but it is to be hoped that this period will not last for too long a time. When all antigens are available in standardized form, a format comparable with that used up to the advent of standardization should allow the physician to proceed as has been described for skin endpoint titration (SET) utilizing five fold dilutions; under the standardized format, this process should be even more reproducible and safer in progression. At present, the best approach, and the one that has been put into the widest use, is to consider 10,000 AU as a #1 dilution for SET, and 30,000 AU, when available, as a concentrate. This does not mean that these concentrations will match the concentrate and #1 dilutions of SET, but that they will probably most closely approximate these concentrations. Successive fivefold dilutions are then made as for SET, and testing and treatment are carried out in the same manner. Although the units described in the w/v table will not match, at least the glycerine concentrations may be compared with those in SET, making control testing on the skin reliable after appropriate conversion factors have been used.

After these new serial dilutions have been made, they should be compared with the w/v SET dilutions. The allergen extract supplier can be of considerable help in this, providing a basic conversion factor for each antigen, but final comparison should be made directly. This at present will require cautious skin testing of the serially diluted standardized extract, starting with a #6 dilution, until the skin reaction parallels that seen when the patient has been tested by conventional SET. At this point, it should be possible to construct a chart showing the parallel between the w/v and standardized antigens. An appropriate conversion factor can then be established for each antigen. This conversion should hold for other patients sensitive to the same antigens, as it is by such parallel tests that standardization has been developed. Applying the conversion factor will allow the physician to prepare appropriate treatment vials during the transition period, and when all antigens are available in standardized form, the standardized test results will already be available and no further conversion will be required.

In the interest of completeness, it should be mentioned that there are a variety of methods by which antigens are measured in regard to potency and purity.[3] These are used primarily in research, however, and this book is designed for the clinician; therefore, only the measurements used in commercial production of allergenic extracts are discussed.

It is unfortunate that at present, and probably for some time in the future, such a transition problem should occur in the formulation of allergenic extracts. The need for standardization has been evident almost since the onset of immunotherapy, and eventually the result should justify the difficulties inherent in the transition. During this period, it will be necessary for allergists to accept the problem and cope with it as best they can. We trust that our suggestions will prove helpful during this rather trying time.

REFERENCES

1. Noon L. Prophylactic inoculation against hay fever. Lancet 1911;1:1572–1573.
2. US Department of Health and Human Services, Food and Drug Administration. Biologic products, allergenic extracts, implementation of efficacy review. Proposed rule. 21 CFR, parts 610, 680. Federal Register 1985 Jan 23.
3. Mason WW, Ward WA. Standardized extracts. Otolaryngol Clin North Am 1992;25: 101–117.

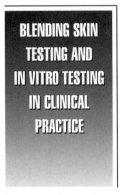

11

BLENDING SKIN TESTING AND IN VITRO TESTING IN CLINICAL PRACTICE

It is a basic axiom of the field that the diagnosis of allergy is made on clinical grounds. Clinical evaluation of the patient, however, does not identify the offenders. The most direct method of confirmation of inhalant offenders is by mucosal challenge, which remains a useful research tool but has not been popular with patients since Leonard Noon first used it in 1911. Skin testing, in several forms, remains the benchmark against which all other allergy tests are measured. However, in vitro testing has become increasingly popular since the characterization of immunoglobulin E (IgE) in 1967. To this day, disagreement continues between proponents of skin testing and in vitro testing about the validity and clinical usefulness of each of these methods. The modern practitioner of otolaryngic allergy should understand both and may actually employ both in the practice. With a firm grasp of the principles of each method, it is actually possible to move back and forth between them, utilizing whichever is most appropriate for the circumstances at hand.

PRINCIPLES COMMON TO SKIN TESTING AND IN VITRO METHODS

Many types of skin test are available. However, undoubtedly the most accurate and reproducible is the method of intradermal testing in which progressively stronger concentrations of antigen are used to determine the endpoint of reactivity. This method, initially known as *skin endpoint titration* (SET) and now sometimes referred to as *progressive intradilutional skin testing*, also presents the advantage of bearing a reproducible relationship with results obtained from in vitro radioallergosorbent testing (RAST). Although variants of RAST have now been introduced, some using radioactive markers and others using enzymatic or fluorometric methods (enzyme-linked immunosorbent assay, or ELISA), only the Fadal-Nalebuff modification of the RAST scoring system (F/N mRAST) parallels SET. In this text, the term *RAST* refers to F/N mRAST, and to other tests that are truly equivalent to F/N mRAST. Whether the system employed by an individual practitioner also bears this relationship will have to be determined.

TABLE 11–1. Principles common to SET and RAST

For testing
 Initial screening is performed with a limited number of antigens.
 Testing is performed with individual antigens rather than mixes.
For treatment
 Treatment is based on clinical judgment, not just test results.
 Endpoint indicates safe starting dose.
 Testing and treatment may safely begin at 1:312,500 w/v.
 Initial treatment is carried out with separate vials for high and low reactors.

Adapted from Mabry RL. Blending skin endpoint titration and in vitro methods in clinical practice. Otolaryngol Clin North Am 1992;25:61–70.

A number of principles of allergy testing and immunotherapy, some initially derived from experience with SET and others based on principles learned using RAST, are equally applicable to both methodologies (Table 11–1). These principles are discussed in the appropriate chapters elsewhere in this text, but they bear repetition here to put in context the relationship between SET and RAST.

PRINCIPLES OF SCREENING

It has been clearly shown, using RAST testing, that an antigen screening panel comprising a significant grass, weed, and tree for the area, plus two molds, housedust mite, and animal danders chosen on the basis of exposure, is effective for inhalant allergy.[1] The effectiveness of this "miniscreen" of six antigens (plus animal danders as necessary) may be enhanced by increasing the number of antigens to provide a "midscreen" of two grasses, one weed, two trees, three molds, and a dust mite (plus animal danders).[2] If the results of such a screen are negative, the chances of the patient being significantly allergic to other inhalants are extremely small. On the other hand, if positive reactors are noted, further testing will probably be needed for additional antigens in these classes. Although this concept was initially developed from RAST as a means of demonstrating a cost-effective in vitro approach, the entire screening concept is equally valid for skin testing.

For many years, skin testing was performed and immunotherapy administered using a series of mixed antigens from the same general family. Thus, it was not uncommon for patients to be tested and treated using "weed mix," "tree mix," or "grass mix." RAST technology and a technique called *RAST inhibition* have shown that it is more effective to test and treat for individual antigens. Patients may not be sensitive to all the antigens contained in the mix, and although a sensitivity to one or more allergens will give a positive response on skin testing, patients will ultimately receive injections containing antigenic material to which they are not allergic but to which they are likely to become allergic through repeated exposure in this fashion. Another factor to be considered is that because of the presence of multiple antigens in the mixture, each one effectively dilutes the concentration of all the other antigens. For this reason, testing and subsequent immunotherapy are recommended with individual antigens, not mixes.

One exception to the above concept is the use of mixtures for screening in patients not strongly suspected of allergy. In the case of skin testing, this involves testing with an antigen mix. A similar RAST screen is the Microscreen, utilizing two RAST disks. The first (seasonal) disk contains antigens for two grasses, two weeds, and two trees. The second (perennial) disk contains antigens for a dust mite and a common mold (*Alternaria*). In either case, if the screening test result is positive, retesting with specific antigens is necessary to make a more definitive diagnosis and prepare for immunotherapy.

Regarding treatment, whether testing is by skin test or RAST, the decision to institute immunotherapy is based on the clinician's evaluation of the patient rather than simply an abnormal laboratory test result. This situation rarely arises in patients undergoing skin testing. However, the temptation is very real for some physicians who depend entirely on RAST for diagnosis to let the laboratory do their thinking for them. The process of blindly ordering immunotherapy for every patient with one or more positive results on inhalant RAST involves no clinical judgment and may subject patients to unnecessary treatment. This dependence on in vitro results instead of clinical judgment has given rise to the pejorative term *in vitro allergist*. Both the American Academy of Otolaryngic Allergy and the American Academy of Allergy, Asthma and Immunology have adopted position statements against this "remote practice of allergy."

TREATMENT VIALS: IN VIVO AND IN VITRO

A concept that is very important when considering the mechanics of mixing treatment vials is that, whether determined by SET or F/N mRAST, the endpoint defines a safe antigen starting dose. More precisely, because of the slight sensitivity differences in the two techniques, immunotherapy based on in vitro results is generally started one dilution weaker than the F/N mRAST class—that is, at the RAST minus one level. This means that an F/N mRAST class III would be equated with an SET endpoint of #4

TABLE 11–2. Relationship of SET and RAST-based* immunotherapy

SET endpoint	Antigen concentration†	RAST 0‡	RAST − 1§
#1	1:100	1:100	1:500
#2	1:500	1:500	1:2500
#3	1:2500	1:2500	1:12,500
#4	1:12,500	1:12,500	1:62,500
#5	1:62,500	1:62,500	1:312,500
#6	1:312,500	1:312,500	1:312,500#

Adapted from Mabry RL. Blending skin endpoint titration and in vitro methods in clinical practice. Otolaryngol Clin North Am 1992;25:61–70.
* F/N mRAST; may be true of other RAST and ELISA systems.
† Weight/volume, if "concentrate" is 1:20.
‡ Aggressive regimen, not recommended for novices, in which vials are prepared using RAST score as "endpoint."
§ Usual regimen, in which "endpoint" is considered one dilution weaker than RAST score (RAST −1).
# It is rarely necessary to begin treatment at strengths weaker than #6 dilution.

(1 : 12,500 w/v). Although this relationship may vary from antigen to antigen, it is sufficiently constant to be a basis for moving freely between the two methodologies.[3] This is discussed more completely in Chapter 9, but it should be evident that it is possible to incorporate into treatment vials antigens whose endpoints have been determined from both SET and RAST. This relationship is depicted in Table 11–2.

Before RAST was commonly used, in an attempt to start at an anticipated nonreacting concentration, SET testing was sometimes begun using extremely dilute antigens. This gave rise to whealing patterns such as the "hourglass," described in the section on bizarre whealing in Chapter 6, Testing Methods for Inhalant Allergy. This pattern caused significant confusion among novice practitioners. After experience with RAST, it was found that it was very rarely necessary to begin skin testing with antigen concentrations weaker than the #6 SET dilution (1 : 312,500 w/v). Likewise, treatment could almost always be started at this strength, even if a skin test wheal at this concentration produced a wheal larger than usual.

Whether testing is done by SET or RAST, the quantitation of results provided by these methods allows treatment to be begun at the highest safe dose. RAST-based immunotherapy confirmed the clinical impression gained from SET-based treatment that patients with very high allergen-specific IgE levels (F/N mRAST levels IV or V) were very labile in their reactions to immunotherapy, requiring low initial antigen doses and cautious advancement.[4] Doses of antigens to which hypersensitivity was lower, on the other hand, could be advanced more rapidly and with less risk for reaction. This

TABLE 11–3. Advantages of skin testing

Accuracy
  May be quantified (intradermal titration)
Safety
  Testing antigen identical to treating antigen
Convenience
  Rapidly performed
  Little equipment required
  Results quickly available

Adapted from Mabry RL. Blending skin end-point titration and in vitro methods in clinical practice. Otolaryngol Clin North Am 1992;25:61–70.

led to the practice of initially splitting treatment vials, whether based on skin tests or in vitro methods, to include highly reacting antigens (RAST classes IV and V; SET endpoint #6, #5, or #4) in one, to be advanced cautiously, and antigens to which the patient is less sensitive in another vial, to be advanced more quickly.

CHARACTERISTICS OF SKIN TESTS

Skin testing (in this context, the term will apply primarily to SET) has both advantages and disadvantages (Tables 11–3 and 11–4). A skin testing session may take about an hour, but at the end of that time the results are available, with no further delay. Because of the effect on skin reactivity of antihistamines, tricyclic antidepressants, and some tranquilizers, patients must omit these for several days before skin testing. Patients whose skin is hyperreactive (dermatographia) may exhibit false-positive results on skin testing. For this

TABLE 11–4. Disadvantages of skin testing

Accuracy
  Placement of accurate wheals depends on skill and experience.
  Reading and interpretation of results are subject to variability.
Safety
  There is risk for anaphylaxis or systemic reaction.
Convenience
  Procedure is time-consuming.
  Multiple sticks are uncomfortable.
  Patient must omit medications (antihistamines, others).

Adapted from Mabry RL. Blending skin endpoint titration and in vitro methods in clinical practice. Otolaryngol Clin North Am 1992;25:61–70.

TABLE 11–5. Advantages of in vitro testing

Accuracy
 Not affected by skin reactivity
 Not affected by drugs
 Fewer false-positives than with skin testing
Safety
 No risk for anaphylaxis
 Safe starting dose determined before first injection
Convenience
 One venipuncture instead of multiple needle sticks

Adapted from Mabry RL. Blending skin endpoint titration and in vitro methods in clinical practice. Otolaryngol Clin North Am 1992;25:61–70.

reason, positive and negative controls must be a part of each skin-testing session. The financial investment required to purchase equipment and supplies for skin testing is modest. However, persons performing the test must be trained, and supervision must be provided until they are experienced. Although prick testing or single-dilution intradermal tests give only a rough approximation of the degree of sensitivity of the patient, dilutional intradermal testing (SET) is quantitative and reproducible. After skin testing, one knows exactly how the patient will react to the antigen that will be used in the treatment vial, as the patient has undergone a bioassay with that exact substance (from the same stock vial).

It is readily apparent that skin testing is good, but not perfect. For this reason, enthusiasm for in vitro testing has steadily increased.

CHARACTERISTICS OF IN VITRO TESTS

The advantages and disadvantages of in vitro tests for allergy are set forth in Tables 11–5 and 11–6. These tests are unaffected by skin reactivity, either

TABLE 11–6. Disadvantages of in vitro tests

Accuracy
 Test may not detect borderline positive reactors.
 Test is subject to system and human errors.
Safety
 Treatment antigen is not the same as test antigen; vial test is required before treatment.
Convenience
 There is a delay of hours to days in availability of results.
 Unusual antigens may not be available for testing.

Adapted from Mabry RL. Blending skin endpoint titration and in vitro methods in clinical practice. Otolaryngol Clin North Am 1992;25:61–70.

the hypersensitive state seen in dermatographia or the suppressed responses noted in patients who have (either inadvertently or to control severe symptoms) failed to discontinue antihistamines or other drugs affecting skin reactivity. Depending on what one chooses as a benchmark, in vitro tests are either praised as being more specific than skin tests (yielding fewer false-positive responses) or condemned as being less sensitive (as some patients may demonstrate positive skin test results with negative in vitro test results). In vitro tests are popular with patients and medical personnel alike because they require only a single needle stick and a minimal investment of time and effort to obtain a blood sample. However, results are not available for hours (for most enzymatic tests) to days (for tests using radioactive markers). If physicians choose to have these tests run in their own office, the cost of equipment and training of personnel can be significant, and compliance with CLIA (Clinical Laboratory Improvement Act) regulations can be onerous. The use of a reference laboratory avoids these problems but necessitates sample preparation and mailing, and a delay waiting for results to be returned. In rare situations, an unusual antigen may be available for skin testing but not for in vitro evaluation. However, even with the large number of antigens available for in vitro tests, the material in the actual treatment mix is not necessarily identical with that used in the in vitro test, so that a confirmatory skin test (''vial test'') is necessary. Although more critical when in vitro testing is used because of the difference in antigens, a vial test is a valuable safety measure even when all testing has been done on the skin.

ROLE OF SKIN TESTS IN IN VITRO TESTING

It is readily apparent that although skin tests and in vitro tests have unique benefits, each has its shortcomings. The practitioner who is able to use both methods, choosing appropriately between them, is uniquely qualified to test and treat for allergy most effectively and efficiently.

There are situations in which skin testing is probably the best choice. For example, if a patient already is on immunotherapy, testing for a few additional antigens may become desirable. In this situation, a few skin tests, administered and interpreted in one visit, can rapidly and effectively check for the presence and degree of sensitivity to other antigens that might need to be added to the mix. If the patient's initial testing was done by RAST only a few months earlier, the balance of the sample may have been frozen and retained by the reference laboratory. If this is the case, additional tests may be run on this specimen without the inconvenience of an additional venipuncture. However, the length of time that reference laboratories retain samples before discarding them is highly variable and must be determined for the laboratory in question. The performance of a few additional skin tests, on the other hand, is always a viable option.

Many physicians find themselves in a quandary regarding borderline sensitivities on in vitro testing (e.g., RAST class O/I) and equivocal allergy histories for these antigens. It is evident that if these patients are sensitive, they are not sensitive to a high degree. Placement of a #2 (1:500) dilution intradermal skin test, followed if necessary by a #1 (1:100) test, may clarify the situation.

At times, patients are referred from a distance for a consultation and want answers that same day. If they have abstained from antihistamines and tricyclic antidepressants for at least 48 to 72 hours and have a few hours to devote to testing with a representative screening panel, the question of allergy can be solved on the spot.

Not all hypersensitivity reactions are IgE-mediated and so are not amenable to in vitro IgE assay. A typical example is delayed fungal hypersensitivity. In these cases, skin testing is mandatory.

Although skin tests are useful, situations may arise in which in vitro testing is more appropriate or efficient. For example, circumstances occasionally arise in which a patient is unable or unwilling to omit drugs that affect skin whealing (e.g., antihistamines, tricyclic antidepressants). Because in vitro tests are unaffected by such medications, they may be performed without regard to such circumstances. In a similar fashion, if patients who are taking antihistamines at the time of their visit find it impractical to return in a few days for skin testing, blood may be drawn for an in vitro study.

Some patients have skin disorders or abnormalities that make skin testing difficult or unreliable. Examples include patients with dermatographia, in whom any trauma to the skin results in a wheal-and-flare reaction that is not immunologically mediated, and patients with chronic eczema, a finding that is not unusual in atopic individuals, especially children. In vitro testing is ideal for these situations.

Patients likely to be more prone than usual to anaphylactic or systemic reactions from skin testing may be tested by in vitro methods with no such risk. This group includes patients with a history of prior anaphylaxis (from any cause), patients with asthma (especially unstable or steroid-dependent cases), and those with a history of angioedema. In these situations, in vitro methods will indicate the presence and degree of IgE-mediated hypersensitivity to tested antigens with no risk; as it has been put so well, "Anaphylaxis does not occur in a test tube."

Even if all allergy testing has been done by in vitro means, the practitioner cannot do without a working knowledge of skin test methods. As has been noted, the antigens employed in in vitro assays are not identical to those in the stock vials, from which treatment vials are made, so that some sort of bioassay in the patient must be carried out to ''fine tune'' the antigenic mixture delivered by subsequent allergy injections. The performance and interpretation of such a ''vial test'' necessitate a knowledge of whealing responses and dilutional intradermal testing.

In other words, the informed practitioner of otolaryngic allergy should be conversant with both skin test and in vitro testing methods. Although it is true that some individuals successfully practice using only one or the other methodology, patient safety and optimum results of immunotherapy are best served by a broader knowledge base.

RELATIONSHIP OF RAST AND SET

As already mentioned, F/N mRAST and SET bear a fairly constant relationship. This was not the case with early RAST systems. The earliest RAST, from Phadebas, utilized scoring against four standards but was found to have a very low sensitivity. A modification of this scoring system by Phadebas only partially rectified the problem, although maintaining a very high specificity. The problem, as discovered by Drs. Fadal, Nalebuff, and Ali, was in the cutoff point for significant levels of allergen-specific IgE. The changes they instituted included an increased incubation time, an increased volume of test serum, removal of disks to clean test tubes before gamma counting, and the development of a scoring system corresponding to fivefold changes in serum concentration.[5] Their efforts resulted in a test with acceptable sensitivity and specificity, and because of its fivefold incremental basis, it gave results parallel to those obtained by SET. Because skin tests tend to be slightly more sensitive than RAST, the in vitro study typically gives a score that is one class lower (weaker) than a corresponding SET endpoint. For example, a modified RAST score of class III is usually equivalent to an SET endpoint of #4 (testing with 1 : 12,500 w/v). This correlation has been well established for the F/N mRAST, which, although generally uniform in pattern, may vary somewhat from allergen to allergen. Most other in vitro testing methods have been designed attempting to maintain this relationship, with responses correlated with F/N mRAST. However, the exact correlation between their results and SET should be established by the practitioner's use of an incremental vial test, which is described below.[6]

NURSE'S NOTE

Do not expect RAST test scores to be identical with SET test results. Because skin reactivity is often the basis for dose advancement or adjustment in immunotherapy, it is necessary to know how RAST results and SET are related. This may be determined by placing individual antigen skin tests at a concentration one dilution weaker than indicated by the RAST score (RAST minus one). Grass and ragweed antigens frequently produce reactions greater than expected at a RAST minus one score, especially when they are pollinating.

UTILIZING SKIN TESTS TO CONFIRM IN VITRO RESULTS (THE VIAL TEST)

No laboratory test is foolproof. This holds true for in vitro allergy tests. Drs. Richard Fadal and Donald Nalebuff have explained it thus: "RAST is a blood test which is prepared by a lab technician and calculated by a gamma counter. The results come off the gamma counter like numbers off a cash register tape. This result is in turn recorded on the report sheet after tube numbers are coded back to the patient's name, antigens, and specific antibody counts. The possibility of mechanical or human error exists; therefore, the skin test serves as a double check for safety."[7]

Even if no errors are made in the sequence described above, numerous opportunities exist for mistakes during compounding of the vial. Added to this is the factor already alluded to, that there is never an exact match between the antigen used on a RAST disk or other in vitro testing device and the antigen in the stock vial from which a treatment vial is prepared.

Performing the Vial Test

For all these reasons, a bioassay of any treatment mixture prepared based on in vitro results must be performed. Several methods are available for vial testing, but all involve a knowledge of incremental whealing gained from practice in SET. In other words, even in vitro allergists must possess some knowledge of skin testing, specifically SET.

In a conventional vial test, one or more treatment vials are prepared in the usual fashion already described elsewhere in this book. A skin test with the vial contents is performed by withdrawing a small amount of fluid from the vial; with a testing syringe, a 4-mm intradermal wheal is created in the fashion described in Chapter 6. For completeness, this vial test should also include a positive and a negative control (histamine and diluent, respectively). An acceptable vial test reaction is generally considered to be enlargement of a 4- or 5-mm wheal to a diameter of 13 mm or less within 10 minutes. If this occurs, immunotherapy using that vial is considered safe. Most practitioners consider that this vial test constitutes the patient's first injection, although if the resultant wheal is quite small (e.g., 7 mm), it is acceptable to inject an additional 0.05 mL subcutaneously that day.

NURSE'S NOTES

Preparing to treat according to RAST scores may be confirmed in one of two ways. Details of each are found in the chapter.

1. Each individual positive antigen, at one dilution weaker than indicated by the RAST score (RAST minus one), is placed as a skin test. The results provide a means for adjusting the eventual score used in making the treatment vial (Table 11–7).

2. A vial is prepared based on the RAST scores, but with each antigen one dilution weaker (RAST minus one). The vial is then skin-tested; depending on the results, treatment is with the vial at that concentration or diluted further. If the resulting wheal is 13 mm in diameter or less, the vial can be used for treatment.

Dealing with an Unacceptable Vial Test Result

If the wheal produced is larger than 13 mm, it is unsafe to start treatment from the vial as it has been prepared. There may be several reasons for the unacceptable wheal, and the cause must be identified and corrected before treatment is undertaken. One possibility is that the vial test result is like the "flash response" seen in SET (see the section on bizarre whealing in Chapter 6), the true endpoint being obscured by a concomitant food reaction or a high antigenic exposure preceding the test. This possibility may be clarified

TABLE 11–7. Technique of incremental vial test (antigen administered at RAST −1 concentration)

Wheal size	Action
<7 mm	Apply stronger concentrations until endpoint is determined.
7–10 mm	Treat at RAST − 1 for this antigen.
11–13 mm	Treat at RAST − 2 for this antigen.
14 mm	Apply RAST − 3 wheal; if acceptable, treat at this level.

Adapted from Mabry RL. The relationship between SET and in vitro testing. In: Emanuel IA, (ed.). In Vitro Testing. New York: Thieme Medical Publishers; 1994: 53–59.

by waiting a few days and repeating the test. If the results of the vial test at that time are still unacceptable, other possibilities must be investigated.

Another common cause of an unacceptable vial test result appears simply to be a heightened potency of the vial, above that indicated by the original in vitro test endpoints. This may be the consequence of a potentiating effect of combining the antigens, making the potency of the sum greater than that of the parts. To test for this possibility, the vial is diluted fivefold and retested. If this test result is still unacceptable, the most commonly recommended course of action is to prepare successive fivefold dilutions from the original treatment vial, and to test the skin with these until a dilution producing an acceptable wheal is reached. This is known as *titrating the vial*. Treatment is then begun at that level and advanced as usual.

There is always a possibility that the person preparing the vial may have made an error. If this appears at all likely, it is often advisable to remake the vial. For safety, it may be wiser to prepare a new vial that is at least five times more dilute than the offending one, but that also is certain to contain the appropriate antigens in proper concentration. It is always better to waste a bit of time and money in remaking a vial than to risk a systemic reaction.

Although more time-consuming, the definitive means of investigating an unacceptable vial test result is checking individual skin responses for each antigenic component at the concentration contained in the vial (generally a RAST minus one level, or one dilution weaker than the RAST endpoint). This is sometimes called an *incremental vial test*. This procedure may reveal a discordance between the skin reaction produced by one or more antigens and the RAST results for these substances, with a significantly greater skin reactivity than that shown in vitro. This is a not uncommon occurrence when the antigen in question is ''in season.'' It may be necessary to test the skin with more dilute antigen concentrations to define an endpoint exactly. It is often possible by extrapolation to determine how much more dilute the antigen should be in the treatment mixture, or at least to come very close. The progression of whealing seen in SET, in which each successive positive wheal is at least 2 mm larger than the preceding wheal (usually very close to 2 mm), can be used to count progressively backward in 2-mm increments from the unacceptable wheal to the probable endpoint. This presumptive endpoint will need a confirming wheal to be considered decisive, but testing in this manner may save unnecessary intermediate test injections. However, keep in mind that treatment at concentrations more dilute than #6 (1:312,500) is very rarely necessary. When a new vial is made using the endpoints determined by the incremental vial test, it can in turn be "vial-tested" and will almost always give an acceptable result.

In general, the results of an incremental vial test may be utilized to alter a treatment vial in a fairly constant fashion (Table 11–7). If the wheal size produced by a RAST minus one antigen level is 7 to 10 mm in diameter, treatment may be given at that level. If the wheal is 11 to 13 mm in diameter, treatment should be at yet one further dilution (RAST minus two level). If a wheal with a diameter of 14 mm or greater results, testing should be performed at a RAST minus three level to confirm the appropriateness of treatment at that level. In these situations, this antigen level generally produces an acceptable wheal size. Again, recall that it should rarely, if ever, be necessary to begin treatment at antigen levels more dilute than a #6 (1: 312,500) concentration.

In the unlikely event that a wheal from an antigen at a RAST minus one concentration does not enlarge to a positive (7 mm diameter or larger) wheal, testing with the next higher concentration of antigen is recommended. Because of the relationship between RAST and skin tests, this scenario is very rarely encountered.

For those just beginning RAST-based immunotherapy, it is recommended that incremental vial tests be performed (at no additional charge to the patient) until the physician is comfortable with the general relationship between RAST results (from the office laboratory or a reference laboratory) and SET. It may even be desirable to construct a correction table based on such testing, until the knowledge gained becomes second-nature. These methods are time-consuming but necessary training steps for the person wishing to become truly skilled at in vitro-based immunotherapy.[8]

PRACTICAL APPLICATION OF THE BLENDING CONCEPT

It should now be readily apparent that even the most devoted proponent of in vitro testing should have a basic knowledge of skin testing and whealing patterns. Or, in the words of our colleague Dr. William King, "If in doubt, SET can bail you out." With this as background, let us consider how the practitioner can use both skin tests and in vitro allergy tests in the office practice of allergy.

The first key is constantly to consider allergy as a primary or contributory factor in the production of the patient's symptoms. Although this discussion is limited to inhalants as triggers, remember that food allergy is also a likely culprit. If it becomes necessary to test for allergy, the degree of testing will vary with one's degree of clinical suspicion. If allergy is a "long shot," a simple and effective approach utilizes a RAST microscreen (one perennial and one seasonal disk, screening for eight antigens), coupled with a total IgE determination (which is not a good screening tool alone but is helpful when coupled with the microscreen). Although not available from all laboratories or with all in vitro allergy testing methodologies, a microscreen can be a very useful screening tool. It is especially suited for physicians considering adding allergy to their practice, who wish to acquire an idea of the prevalence of allergy in their patient population.

If both microscreen results are negative, especially if the total IgE is normal (well below 100 mL), inhalant allergy becomes highly unlikely. It has not been totally ruled out, as it is possible for patients to be atopic to one or more antigens not included on the microscreen disk. However, in the absence of a strongly suggestive history, a negative microscreen result and normal total IgE are strong evidence against the presence of significant inhalant allergy.

If either disk shows positive responses, especially with a total IgE of 100 mL or more, further investigation is necessary. If this occurs, the laboratory (one's own or a reference laboratory) can use the same specimen (which should be kept frozen for several weeks, for just such a purpose) to run allergen-specific IgE determinations for the antigen classes in question. If the seasonal disk (which screens for two grasses, two trees, and two weeds) is positive, then specific index antigens in these classes should be investigated. A positive perennial disk (mold, dust mite) necessitates further investigation in these areas, plus animal danders as indicated by history. The results of this testing should allow one to proceed with appropriate treatment, including immunotherapy for relevant positive antigens if indicated. The confirmatory vial test constitutes the only skin test involved. Otherwise, all this has been accomplished with one needle stick, at the cost of additional time for running the various tests.

If allergy is more likely to be present, the screening can be done with a miniscreen (about nine antigens) or a midiscreen (12 to 15 antigens) and immunotherapy based on these results. If specific IgE determinations are made, a total IgE determination is unnecessary. If treatment with key positive antigens fails to control symptoms adequately, more antigens may be investigated and added to the mix. Although the initial serum sample may be checked for other possible culprits, it may be more expedient to perform limited SET for these antigens. The initial RAST results give some indication of the degree of hypersensitivity one may expect for the various antigen classes, and it may be possible to start with a higher antigen concentration than the #6 strength in these cases (if the patient is not brittle, and if testing for antigens out of season). Once the endpoint has been determined, these antigens can be added to the treatment mix at the endpoint concentration. Because the relationship of results from the mRAST and SET is fairly constant, a treatment mix prepared from some SET and some mRAST results is feasible. If doubt exists as to the patient's tolerance of the new antigens in the treatment vial, a vial test will settle the question.

Although third-party payers often place unrealistic restrictions and prohibitions on the use of in vitro allergy tests, there is no doubt that they remain a safe, convenient, and accurate diagnostic tool. Unfortunately, when they cannot be used, the practitioner who has no knowledge of skin testing is left with no viable treatment options except pharmacotherapy. On the other hand, if one has the ability to diagnose by either SET or RAST, there will be very few situations in which the identity of triggers of inhalant allergy cannot be accurately determined and immunotherapy cannot be safely and effectively begun.

SUMMARY

Confirmation of offending antigens may be obtained by either skin testing or in vitro methodologies. The most quantitative and reproducible method of skin testing is SET. The gold standard for in vitro tests is generally considered the F/N mRAST, and other in vitro methodologies and improvements generally try to match the correlation between this in vitro test and the fivefold increments of SET. Whatever one's method of choice, it is extremely useful to be familiar with the technique and interpretation of results obtained in either fashion. This allows the choice of the most appropriate testing technique for the particular situation at hand, and further permits the practitioner to move back and forth between the two, testing and treating based on the results of either or both methods.

Moreover, for reasons of safety and enhanced patient care, all treatment vials based in vitro results must be subjected to a bioassay by skin testing, requiring even the most confirmed devotee of RAST to understand skin test methods and whealing responses.[9]

REFERENCES

1. King WP. Efficacy of a screening radioallergosorbent test. Arch Otolaryngol 1982;108: 781–786.
2. Lehr AJ, Mabry RL, Mabry CS. The screening RAST: is it a valid concept? Otolaryngol Head Neck Surg 1997;117:54–55.
3. Tandy JR, Mabry RL, Mabry CS. Correlation of modified radioallergosorbent test scores and skin test results. Otolaryngol Head Neck Surg 1996;115:42–45.

4. Nalebuff DJ. In vitro tests and immunotherapy. Ear Nose Throat J 1988;67:33–40.
5. Nalebuff DJ, Fadal RG, Ali M. Development of the modified RAST. In: Fadal RG, Nalebuff DJ, (eds.): RAST in Clinical Allergy. Carlsbad, CA: Symposium Foundation; 1989:35–48.
6. Mabry RL. The relationship between SET and in vitro testing. In: Emanuel IA, (ed.) In Vitro Testing. New York: Thieme Medical Publishers; 1994:53–59.
7. Fadal RG, Nalebuff DJ. Procedure Manual. Waco, TX: The Allergy and Immunology Center; 1985.
8. Mabry RL. Blending skin endpoint titration and in vitro methods in clinical practice. Otolaryngol Clin North Am 1992;25:61–70.
9. Willoughby JW. Inhalant allergy immunotherapy with standardized and non-standardized allergenic extracts. In: Johnson JT, Blitzer A, Ossoff RH, et al, (eds.). Instructional Courses. St. Louis: Mosby; 1988:151–171 (Vol 1).

12

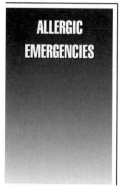

ALLERGIC EMERGENCIES

The practice of office allergy has been compared with flying: hours of calm interspersed with occasional moments of stark terror. Those engaging in this practice must be constantly mindful that they are injecting patients with an antigen that may at any time potentially precipitate a life-threatening anaphylactic reaction. Obviously, the preferred approach is the prevention of such an emergency situation, and this chapter outlines steps aimed at just such a purpose.

However, because bad things sometimes happen to good people despite our best efforts, the appropriate management of an allergic emergency is also discussed. In the same fashion as a flight attendant calling your attention to the emergency procedure card located in the airplane seat pocket, we suggest you read this information carefully and hope you never need to use it.

PREVENTION OF ALLERGIC EMERGENCIES

Although it is mandatory that every health care provider who deals with allergy immunotherapy be well versed in the management of allergic emergencies, it is much better to avoid the occurrence of such crises altogether. Thus, it is worthwhile to devote some attention to measures that minimize the risk for anaphylaxis associated with allergy immunotherapy. Happily, the authors can attest to the effectiveness of these safeguards in their own practice of otolaryngic allergy.

Initial Testing Methods

The first important measure is the use of quantitative testing methods as a basis for immunotherapy. With skin endpoint titration (SET), skin testing is begun at an anticipated nonreactive antigen dilution, and concentrations are advanced in fivefold steps until reactivity is observed and confirmed. This methodology immediately identifies the threshold of reactivity for each antigen to which the patient is sensitive, and allows the practitioner to avoid the introduction through testing or treatment of excessive amounts of that antigen.

Testing by in vitro methods, such as radioallergosorbent testing (RAST) or enzyme-linked immunosorbent assays (ELISA), not only provides quantitative information in a fashion similar to testing with SET, but avoids altogether the introduction of antigen into the patient's system for testing purposes. With the diagnostic information provided by a quantitative in vitro assay, it is possible to know the degree of sensitivity of patients to any antigen long before a therapeutic injection is administered. In vitro tests are always safer than skin tests.

In either case, the immunotherapy treatment mixture formulated from SET or RAST can be adjusted so that every antigen is initially administered at the threshold concentration of reactivity. Antigens to which the patient is highly sensitive are placed into the mix in very dilute concentrations, whereas those to which the patient has only a limited degree of sensitivity can be introduced at stronger concentrations, providing treatment that is both efficient and safe.

Vial Testing

The final test to ensure safety is the initial in vivo test of the treatment vial. If no errors in compounding have occurred, this may be unnecessary in the case of SET-based therapy, as testing and treatment vials have come from identical antigen sources in the stock vials. However, vial testing remains an excellent "fail-safe" measure to avoid any possible reactions resulting from errors in compounding the treatment vial. RAST-based therapy must always include a vial test, as it is not certain that the antigens in the treatment vial are antigenically the same as those on the RAST disk used in testing. Details of the vial test concept are presented in Chapter 11.

When a new stock vial of an antigen is obtained, even though it comes from the same manufacturer who provided the previous vial, it may not have the same antigenic potency as the one it is replacing. In this situation, vial tests of new treatment mixes made after such a change are a valid safety measure. However, as a practical matter, it is not always necessary to perform such vial testing if the antigen manufacturer is the same. On the other hand, if antigen is obtained from a new manufacturer, vial tests or even parallel SET determinations using the old and new material may be necessary to avoid unnecessary reactions. An additional safety measure is to combine initially equal parts from the old and new lots to give the required amount of antigen. Observation of the responses of a number of patients to this mix of old and new will soon provide an idea of whether the new antigen differs substantially in biologic potency from the old.

Recognition of Potential Hazards

Some antigens are known to present a significant potential for severe systemic reactions and should be used in skin tests with caution. The generally recognized examples of cottonseed, flaxseed, castor bean, and peanut will probably never concern the novice allergist, and if it is necessary to test for these, RAST is a safe choice. Among the more common inhalant antigens, grass is recognized as being the most antigenically potent material, milligram for milligram, of any in the allergist's armamenterium. Skin testing for any antigen while it is in season and/or in an individual whose history suggests a high degree of sensitivity should never be begun at a level more concentrated than the #6 (1:312,500 w/v) dilution.

Some patients are recognized as "brittle," or highly sensitive, with a high potential for reactions to skin testing or injections. The prime examples of such high-risk patients are those with asthma.[1] Others in this category include patients with urticaria, those with a history of prior severe reactions to allergy skin testing or injections, and patients suspected of having sensitivities to a great many allergens. These patients should be tested by in vitro means when possible, and if skin testing is required, they should have tests administered beginning at a very low concentration (#6 SET). Furthermore, it may be wise to limit the number of antigens tested for at any one sitting, to avoid a cumulative effect of numerous positive reactions in possibly producing a systemic reaction. A more common error is testing for numerous antigens in the same or cross-reacting families (e.g., multiple grasses), which effectively administers a higher dose of that antigen. Placing additional wheals at higher concentrations after the confirming wheal has occurred is another way in which an unacceptable antigen load may be administered during testing. As a practical matter, if SET is correctly performed (including proper antigen selection and not progressing past a confirming wheal), a reaction is unlikely to occur. However, unless individual circumstances dictate otherwise, testing should probably be limited to 12 to 15 antigens per sitting.

Reactions are more likely to occur during advancement immunotherapy than during skin testing, and this risk is heightened when the antigens in question are "in season."[2]

Dose Advancement

The first injection from any new treatment vial should ideally be administered in the physician's office. Thereafter, dose advancement should be modified as circumstances change. One can never completely place a patient on a routine "schedule" for dose advancement without consideration of changes in allergic load, complicating infections, and similar modifying factors. The dose should be advanced to the maximally tolerated dose, with the realization that local (and systemic) reactions will indicate the need for modification of dose schedules. If continued reactions occur despite appropriate dose adjustments, it is often best to discard the treatment vial in use and begin again. The effort involved in remaking a vial is small, whereas the costs of dealing with anaphylaxis are large and not simply measured in units of time and money.

Human Errors

The possibility for error in the allergy office exists at every step, from testing to vial formulation to administration of immunotherapy. If properly performed, SET is a safe means of skin testing for inhalant allergy. However, if additional wheals are placed beyond the "confirming wheal," overdosing is possible. Correct interpretation of the test results is necessary to assess accurately the antigen concentration that will be included in the initial treatment vial. Once endpoints have been determined (either from SET or RAST), accurate calculations and mixing are necessary to prepare the treatment vial, and errors in this process can have disastrous results. One of the most common (and potentially catastrophic errors) is a misplaced decimal point, either in calculations of dose or in drawing up the appropriate volume for injection.

The administration of injections from the treatment vial requires that the vial of the correct patient be chosen from all the available vials (Fig. 12–1) and that the proper dose be given. The opportunities for disastrous consequences of a mistake in this process are obvious. To avoid any such misidentification, the authors advise that the treatment vial be shown to the patient, who is asked to confirm its identity (Fig. 12–2).

Measures to avoid allergic reactions begin with adequate training of the person responsible for testing, so that proper technique and procedure are followed. It is a good idea to have the physician or another member of the allergy team double-check the determination of endpoints and the mathematics of vial preparation from the data obtained. It must be emphasized that the person preparing vials should do so in an environment totally free from interruptions and distractions, to minimize lapses in concentration and possible compounding of errors. During mixing, labels should be checked and double-checked. When an injection is administered, the patient's identity should be checked against the vial label, and the dose administered should be carefully scrutinized. Many reactions have ensued after a dose of 0.05

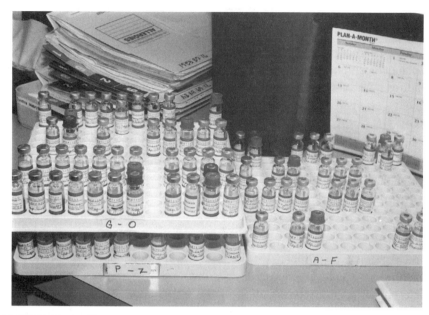

FIGURE 12–1. The correct patient's vial must be carefully selected from all those available.

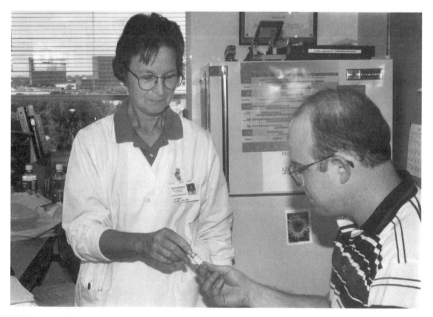

FIGURE 12–2. Both the person giving the injection and the patient should make sure that the proper treatment vial has been chosen.

mL has been confused with one of 0.5 mL, providing a 10-fold overdose of antigen.

In short, allergy testing and treatment present numerous opportunities for errors that can possibly result in anaphylaxis. The prevention of these errors requires constant and meticulous attention on the part of the allergy nurse or assistant.

NURSE'S NOTES

A number of points should be emphasized for safety:

1. When making an initial treatment vial, have a second person check the calculations, including the strengths of each antigen to be placed in the vial.
2. Carefully check the decimal point when drawing up a dose.
3. Have patients identify treatment vials as their own.

TYPES OF ALLERGIC REACTIONS

True allergic reactions may be immediate or delayed. These should be differentiated from nonallergic, vasovagal reactions, which are (fortunately) much more common than true allergic reactions. Both immediate and delayed reactions may be local or systemic. Local reactions are characterized by induration (wheal) surrounded by erythema (flare) (Fig. 12–3). The size of the wheal (not the flare) is the determining factor in altering subsequent immunotherapy doses.

Delayed allergic reactions may be either local or systemic, and the former are much more common than the latter. A significant delayed local reaction is characterized by an area of induration and redness greater than 30 mm in diameter (i.e., larger than a half-dollar) at the site of a previous injection. Delayed systemic reactions are generally manifested as an increase in the patient's usual allergic symptoms, but symptoms may also include urticaria, arthralgias, or constitutional symptoms involving almost any organ system.

Delayed allergic reactions are generally of the Gell and Coombs type III. They are most often seen in association with allergy to molds. These reactions typically occur from 6 to 36 hours after an injection (or skin test) and thus do not occur while the patient is in the office or has just had the injection or test. It is therefore important not only to educate patients about the possible occurrence of such reactions, but also to advise them regarding proper treatment measures. The treatment of a delayed local reaction generally requires only the administration of one or more doses of an antihistamine, sometimes

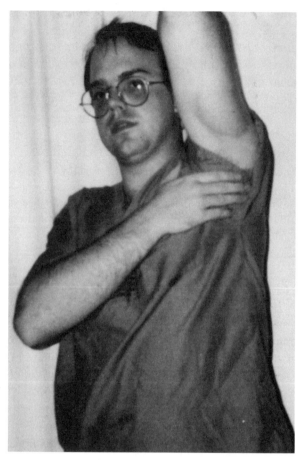

FIGURE 12–3. Large delayed local reaction, with central induration (wheal) and surrounding erythema (flare), indicating a need for dose adjustment.

augmented by application of ice to the reaction site followed by a topical steroid cream or ointment. However, it is important that these reactions be reported so that appropriate adjustment of the immunotherapy dose can be made if they occur regularly.

Delayed general reactions are extremely uncommon. Treatment consists of the administration of antihistamines, augmented by systemic corticosteroids for a few days (such as a tapered-dose pack) if the severity of symptoms warrants. As with delayed local reactions, a decrease in dose to prevent a recurrence is prudent.

Acute local reactions display the same characteristics as delayed local reactions, except that they occur within an hour or less of the test or injection. They are treated in the same fashion: a systemic antihistamine (by mouth), local application of ice to the affected area followed by a steroid ointment or cream if necessary, and subsequent adjustment of the immunotherapy dose.

Vasovagal reactions, in which symptoms range from sweating and pallor to syncope, do not present the same potential for severe consequences as anaphylaxis. However, it is important to differentiate between these types of reaction rapidly and accurately, to avoid either undertreatment or over-treatment. Patients with vasovagal reactions typically complain of "feeling faint" and manifest both pallor and sweating (the classic "cold sweat"). Their pulse is slow. In vasovagal episodes, the blood pressure may be slightly low in the sitting position but is normal when the patient is placed in a recumbent position. These patients may lose consciousness, although generally for a minute or less. This event is frequently initiated by a brief episode of twitching or even tonic movements and must be differentiated from a true seizure. Patients undergoing vasovagal syncope do not lose bowel or bladder control, do not chew their tongues, and do not demonstrate the persistent or prolonged tonic or clonic motions that characterize a seizure. They usually awaken rapidly, with no sequelae.

The treatment of vasovagal reactions is recumbency, reassurance, and time. This is generally augmented by placing a cold cloth to the forehead and administering a whiff of an ammonia ampoule. Although not a required therapeutic maneuver, oxygen administered by a mask is sometimes reassuring. The most important part of managing a vasovagal reaction is differentiating it from anaphylaxis.

Anaphylactic reactions are of the immediate type and represent a Gell and Coombs type I event. Their importance lies in their potential for rapid progression to an ultimately fatal outcome. Therefore, it is important to recognize their characteristic signs and symptoms (Table 12–1). In anaphylaxis, the organs richest in mast cells (respiratory tract, blood vessels, skin) are primarily affected. The onset of anaphylaxis is generally seen within 15 to 20 minutes of the allergic event and almost never begins after 45 to 60 minutes have passed.[3]

From a cardiovascular standpoint, the pulse in anaphylaxis is rapid (except in patients receiving beta-adrenergic blockers) and is associated with a falling blood pressure. These changes may progress to an arrhythmia in the later stages of the reaction. Circulatory support is important in treating anaphylaxis. However, more deaths associated with anaphylaxis are caused by respiratory obstruction than by cardiovascular problems.

TABLE 12–1. Anaphylaxis versus vasovagal reaction

Signs and symptoms	Vasovagal reaction	Anaphylaxis
Cardiovascular system		
Pulse	Slow	Rapid
Blood pressure (recumbent)	Normal	Low
Skin		
Color	Pale	Red (cyanosis late)
	No rash	Angioedema
Temperature	Cool	Warm
Perspiration	Profuse	Little
Respiratory system		
Itching	None	Itching mucous membranes
Secretions	No change	Increased
Nasal congestion	No change	Increased
Hoarseness	None	Progressive
Cough, wheezing	No change	Present
Dyspnea	None	Progressive (retractions late)
Central nervous system		
Loss of consciousness	Transient	Late
Apprehension	Anxious	Angor animi
Gastrointestinal system		
Nausea, diarrhea	Generally absent	Present late
Genitourinary system		
Urinary urgency	Generally absent	Present late
Uterine cramps	Generally absent	Present late

The signs and symptoms of anaphylaxis involving the respiratory tree include itching membranes, increased respiratory secretions (especially from the tracheobronchial tree), nasal congestion, a sense of the throat closing, hoarseness, cough, wheezing, and eventual stridor.

Cutaneous manifestations of anaphylaxis begin with a flushed, warm skin, with subsequent development of erythema or urticaria that sometimes progresses to angioneurotic edema (Fig. 12–4). Cyanosis may occur in the late stages of cardiorespiratory collapse.

Patients with anaphylaxis typically manifest a feeling of impending doom, or angor animi, also seen in acute myocardial infarction. They may experience nausea, vomiting, and diarrhea. Urinary urgency and uterine cramps are also a result of the massive histamine release that occurs in anaphylaxis.

TREATMENT OF ANAPHYLAXIS

The treatment of anaphylaxis requires three things: equipment, drugs, and expertise in their use. It is mandatory that any office administering allergy

NURSE'S NOTE

Differentiating a "faint" from anaphylaxis:

	Faint	*Anaphylaxis*
Pulse	Slow	Rapid
Blood pressure	Normal (recumbent)	Low
Skin	Pale, clammy, cool	Flushed, warm

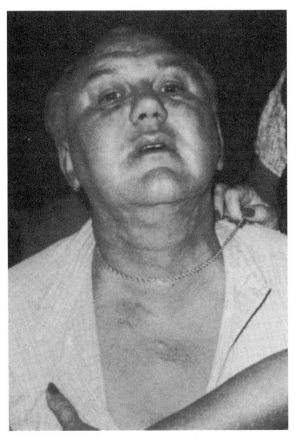

FIGURE 12–4. Patient with anaphylaxis, demonstrating urticaria, angioedema, and respiratory distress with angor animi.

TABLE 12–2. Protocol for treating a systemic reaction

1. Call for help!
2. Place patient in a recumbent position, loosen tight clothing.
3. Apply BP cuff, check pulse and BP.
   A. For vasovagal reactions, treat supportively and observe.
   B. For anaphylaxis, start procedure as noted and call for medical assistance!
4. Apply tourniquet above injection site (loosen every 20 minutes).
5. Give epinephrine, 0.3 mL SC or IM (adult dose), in the arm opposite the tourniquet. (Dose may be altered for age, size, and circumstance; a usual dose for a child is 0.1 mL.)
6. Suction airway if needed; give oxygen by mask if no airway obstruction is present.
   A. For wheezing, give albuterol inhaler, two puffs; repeat in 5 minutes if needed.
   B. If airway becomes obstructed, insert oral airway and deliver oxygen via Ambu or other positive-pressure bag.
   C. If glottis is obstructed, intubate or perform cricothyrotomy (or tracheotomy).
7. Start IV with large-bore needle (arm opposite injection site, using BP cuff as tourniquet). Run at keep-open rate unless BP falls.
8. Monitor BP, and if patient is hypotensive, increase IV infusion rate and prepare dopamine to administer IV. Run dopamine to maintain adequate BP.
9. Repeat epinephrine if needed (may be given by slow IV or injected into tongue if urgent).
10. Give the following medications IV:
    A. H_1 blocker (diphenhydramine, 50 mg IV)
    B. H_2 blocker (ranitidine, 50 mg, or cimetidine, 300 mg, slow IV)
    C. Corticosteroid (dexamethasone, 20 mg, or prednisone, 40 mg IV)
11. Transport patient as soon as possible to a hospital, where patient should be observed for at least 24 hours, watching for late-phase reactions, and other complications. Continue antihistamines and corticosteroids for 24 to 48 hours after the initial reaction.

immunotherapy be prepared to deal with anaphylaxis. Because it is often difficult to collect one's thoughts and act in a coherent manner under the stress of such a situation, regular "practice runs" are advisable. These not only serve to keep the members of the allergy team sharp, but also point out deficiencies in the ready availability of equipment and drugs that can be corrected before a need for them arises. A suggested emergency protocol is given in Table 12–2.

Even though the office may choose to purchase a commercially available kit that purports to contain the necessary supplies for dealing with medical emergencies, it is nevertheless a good idea to "personalize" it by adding other drugs and supplies after careful consideration of the material that follows.

Equipment

Whether suffering from syncope or early anaphylaxis, the patient must be placed in a recumbent position, which means that a *cot or table* must be

---

NURSE'S NOTES

The management of anaphylaxis begins with having a plan in mind. If a reaction is suspected, proceed as follows (for details, consult Table 12–1):

1. Have the patient lie flat. Check pulse, blood pressure, and skin to differentiate faint from anaphylaxis.

2. Call for help! For a faint, administer ammonia ampoule.

3. For anaphylaxis, have 1 : 1000 epinephrine ready for injection. If a physician is unavailable and anaphylaxis is evident, administer subcutaneously.

Normal adult dose: 0.3 mL

Usual pediatric dose: 0.1 mL

(The effect of these doses lasts about 5 to 10 minutes; be prepared to repeat.)

4. Place tourniquet above injection site.

5. Start oxygen and prepare equipment to start IV.

6. Have albuterol inhaler ready if bronchospasm occurs.

---

available for this purpose. This in turn necessitates that the office space devoted to allergy tests and injections be large enough to allow placing a patient in a recumbent position and performing the various maneuvers that may be necessary in treating an allergic reaction. Although cots and beds are softer and more comfortable, if actual cardiopulmonary resuscitation becomes necessary, the patient should be on a hard surface, such as a table or the floor.

Because the best means of differentiating vasovagal responses from anaphylaxis are measurements of pulse and blood pressure, a *sphygmomanometer* and a *stethoscope* should be close at hand. In addition, a *tourniquet* should be available, to be applied above the injection site, to slow absorption of the antigen. The blood pressure cuff will therefore be placed on the arm opposite the injection site.

The maintenance of an airway is extremely important, so a small *oxygen tank* with a mask should be readily available. This should be checked periodically to ensure that it is properly charged. To deliver oxygen under pressure requires *airways* and an *Ambu (or similar positive-pressure) bag*; the possibility of laryngeal obstruction requires the availability of a *laryngoscope* and *endotracheal tubes* or a *cricothyrotomy* or *tracheotomy tray*.

Because one of the characteristics of an anaphylactic reaction is an overproduction of upper and lower airway secretions, a *suction apparatus* and *catheters* must be available to clear these from the airway.

Establishing an intravenous line should be performed as rapidly as practical. This serves to administer fluids and drugs, and because the development of vascular collapse may make starting an intravenous line difficult, it should be done as quickly as possible after the diagnosis of anaphylaxis is confirmed. The equipment necessary includes not only *intravenous fluids*, but also a *pole, tourniquet, needles, alcohol sponges,* and *tape.* Because the tourniquet is placed on the arm where the injection was given, the intravenous infusion should be started in the opposite arm. The blood pressure cuff, which should have already been applied, may be partially inflated to act as a tourniquet in starting the intravenous infusion.

Although allergy syringes and needles are present in the allergy room, they are not helpful in administering the medications generally given to treat anaphylaxis. Therefore, a supply of *needles* and *syringes for intramuscular/intravenous injections* should be readily available. These should include several 1-mL syringes with 25-gauge needles and 2.5-mL syringes with 22-gauge needles. A few 5-mL syringes should also be available.

Drugs

The only "drug" necessary for the treatment of vasovagal syncope is an ampoule of *ammonia*. A supply of these ampoules should be readily available in the allergy room (and in the other office treatment rooms as well), as ammonia inhalation is a highly effective adjunctive measure in the treatment of fainting spells.

The primary drug for the treatment of anaphylaxis is *epinephrine.*[4] The subcutaneous administration of 0.3 to 0.5 mL of a 1:1000 dilution of epinephrine should be one of the first responses to a developing anaphylactic reaction. The subcutaneous route of injection is preferred to intramuscular administration, although either avenue is acceptable. In dire circumstances, the medication may be injected into the tongue, which is a very vascular organ providing almost immediate uptake into the systemic circulation. Epinephrine is available in a 1:1000 w/v concentration in 1-mL ampoules and multidose vials (Adrenalin). It is also available as preloaded cartridge-syringe units (EpiPen, EpiPen Jr., Ana-Kit) that dispense a measured dose (generally 0.3 mL for adults and 0.15 mL for children). In the unusual situation requiring intravenous administration of epinephrine, it should be diluted to at least a 1:10,000 concentration if this concentration is not already available (as it is on most commercially stocked "crash carts"). The availability of both 1:1000 (for intramuscular and subcutaneous injection) and 1:10,000 (for intravenous use) concentrations of epinephrine requires the health care provider to be absolutely certain that the proper dose form is chosen.

The authors are sometimes asked about the use of epinephrine (which contains sodium metabisulfite as a stabilizer) to treat allergic reactions in patients who are sulfite-sensitive. Although a formulation of epinephrine is available (Sus-Phrine) that does not contain sulfites, this is a delayed-release preparation that has been recommended to treat asthma and is not appropriate for the management of anaphylaxis. In treating sulfite-sensitive patients for a systemic reaction, it is probably best to utilize conventional epinephrine and trust that the additional measures discussed later (antihistamines, corticosteroids) will afford some degree of protection against a sulfite reaction.

Because epinephrine is rapidly inactivated in the body, with one dose said to be effective for only about 5 minutes, doses may be repeated every 5 to 10 minutes as long as necessary, so long as careful monitoring of vital signs accompanies the continued administration.[5]

The dose of epinephrine may be lessened or increased, depending on the patient's size, age, and other factors. The usual pediatric dose of subcutaneous 1:1000 epinephrine is 0.01 mL/kg up to a maximum of 0.5 mL. Patients receiving beta-adrenergic blockers may experience augmented hypertensive responses to epinephrine resulting from unopposed alpha-adrenergic stimulation. This may in turn stimulate carotid sinus baroreceptors, resulting in a slowing of the pulse and possible asystole. Patients who are receiving monoamine oxidase (MAO) inhibitors or tricyclic antidepressants are more sensitive to the cardiovascular stimulatory effects of epinephrine. This effect of MAO inhibitors may persist for up to 14 days after the compounds have been discontinued. In those instances in which patients are taking beta blockers, tricyclic antidepressants, or MAO inhibitors, a somewhat lower initial dose of epinephrine (0.2 mL) should be considered.

Tachycardia and hypotension are early signs of anaphylaxis. If hypotension does not immediately respond to an injection of epinephrine and the administration of intravenous fluids, *dopamine* should be administered intravenously to maintain an adequate blood pressure. This is available for addition to intravenous fluids in 5-mL syringes at concentrations of 40, 60, and 80 μg/mL. For cardiovascular support, it is recommended that dopamine be infused at a dose of 5 to 20 μg/kg per minute.[6] As a practical matter, a 5-mL syringe of the 80-μg strength is added to 250 mL of intravenous fluid, and the rate of administration is adjusted as determined by the blood pressure response. Because dopamine forms a precipitate with some other medications, this infusion should have a separate intravenous line.

Bronchospasm is part of the picture of full-blown anaphylaxis. If this occurs, it should be treated with an *inhaled bronchodilator* such as albuterol (Proventil, Ventolin). Two puffs should produce relief of the bronchospasm, especially when combined with the bronchodilator effect of the epinephrine already administered. However, an additional two puffs may be given if the spasm does not break or if it recurs. Salmeterol (Serevent), a long-acting bronchdilator preparation with a slow onset of action, is not appropriate for use in these circumstances.

Some authors have recommended the use of intravenous aminophylline to treat bronchospasm. Although it is effective in this regard, it may cause hypotension, further compounding an existing problem. Thus, it should be employed to treat only bronchospasm that has failed to resolve with the administration of inhaled alpha-adrenergic agonists and the systemic administration of epinephrine.

An alternative treatment for unrelenting bronchospasm, shown in experimental studies to be effective, is inhaled ipratropium hydrobromide (Atrovent inhaler) in very high doses (e.g., 15 to 30 inhalations every 4 hours).[7]

The use of H_1 and H_2 blockers is recommended in the treatment of anaphylaxis. Actually, the amount of histamine generated by such a reaction is so large that it would require near-toxic amounts of these drugs to saturate all the potential histamine-binding sites. Furthermore, other mediators in addition to histamine are generated during anaphylaxis. Nevertheless, these measures are firmly entrenched in the scheme of treating anaphylaxis and should not be omitted. An antihistamine, such as 50 mg of diphenhydramine (Benadryl), and an H_2 blocker, such as 50 mg of ranitidine (Zantac) or 300 mg of cimetidine (Tagamet), are administered intravenously. The H_2 blockers should be diluted to a volume of 20 mL or more and administered slowly (2 to 5 minutes) to avoid producing hypotension. Both these medications remain effective for 4 hours or more, so repeated dosing in the acute management of anaphylaxis is unnecessary.

The role of *corticosteroids* in the management of anaphylaxis is a secondary one. Corticosteroids have no affect on the acute portion of the Gell and Coombs type I reaction, instead exerting their influence on the late phase, which follows after 4 to 6 hours. High doses of intravenous corticosteroids have also been recommended as an empiric therapy for shock. The intravenous administration of an aqueous corticosteroid, such as 20 mg of dexamethasone (Decadron) or 40 mg of methylprednisolone (Solu-Medrol),[8] is aimed at preventing delayed symptoms that might otherwise occur after apparent control of the reaction. After stabilization of the patient (and transport to the hospital for observation), oral corticosteroids should be continued in usual doses for at least 24 hours after an anaphylactic reaction. Although probably less important, the same is true of oral H_1 and H_2 blockers.

Although not recognized as a first-line therapeutic measure in the treatment of anaphylaxis, *heparin* has a well-documented ability to neutralize histamine.[9] The use of heparin in the treatment of anaphylaxis has a basis both in anecdotal experience[10] and in clinical studies.[11] Nevertheless, heparin should be used in the treatment of refractory anaphylaxis only after standard measures have been implemented. When given, a bolus of 10,000 units is administered intravenously. Heparin should not be given if the patient has a history of a bleeding problem, is already on an anticoagulant (including aspirin), or has had recent surgery.

OTHER CONSIDERATIONS IN MANAGING REACTIONS

As already noted, some patients may be vulnerable to the development of hypertension during the administration of epinephrine in the treatment of anaphylaxis. To control this, one should have available phentolamine (Regitine), which is a pure, nonselective alpha-adrenergic blocker. It is administered intravenously in 5- to 10-mg increments every 5 to 15 minutes,[12] with care taken not to "overshoot" and produce hypotension. An alternative medication is sodium nitroprusside (Nipride). If neither of these is available, sublingual nitroglycerin may be administered to produce peripheral vasodilation and lower blood pressure. Nitroglycerin has the added benefit of protecting from coronary vasospasm, but it is less effective in controlling blood pressure than the agents listed. Yet another alternative is to puncture a soft gelatin 10-mg capsule of the calcium channel blocker nifedipine (Procardia) and squeeze the contents into the sublingual area for rapid absorption into the circulation.

The development of angina during an episode of anaphylaxis is not unheard of. This may be treated with the sublingual administration of nitroglycerin tablets, 0.4 mg every 5 minutes, until relief is obtained or to a maximum of three tablets.

Although not available in every physician's office, devices such as pulse oximeters and electrocardiographic monitors provide helpful information during the treatment of an episode of anaphylaxis. The details of management of arrhythmias and cardiac problems that may accompany or follow anaphylaxis are beyond the scope of this text. However, every member of the allergy team should receive basic training (and recertification at appropriate intervals) in basic cardiopulmonary life-support techniques. It is beneficial if the medical members of the team are also certified in advanced cardiac life support.

The setting in which allergy care is delivered may be an office that is far removed from a hospital or medical support facility, or it may be within such a medical center. Thus, backup facilities and assistance may be near at hand or may require quite some time to reach. The farther one is from such a source of assistance and advanced care, the greater the need for the office and staff to be self-sufficient in dealing with an allergic emergency. Although the details will vary from office to office, it is accepted that the basic equipment, drugs, and expertise required for the initial management of anaphylaxis should be available in every office in which allergy testing and immunotherapy injections are carried out. The arrangement may vary from a very basic kit of drugs and equipment (Fig. 12–5) to a crash cart (Fig. 12–6). Whatever the level of equipment provided, the material should be kept close to the site of allergy testing and treatment. Expiration dates of drugs should be regularly checked, the oxygen tank should always be fully charged, and regular drills in the management of anaphylaxis should be carried out to keep the allergy personnel ready to deal with a problem that everyone hopes will never occur.

CONFIRMING AN ANAPHYLACTIC REACTION

In rare instances, a patient may present in the office or emergency department with symptoms suggesting anaphylaxis, but under circumstances that make the diagnosis less than clear. For example, consider the patient who returns 30 minutes after an allergy injection (or the ingestion of a penicillin tablet) with dyspnea, tachycardia, and hypotension, but no wheezing or rash. The question arises whether this is a cardiac event or an anaphylactic reaction. Although not of immediate help, the determination of *serum tryptase*, which is a very specific marker for systemic mast cell activity, may give an eventual answer. A reaction such as symptomatic allergic rhinitis or asthma will not cause enough mast cell degranulation to raise serum tryptase values to abnormal levels, but anaphylaxis will. Unlike histamine, which is cleared from the circulation in a matter of minutes after its release, tryptase has a serum half-life of about 2 hours. In anaphylaxis, the level will rise after 15 to 30 minutes, peak at 1 to 2 hours, and remain elevated for a total of about 4 to 8 hours.[13] Patients with systemic mastocytosis may have elevated levels of this enzyme in about 35 to 65% of cases, but that disorder has other characteristics that readily distinguish it from anaphylaxis.[14] Unfortunately, serum tryptase determinations are available only at regional reference laboratories

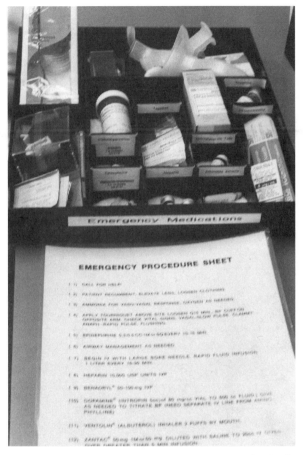

FIGURE 12–5. A simple divided box contains the basic drugs for dealing with anaphylaxis, all readily identified for immediate use.

and large medical centers, so results may not be available for several days. This determination is mainly of benefit in documenting the occurrence of a true anaphylactic reaction and confirming the diagnosis retrospectively.

NURSE'S NOTE

After an anaphylactic reaction, it is wise to wait at least a week before administering another allergy injection. In the interim, a determination should be made of the probable cause of the reaction and steps taken to correct the situation.

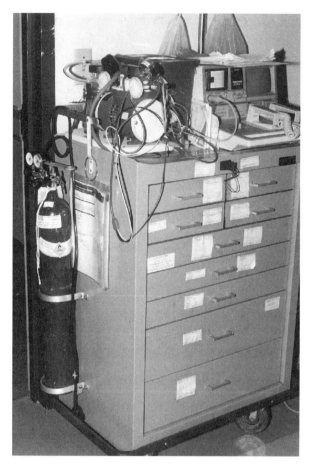

FIGURE 12–6. A fully stocked crash cart provides the necessary equipment for dealing with virtually all degrees of allergic emergencies.

WAITING AFTER INJECTIONS; SAFETY OF IMMUNOTHERAPY AT HOME

In a survey of 17 fatalities associated with immunotherapy for the years 1985 through 1989, the American Academy of Allergy, Asthma and Immunology (AAAAI) found two instances in which it was felt that not waiting after an injection was a contributory factor; one death occurred following a home injection. No fatalities were recorded in association with skin testing during this same period.[15] At about that same time, the AAAAI revised its previous position statement to go on record saying that "allergen immunotherapy should be given only in settings where emergency resuscitative equipment and trained personnel are immediately available to treat systemic reactions under the direct supervision of a physician.'' That same statement went on to say that ''the patient should be kept under observation for an appropriate period of time after the injection, which will ordinarily be 20 minutes.''[16] This proscription of at-home injections caused a division between those members of the AAAAI who had for years allowed maintenance immunotherapy injections to be given outside the office[17,18] and other members who supported the new position prohibiting at-home injections.[19,20] The debate goes on, but the policy has not changed.

In a study supported by the American Academy of Otolaryngic Allergy (AAOA), an analysis was made of immunotherapy administered to 450,512 patients by 592 of its members. The overall reaction rate after injections was 0.3%. In this total of 215 reportable reactions, symptoms limited to increased sneezing and nasal congestion constituted about one third and urticaria another third; wheezing with throat tightness occurred in about a fourth. Two patients demonstrated true shock. No fatalities occurred in the study population.[21] The position of the AAOA, as reflected in its most recent practice guidelines, is that immunotherapy should be ''prescribed by specially trained physician practitioners and administered under the supervision of physicians trained to manage systemic reactions and with the immediate availability of adrenalin (epinephrine) should anaphylaxis occur. Patients should be observed for at least 20 minutes after injections when the dosage of antigen is being increased.''[22] As a practical matter, with the safeguards inherent in quantitative testing (using SET or RAST) and when proper precautions are taken, maintenance immunotherapy may be administered outside the treating physician's office. This includes not only administration of antigen in another physician's office, but maintenance immunotherapy given at home.

The precautions to be taken when considering at-home immunotherapy include an evaluation for risk factors: beta-blocker therapy, the presence of asthma (and especially steroid-dependent asthma), and a history of prior severe reactions. The responsibility and cooperativeness of the patient and any other care givers involved in the process must be assessed. If no contraindications are found, the patient and the person who will administer the injections (if other than the patient) are counseled by the allergy nurse or assistant. They are provided with a set of single-dose vials so that there is no question of dose adjustment involved. The person designated to give injections is taught the proper technique. Counseling includes the admonition to omit the injection in the face of active infection and to call immediately if an unacceptable local reaction follows an injection. The patient and care giver

TABLE 12–3. Instructions for patients receiving vials outside the office

REACTIONS TO ALLERGY SHOTS:

The techniques we use for testing for the presence and degree of sensitivity to an allergen, and the way in which doses are advanced, make a reaction to an allergy injection unlikely. However, this information is furnished to make your treatment even safer. Please read it carefully, call us if you have questions, and *keep this sheet where it can be easily found if you need it.*

To treat a possible reaction, you will need an *antihistamine* and *epinephrine.* Any antihistamine, either prescription or over-the-counter, will do. Examples are Allegra, Zyrtec, Claritin, Chlor-Trimeton, or Benadryl. Epinephrine is available in an automatic injection form called EpiPen, EpiPen Jr., or Ana-Kit. You will receive a prescription to purchase one of these. It is unlikely that you will ever need it, but *it must be available when you receive your allergy shot.* Don't forget to check the expiration date from time to time.

The combination of an allergy shot with higher-than-usual allergen exposure may sometimes result in a *local reaction,* which is an area of firmness (not necessarily redness) at the injection site that is larger than a 50-cent piece and that persists for at least 24 hours. Redness and/or firmness can also be caused by a complicating infection, or by a reaction to glycerine in the mixture. If a local reaction around an injection site occurs, take an antihistamine and apply a cool compress, but *report this to the nurse before your next injection, for dose adjustment if necessary.*

A true *severe reaction* must be treated immediately. It usually begins within 5 or 10 minutes of the injection with intense itching of the throat, nose, and chest membranes. If this occurs, take an antihistamine immediately and apply a cold compress to the injection site. If the reaction progresses to any swelling of the face, swelling of the throat, difficulty swallowing or breathing, or generalized itching or redness of the body accompanied by a feeling of distress, *immediately administer one dose of epinephrine,* injecting into the soft tissue of the arm opposite the site of your allergy shot. Put a tourniquet (belt or similar object) above the place where the allergy shot was given to slow the absorption of the material into the system. *If it is necessary to administer epinephrine, go immediately to the emergency department of XXXX Hospital,* where you can receive medical attention while contact is made with the doctor on call.

---

are provided with written instructions and precautions (Table 12–3) as well as a prescription for an epinephrine self-injector (Epi-Pen, Ana-Kit) (Fig. 12–7) and instructions in its proper use. The record of injections (Table 12–4), which is returned before new vials are dispensed, is reviewed by the allergy nurse or assistant, who watch for any complications or untoward reactions. Finally, the patient must return on a regular basis, not only for new single-dose vials, but for evaluation by the physician, to monitor the success of the at-home injections.

CONCLUSION

The last word about allergy emergencies has not yet been written, nor will it be until further advances in medical science totally remove the possibility

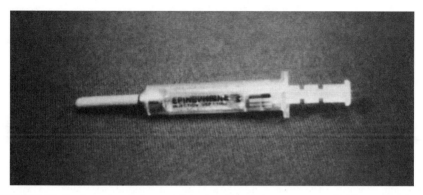

FIGURE 12–7. An epinephrine autoinjector. Several types are available, and patients receiving immunotherapy outside the office must have one available and be instructed in their appropriate use.

TABLE 12–4. Monitoring form for patients receiving vials outside the office

(Physician's name, address, phone, fax)

PATIENT: _____
INSTRUCTIONS:
    TAKE ALL OF ONE VIAL AT _____ INTERVALS. KEEP THIS FORM WITH
YOUR VIALS AND COMPLETE WHEN INJECTION IS GIVEN. RECORD ANY
SYMPTOMS OR LOCAL REACTION IN SPACE NEXT TO DATE OF INJECTION.

        DATE OF INJECTION   SYMPTOMS/LOCAL REACTION

DATE OF INJECTION	SYMPTOMS/LOCAL REACTION

WHEN YOU HAVE TAKEN ALL VIALS, RETURN THIS FORM **IMMEDIATELY** TO
THE CLINIC. YOU MAY MAIL IT TO THE ADDRESS ABOVE, OR FAX IT TO THE
NUMBER ABOVE. **THIS FORM MUST BE RETURNED BEFORE YOU CAN
RECEIVE MORE VIALS!!** AFTER RETURNING THE FORM, PLEASE CALL TO
MAKE YOUR NEXT APPOINTMENT FOR AN INJECTION AND TO PICK UP
YOUR VIALS.

NURSE'S NOTE

Before patients are allowed to take their injections outside the office, they must be thoroughly instructed in the management of any possible anaphylactic reaction, which includes being provided with epinephrine and taught how to use it.

---

of such reactions. Other authors have written effectively about the prevention and management of allergic emergencies, and the reader may wish to consult their work for additional information.[23,24]

Allergy skin testing and immunotherapy always carry the risk for producing a reaction, which may be local or systemic. The most catastrophic systemic reaction is anaphylaxis, which may culminate in death. Prevention of reactions is always preferable to treating them. The allergy team should remain constantly aware of the risks involved in the treatment they render and be prepared to deal with reactions should they occur. However, careful attention to technique and a cautious approach can significantly minimize the likelihood of a severe allergic reaction.

REFERENCES

1. Greineder DK. Risk management in allergen immunotherapy. J Allergy Clin Immunol 1996;98:330–334.
2. Tinkelman DG, Cole WQ III, Tunno J. Immunotherapy: a one-year prospective study to evaluate risk factors of systemic reactions. J Allergy Clin Immunol 1995;95:8–14.
3. Greenberg MA, Kantman CR, Gonzalez GE, et al. Late systemic-allergic reactions to inhalant allergen immunotherapy. J Allergy Clin Immunol 1988;82:287–290.
4. Valentine MD. Anaphylaxis and stinging insect hypersensitivity. JAMA 1992;268: 2830–2833.
5. American Heart Association. Textbook of Advanced Cardiac Life Support. Dallas: American Heart Association; 1987.
6. Drug Information for the Health Care Professional. 17th ed. Sympathomimetic agents (parenteral-systemic). Rockville, MD: US Pharmacopeial Convention; 1997:2729–2739.
7. Murphy S, Kelly HW. Acute asthma in children: when first-line therapy isn't enough. J Respir Dis 1990;11:589.
8. Drug Information for the Health Care Professional. 17th ed. Corticosteroids-glucocorticoid effects (systemic). Rockville, MD: US Pharmacopeial Convention; 1997:958–983.
9. Dolowitz DA. Drug treatment in allergic disorders. Otolaryngol Clin North Am 1971;4: 591–598.
10. Dolowitz DA, Dougherty TF. The use of heparin as an anti-inflammatory agent. Laryngoscope 1960;70:873–884.
11. Dolowitz DA, Dougherty TF. The use of heparin in the control of allergies. Ann Allergy 1965;23:309–313.

12. Calhoun DA, Oparil S. Treatment of hypertensive crisis. N Engl J Med 1990;323: 1177–1183.
13. Schwartz LB, Yunginger JW, Miller JS, et al. Time course of appearance and disappearance of human mast cell tryptase in the circulation after anaphylaxis. J Clin Invest 1989; 83:1551–1561.
14. Schwartz LB, Metcalfe DD, Miller JS, et al. Tryptase levels as an indicator of mast-cell activation in systemic anaphylaxis and mastocytosis. N Engl J Med 1987;31:1622–1626.
15. Reid MJ, Lockey RF, Turkeltaub PC, Platts-Mills TAE. Survey of fatalities from skin testing and immunotherapy 1985–1989. J Allergy Clin Immunol 1993;92:6–15.
16. AAAAI Board of Directors. Guidelines to minimize the risk from systemic reactions caused by immunotherapy with allergenic extracts. J Allergy Clin Immunol 1994;93: 811–812.
17. Falliers CJ. At-home administration of allergenic extracts. J Allergy Clin Immunol 1995; 95:1061.
18. Wells JH. Home allergenic extract administration. J Allergy Clin Immunol 1995;95: 1061–1062.
19. Lockey RF. Reply (to Drs. Falliers and Wells). J Allergy Clin Immunol 1995;95: 1062–1063.
20. Rumbyrt JS, Borish LC. Home administration of allergen extracts. JAMA 1995;273:897.
21. Cook PR, Bryant JL II, David WE, Benke TT, Rapoport AS. Systemic reactions to immunotherapy: the American Academy of Otolaryngic Allergy morbidity and mortality survey. Otolaryngol Head Neck Surg 1994;110:487–493.
22. Fornadley JA, Corey JP, Osguthorpe JD, et al. Allergic rhinitis: clinical practice guideline. Otolaryngol Head Neck Surg 1996;115:115–122.
23. Anon JB. Emergencies in the allergy office. In: Mabry RL, (ed). Skin Endpoint Titration. 2nd ed. New York: Thieme Medical Publishers; 1994:46–54.
24. Gordon BR. Prevention and management of office allergy emergencies. Otolaryngol Clin North Am 1992;25:119–134.

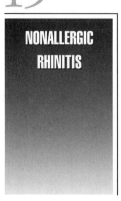

13

NONALLERGIC RHINITIS

Perhaps the most frequent question encountered by the authors during decades of courses and lectures has been, ''What do I do when the allergy test results are negative?'' Although there is no single answer to the question, the possibilities are by no means infinite. In this chapter, we present our thoughts on how to handle this perplexing situation. Here are some of the questions to be asked.

DIAGNOSTIC QUESTIONS TO BE ANSWERED

Has Inhalant Allergy Really Been Ruled Out?

When one says, ''The allergy test results are negative,'' the usual implication is that inhalant testing has been carried out, with negative results. As has been emphasized in earlier chapters, the diagnosis of allergy is initially made by history, and then confirmed by testing to identify antigenic triggers. To avoid needless expenditure of time and money, the ''screening'' concept was introduced. Testing with a limited number of inhalant antigens (generally from nine to 15) gives a specificity and sensitivity well over 90%, but not 100%. Therefore, even though a patient's history is strongly suggestive of (for example) fall weed symptoms, if results of testing for the index antigen (in this case, ragweed) are negative, additional testing may be justified, based on strong clinical suspicion. In the example cited, this might include marsh elder, lamb's quarters, pigweed, or other significant fall weeds in the local area. Results of tests for these will not always be positive, but in a few instances these additional tests will uncover allergies missed in a screening evaluation. It should be strongly emphasized that this is not a carte blanche to perform numerous other tests on every patient with a negative allergy screen result. Only if the history is strongly suggestive is such further testing justified.

A related situation occurs when the patient has allergic symptoms triggered by unusual antigens that are not routinely included in the screening panel, and that do not cross-react significantly with antigens in that group. Again, the history is all-important in this case, and the allergy team members are called upon to be detectives. The culprit may be an animal (e.g., rabbit, horse), an unusual pollen (e.g., *Malaleuca* in certain regions of Florida), or a perennial allergen not generally tested for (e.g., cockroach). If the history is strongly suggestive of atopy to such an antigen, additional testing is justified, although again, this will not be necessary or appropriate in every case. A strong historical suggestion of sensitivity to the unusual antigen should be present.

Does the Patient Have Noninhalant Allergy?

Not all allergy that affects the ear, nose, and throat is caused by inhalants. Foods may play either a primary or secondary role in producing such symptoms. Thus, a negative evaluation for inhalants does not mean that food allergy has been ruled out. The simplest means of doing this is through an assessment of a patient's dietary habits, followed by omission of suspected foods and a challenge refeeding of the individual foods in question. Although this technique requires cooperation on the part of patients, it is fairly simple and is nonetheless probably the most accurate means of diagnosing food allergy. Furthermore, the experience serves to demonstrate forcefully to patients the relationship of their symptoms (as produced by the challenge refeeding) to food ingestion. Dietary modification requires effort by patients and those who will not attempt diagnostic manipulation will probably not be cooperative in efforts to alleviate symptoms by omission of foods. Most of these patients are instead looking for a "quick fix" that is effortless (on their part) and permanent. Details of evaluating and treating for food allergy are found in Chapter 14.

Are Nonallergic Triggers at Work?

Although debate continues as to whether chemicals cause a true "allergic" reaction or simply act as irritants, there is no doubt that these substances do produce symptoms that may include nasal congestion, rhinorrhea, drainage, and headache. Most, if not all, chemicals are not primarily antigens, but some may act as haptens. These are small molecules that, although not antigenic in themselves, bind to a protein carrier to form an immunologically active conjugate. The question of whether "immunotherapy" for chemicals is appropriate is beyond the scope of this text. What is indisputable, however, is that exposure to tobacco smoke, perfumes, hairsprays, colognes, soaps, dyes, paints, inks, and numerous other chemicals produces undesirable upper respiratory symptoms in a significant number of patients. Important nonallergic, irritant causes of nasal symptoms are ozone and air pollution, which are products of high temperatures and calm winds. A good history, in which the patient is involved as a partner in detecting such exposure, is the best method for making the diagnosis of rhinitis caused by chemicals and irritants. Avoidance, if possible, remains the best treatment.

Does the Patient Have Vasomotor Rhinitis?

Although it has been suggested that the term *idiopathic rhinitis* should replace the more time-honored designation of *vasomotor rhinitis*, we have chosen to continue to use the more familiar term. The entity of true vasomotor rhinitis implies an autonomic instability, in which the normal balance of sympathetic and parasympathetic innervation to the nose is disturbed, resulting in an excess of cholinergic stimulation. This in turn produces nasal congestion and/or profuse rhinorrhea and postnasal drainage. The classic example of this problem is the "skier's nose," represented by profuse rhinorrhea on exposure to cold weather.

Other patients react to the stimulus of eating. This latter trigger is not limited to spicy foods, which stimulate trigeminal nerve fibers to produce rhinorrhea, but may involve any food or beverage. Hot or cold foods are especially common triggers in this regard. Unfortunately, results of a search for a true "food allergy" are usually negative, confirming the diagnosis of vasomotor rhinitis. This problem is a source of extreme embarrassment, and many patients will volunteer that they no longer eat out as a result.

It has been long recognized that emotional stress can produce nasal congestion and obstruction.[1] This is an altogether too common cause of nasal symptoms in patients with negative allergy test results. Rhinorrhea is less often associated with this problem, but postnasal drainage and chronic throat clearing may frequently be seen in association with stress-induced rhinitis.

The question of NARES, the non-allergic rhinitis with eosinophilia syndrome, generally is raised when patients are encountered who have symptoms of rhinitis, negative allergy test results, and large numbers of eosinophils in their nasal secretions. The original description of this syndrome[2] included a very small group of patients with symptoms of sporadic episodes of sneezing, watery rhinorrhea, and itching ocular and pharyngeal mucosa. None had nasal obstruction, nor did they experience the consequences of sinusitis, otitis media, or lower respiratory tract symptoms, which often accompany allergic rhinitis. Although they had high numbers of eosinophils in their nasal secretions during periods of symptoms, this level decreased when they were symptom-free. Results of allergy tests, in the form of skin tests, allergen-specific radioallergosorbent testing (RAST), and determination of total immunoglobulin E (IgE), were all negative.

A meta-analysis of all reported series of NARES by Carney and Jones pointed out that the criteria for making this diagnosis have varied significantly with individual investigators, with a range of nasal eosinophilia of from 10 to 25% being considered abnormal. It is their opinion that NARES is probably not a single, clearly defined clinical entity. They further postulate that NARES may represent allergy limited to the mucosal tissue, without systemic IgE-mediated disease.[3]

As a practical matter, from the standpoint of therapy, patients thought to have NARES can be treated in a similar fashion as those with more classic vasomotor or idiopathic rhinitis.

Are We Dealing with a Rhinitis Medicamentous?

The most common form of rhinitis medicamentous is rebound rhinitis, which follows the use of topical nasal decongestants for a period exceeding a week or more. This occurs as the initial decongestion with closure of blood-filled spaces in the turbinates is followed by a reactive vasodilation, resulting in recurrent congestion and the need for more decongestants, setting up a vicious cycle. This rebound congestion may follow treatment with any of the topical decongestants currently available, including phenylephrine (Neo-Synephrine) and oxymetazoline (Afrin). The incidence of rebound rhinitis is higher than might be imagined. In one series of 100 consecutive patients seen for the first time in an otolaryngologist's office with the chief complaint of nasal congestion (excluding only patients with infection), more than half had used decongesting drops or sprays for 14 days or more.[4] Correction of rebound rhinitis begins with making the diagnosis, which in turn means that all patients with the complaint of nasal congestion must be specifically asked about their use of nose drops or nasal sprays. It may take some effort on the part of the clinician to differentiate between decongestant use and use of other nasal sprays, such as corticosteroids, anticholinergics, and cromolyn. However, it is an effort that will be well rewarded.

Although most cases of rhinitis medicamentous are forms of rebound rhinitis, a variety of systemically administered medications may also produce the side effect of nasal stuffiness. The most common cause of this congestion was once a variety of antihypertensive medications, such as reserpine (Serpasil), hydralazine (Apresoline), guanethidine (Ismelin), methyldopa (Aldomet), and prazosin (Minipress). The more frequent cause in recent times has been a noncardioselective beta-adrenergic blocker, such as propranolol (Inderal) or nadolol (Corgard). Finally, nasal congestion may be a side effect of some antidepressants and anxiolytic medications, such as thioridazine (Mellaril), chlordiazepoxide-amitriptyline (Limbitrol), perphenazine (Trilafon), and alprazolam (Xanax). The only way to rule out rhinitis medicamentous effectively as a contributory (or primary) cause of a patient's nasal symptoms is by obtaining a complete history detailing all systemic medications taken. If doubt exists as to the ability of any given drug to produce nasal congestion, one should examine the list of side effects for that drug as printed in the Physician's Desk Reference (Medical Economics Publishers, Montvale, NJ) or Drug Information for the Health Care Professional (US Pharmacopeial Convention, Rockville, MD).

NURSE'S NOTE

Although at the time they begin allergy care patients may not have been receiving a medication that can produce nasal congestion, this situation will often change during the 3 to 5 years they are receiving such treatment. Because of the frequent contact the allergy nurse or assistant has with these patients, the allergy care provider should regularly question patients about their current regimen of medications, note any changes on the chart, and inform the physician if these may affect the patient's allergy care.

Is a Hormonally Mediated Rhinitis Present?

A cause of nasal congestion that is often cited but rarely encountered is hypothyroidism. Nevertheless, patients with hypothyroidism can have boggy, pale nasal mucosa, with the production of clear mucus. If a question exists in this regard, appropriate evaluation for hypothyroidism is not inappropriate.

A more common cause of nasal congestion (or exacerbation of pre-existing nasal symptoms) is the rhinitis that occurs during pregnancy. Estrogen, which is produced in larger-than-usual amounts during pregnancy, exerts a cholinergic action on the nasal mucosa, resulting in edema and turbinate congestion. This may occur to a lesser degree when high estrogen levels, either occurring naturally in the last portion of the menstrual cycle or exogenously administered, produce vasomotor rhinitis in some women. Other factors that may contribute to rhinitis of pregnancy (or rhinitis during pregnancy) are emotional stress, unrecognized sinusitis, and rebound rhinitis caused by a dependence on nasal sprays.[5]

Does the Patient Have an Infection?

A very important concept to communicate to patients, second only to "not everything that sneezes is allergic," is the idea that "allergy does not 'go into' infection." The initial symptoms of an allergic flare and an acute upper respiratory infection may be almost the same: profuse rhinorrhea and post-nasal drainage, nasal congestion, head pressure, and malaise. However, in the case of infection, this first phase soon passes into one marked by sore throat, thick and often purulent nasal and postnasal secretions, ear plugging, and cough. Allergy, on the other hand, does not progress in this fashion; instead, the symptoms already described continue, although sometimes increasing or decreasing in severity.

Despite lay misconceptions to the contrary, the one to two liters of secretions produced by the sinonasal mucosa for humidification of inspired air does not "drain into the chest." If this were so, many of us would experience a near-drowning episode each day. However, the pathogens (either bacterial or viral) responsible for upper respiratory symptoms often inexorably follow a path downward into the lower respiratory tract, giving rise to the conception that the mucus associated with the infection caused this progression.

It is not usually difficult for the experienced clinician to differentiate an active, full-blown infection from an allergic episode. A greater problem is to determine the exact contribution of allergy and/or infection to repeated respiratory symptoms. This requires painstaking history taking and examining the patient at the time of one or more of the episodes in question. In addition to appropriate allergy tests, cultures of the nasopharynx or from the middle meatus may give a clue to the presence of bacterial pathogens.[6] The clarification of whether an ongoing sinusitis might be contributing to the patient's symptom complex may depend on computerized tomography (CT scan) of the sinuses, but this should be done only after 2 to 4 weeks of intensive medical management. Otherwise, false-positive responses may occur, resulting in unnecessary surgical interventions. For more details, consult Chapter 16, Allergy and Sinus Disease.

Although the treatment of allergy should not have a direct effect on the frequency and severity of respiratory infections suffered by patients, experience has repeatedly shown that it often has a salutary effect. Theoretically, this may be explained in three ways. First, the exact mechanism by which allergy injections work remains in question. It well may be that in addition to their effect on IgE and IgG, they affect IgM, which is the first immunologic line of defense against bacterial invaders. Furthermore, if the body's immune system need not be constantly occupied with responding to allergic invaders, it may be able to deal with infections more efficiently. Finally, a decrease in tissue congestion minimizes obstruction of the ostiomeatal complex, making secondary sinusitis less likely. Although all these explanations are appealing in theory, it must be emphasized that their accuracy remains unproven.

THERAPEUTIC APPROACHES TO NONALLERGIC RHINITIS

The treatment of nonallergic rhinitis caused by chemical hypersensitivity is obviously predicated on avoidance of inciting substances, insofar as possible. Beyond this, a few pharmacotherapeutic measures may be helpful. Although the primary therapeutic indication for intranasal cromolyn is IgE-mediated allergic rhinitis, it has been shown (at least experimentally) also to inhibit mast cell degranulation caused by various chemical triggers, such as sulfur dioxide.[7] Likewise, inhaled cromolyn has been shown to be an effective preventive for bronchospasm triggered by exercise or inhalation of cold air. A trial of nasal cromolyn, which is now available over the counter, is worthwhile in the patient who is unable to tolerate being around perfumes, dyes, and similar chemical triggers. Although cromolyn is approved by the Food and Drug Administration only for the treatment of IgE-mediated inhalant allergy, the clinical experience of the authors and many other physicians support this off-label usage.

If the patient's primary symptomatology produced by chemicals is rhinorrhea, nasal ipratropium spray, 0.03%, can be tried. If neither cromolyn nor ipratropium is effective, nasal corticosteroid sprays may deserve a therapeutic trial. However, these preparations are often less effective in alleviating rhinitis resulting from chemical sensitivity than in treating allergic rhinitis.

The best treatment currently available for true vasomotor rhinitis is topical nasal ipratropium hydrobromide. This is available in two strengths, 0.03% and 0.06%. The former is the more appropriate for the patient with vasomotor rhinitis, whereas the latter provides symptomatic relief of the profuse rhinorrhea that often marks the start of a common cold or upper respiratory infection. For vasomotor rhinitis, the patient should begin with two sprays of the 0.03% formulation in each nostril in the morning, and repeat this dose again in midafternoon and in the evening. If control of symptoms is to be obtained from this medication, it will become evident within a week or less. When symptoms abate (or diminish to what is obviously the best level obtainable), the morning dose should be maintained and the afternoon and evening doses halved (i.e., one spray in each nostril in the afternoon and at bedtime). If symptom control continues to be adequate, the morning dose may also be halved, so that the patient is using one spray in each nostril three times daily.

It is sometimes possible to decrease this further to one spray twice daily, but this is about the lowest effective maintenance dose. It appears that the most important factor in this treatment is the use of a substantial "loading dose" early in the day, with subsequent doses to maintain the effect.[8] Although it is sometimes possible to utilize this medication on an as-needed basis, such as before activities known to produce rhinorrhea (e.g., skiing, eating), many patients require regular medication to prevent a recurrence of their symptoms.

In the case of rebound rhinitis, the patient should immediately and permanently discontinue the use of all topical nasal decongestants. This, along with symptomatic treatment of nasal congestion until turbinate edema reverses, is usually sufficient. Such treatment will generally include systemic decongestants, plus nasal steroids (either topically or as an intranasal injection) or a brief burst of systemic corticosteroids.

If rhinitis medicamentous, caused by a systemic medication, is felt to be present, a change to a different compound instead of the suspected offending preparation as a therapeutic trial will usually provide an answer. Unfortunately, in some situations this is impossible, in which case one must simply accept that a very necessary medication may have an undesirable side effect and attempt to provide symptomatic relief insofar as possible.

Rhinitis occurring during pregnancy is a complex problem that may have several components. Symptomatic and supportive treatment should be given during the pregnancy and the patient reassured that the symptoms will almost certainly cease within 2 to 4 weeks of the time of delivery of the child. A number of therapeutic measures have been recommended, but any treatment should be approved by the obstetrician. Intraturbinal steroid injection has been an effective means of treating many of these patients, but the interested reader should carefully consult the appropriate references for details before attempting this procedure.[9]

If infection is complicating the clinical picture of the patient with rhinitis, appropriate antibiotic therapy together with systemic administration of decongestants (often with mucolytics) should be carried out. The details of treating infections of the nose and paranasal sinuses are found in numerous sources, and will not be repeated here.[10]

CONCLUSION

When "the tests are negative," it is possible that not all the right tests have been done. On the other hand, in some instances negative allergy test results are an accurate reflection of the state that exists, and the cause of the patient's symptoms is not allergy. The number of negative test results encountered in one's practice will vary with the clinician's experience, but the physician need not be embarrassed by negative results, as no one's clinical judgment has been shown to be foolproof. It is always appropriate to rule out allergy adequately when it is a legitimate consideration, and many patients appreciate having their self-diagnosis upheld or corrected by an accurate assessment of their problems.

REFERENCES

1. Wolff HG, Wolf S, Grace WJ, et al. Changes in form and function of mucous membranes occurring as part of protective reaction patterns in man during periods of life stress and emotional conflict. Trans Assoc Am Physicians 1948;61:313–334.
2. Mullarkey MF, Hiss JS, Webb DR. Allergic and nonallergic rhinitis: their characterization with attention to the meaning of nasal eosinophilia. J Allergy Clin Immunol 1980;65: 122–126.
3. Carney AS, Jones NS. Idiopathic rhinitis: idiopathic or not? Clin Otolaryngol 1996;21: 198–202.
4. Mabry RL. Rhinitis medicamentosa: the forgotten factor in nasal obstruction. South Med J 1982;75:817–819.
5. Mabry RL. Rhinitis of pregnancy. South Med J 1986;79:965–971.
6. Mabry RL. Allergic and infective rhinosinusitis: differential diagnosis and interrelationship. Otolaryngol Head Neck Surg 1994;111:335–339.
7. Schwartz HJ. Cromolyn sodium and its effect on nasal disease. Am J Rhinol 1988;2: 129–133.
8. Mygind N, Borum P. Anticholinergic treatment of watery rhinorrhea. Am J Rhinol 1990; 4:1–5.
9. Mabry RL. Intranasal steroid injection during pregnancy. South Med J 1980;73: 1176–1179.
10. Calhoun K. Diagnosis and management of sinusitis in the allergic patient. Otolaryngol Head Neck Surg 1992;107:850–854.

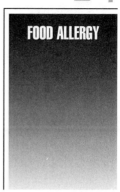

14

FOOD ALLERGY

Up to this point, this book has been concerned primarily with the diagnosis and treatment of inhalant allergy. As a semantic reminder, allergy is divided clinically into inhalant allergy (sensitivity to substances inhaled), ingestant allergy (sensitivity to substances ingested), and contact allergy (sensitivity to items that contact the skin or mucous membranes). These terms are bandied about so freely by the allergist that it is easy to forget that the patient frequently does not understand the distinction and hesitates to ask for fear of appearing stupid. Most aspiring allergists start their program by treating only inhalant allergy, and in many cases only allergic rhinitis, as lower respiratory tract disease is prone to involve additional problems other than allergy. Starting with the management of inhalant allergic rhinitis is quite a realistic approach. The success quotient for those treating this condition is high, and a series of successes both boosts confidence and helps in establishing a reputation for competence. It will not be too long, however, before a situation arises that simply does not fall within the parameters of allergic rhinitis caused by inhalants. It may be that all the symptoms of allergic rhinitis are present, but there appears to be no seasonal or exposure pattern. Alternatively, all the symptoms of allergic rhinitis are present but all the test results are negative. There are several possible explanations for this situation (Chapter 13 is devoted to these), but one possible condition that should immediately be considered is food sensitivity.

For the rhinitis sufferer with negative inhalant test findings, the usual reaction to suggesting the possibility of food sensitivity is, "I'm not allergic to any foods!" This may be translated as, "I don't have any gastrointestinal symptoms." It may take a bit of convincing before the patient accepts the fact that an offender may produce symptoms in body locations other than that by which it entered the body. One explanation that is frequently accepted by patients is to remind them that the antihistamine-decongestant tablet taken to relieve nasal symptoms was ingested, not inserted in the nose, yet the result did not surprise the patient at all. In other words, the route of entry frequently has little to do with the response.

THE CONFUSING REALM OF FOOD SENSITIVITY

To educate the patient to understanding and coping with food sensitivity, the physician must in turn understand the situation, and this is no task for the timid. Many physicians have settled for the degree of success possible in treating only inhalant allergy, electing not to pursue the management of difficult cases. For those to whom less than the best possible result is unacceptable, however, the field of food sensitivity is a fascinating, frustrating, and rewarding one. There is a great sense of accomplishment when a patient, previously written off as hopeless by other practitioners, responds to simple dietary control.

Achieving such control requires an understanding of the many factors involved in food sensitivity. Allergists are justifiably proud of their accomplishments during the past several decades in objectively identifying inhalant allergens and providing predictable results in care. To many physicians, and a majority of third-party payers, it seems incomprehensible that a simple, reliable test for food sensitivity is not even on the horizon. Were such a test available, it would be a fairly simple task to have the patient remove the offenders from the diet, thereby controlling the symptoms. Why does such a test not exist? Careful consideration of several points is necessary to understand the magnitude of the problem.

Definition

The first source of confusion is that there is not even a universally accepted definition of food allergy today.[1] To the layperson, and even the nonallergist physician, food "allergy" is usually defined as an adverse reaction by the patient to a food that does not occur in most people consuming that food. To the allergist, this definition is too simple. The definition of food allergy depends on the mechanism producing the reaction, and even this definition is not uniform throughout the medical world.

Food sensitivity is known to involve all parts of the immune system, as well as mechanisms entirely outside the immune system. Among most general allergists in the United States, *allergy* (of whatever type) is defined as an adverse reaction mediated by immunoglobulin E (IgE). This is a Gell and Coombs type I reaction. Reactions of this type represent only a very small percentage of adverse reactions to food, but because of their nature, they have a high degree of visibility. Also, they are the reactions most easily identified by either skin testing or radioallergosorbent testing (RAST). Such tests are rarely needed, however, as the reaction to a food that falls within this category is prompt, obvious, and frequently violent. A type I (anaphylactic) reaction is the only form of allergy easily capable of producing fatal results. The anaphylactic form of food sensitivity usually persists throughout life, so that it is often referred to as *fixed* form of food allergy. Although the patient's sensitivity to a provoking food may diminish if avoidance is practiced during a period of years, it is easily reactivated with future exposure and may remain fully active at all times.

Fixed, anaphylactic, or type I food sensitivity has been estimated to represent between 5 and 20% of all food hypersensitivity. The broad range of estimates stems not from any question of the presence of this form of response, but from the limitations that exist in recognizing the extent of other types of food hypersensitivity, which will be discussed shortly. In the United States, allergic food reactions other than the anaphylactic type are usually designated *hypersensitivity*, and reactions outside the immune system are simply *adverse reactions*. To complicate matters further, in Europe, adverse reactions involving any or all Gell and Coombs categories are usually considered *allergy*, whereas specific adverse reactions outside the immune system are considered *hypersensitivity*. These definitions are by no means universally adhered to, however, and rarely does a contributor to the literature bother to define the terms being used when writing an article. This further compounds the difficulty of interpreting the significance of any study. In 1994, at a major pediatric conference, three articles were presented lamenting the lack of uniformity in defining food sensitivity and proposing carefully thought out definition formats. Unfortunately, no two of the articles were in agreement in their choice of terminology.[2] Thus, it is not difficult to see why confusion reigns concerning the subject of food allergy when the parameters of the problem have not even been adequately defined.

Because this book is designed for clinicians, and especially for physicians newly adding allergy to their practice, the fine points of immunologic definitions of allergy will not be scrupulously observed further in this chapter. For adverse reactions to foods, *allergy*, *sensitivity*, and *hypersensitivity* will be taken to mean an abnormal reaction to a food in one person that is not seen in the general population. The bottom line, after all, is relieving the patient's symptoms. As will be evident in the portion on treating food reactions, this involves dietary manipulation, which serves to treat both immunologic and nonimmunologic reactions alike.

BIOLOGIC PATHWAYS OF FOOD REACTIONS

Immunologic Reactions

Food may act on the body through any of the four immunologic mechanisms defined by Gell and Coombs (which are explained in detail in Chapter 3).[3]

TABLE 14–1. **Mechanisms of immunologic food reactions**

Gell and Coombs type	Mediators
I (anaphylactic)	IgE
II (cytotoxic)	IgG, IgM, complement
III (immune complex)	IgG, complement
IV (cellular)	Sensitized T lymphocytes

In addition to the type I reaction already described, types II, III, and IV have been demonstrated to occur in food allergy. It is felt that the type III reaction is the most common mechanism in food allergy, but actual determinations of the degree to which each Gell and Coombs type occurs have not been made, as accurately identifying such reactions on a clinical basis has not as yet proved practical. It is felt that type II food reactions are probably quite rare. Type IV (cell-mediated) reactions may actually be fairly common in food allergy, but the delay in appearance of symptoms in such reactions makes clinical correlation extremely difficult. The underlying mechanism of the immunologic reactions is shown in Table 14–1.

Clinical Categories

While each division of the immune system may provide a route by which a food may produce an allergic reaction in a patient, the reactions have been clinically divided into *fixed* and *cyclic* types. Fixed food reactions are defined as those that occur regularly when the offending food is ingested in any quantity (even minute amounts). These reactions are rapid in onset and may be severe. As previously noted, such sensitivity is normally sustained throughout life, although it may weaken somewhat during several years if there has been no exposure. Fixed reactions are now considered synonymous with IgE-mediated type I reactions.

   Fixed reactions are always immediate; cyclic food reactions may be immediate or delayed, with the delay ranging from a few hours to as much as 1 to 2 days or more. These reactions, unlike fixed food reactions, are dose- and frequency-related. This means that the food may be eaten on occasion without the patient sustaining a reaction, but if the food is eaten regularly at every meal, or even every day or so, a reaction will occur. The more frequently the food is eaten, the more rapid and pronounced the response may be expected to be. Similarly, a small quantity of an offending food may be eaten without the patient suffering any ill effects, but if a large quantity of the food is consumed, the symptoms will appear. Cyclic food sensitivity is mediated by any component of the immune system other than that involved in the type I Gell and Coombs mechanism.

It is easy to see why identification of a cyclic food offender can be difficult for the physician and virtually impossible for the layperson. In the instance of a delayed reaction, it might be necessary to recall every food eaten during a period of a day or more and make the relevant connection to the reaction. For the average individual, this is not a practical approach. Fortunately, other methods exist for identifying offenders, and these will be discussed later.

Masking

An interesting, and very common, aspect of cyclic food sensitivity is the development of *masking*. In many patients with low-grade but persistent cyclic food allergies, a tendency develops to eat the offending food at every meal, and frequently between meals. Like narcotics addicts, they "crave" the food because a regular dose of the offending substance temporarily relieves some of their symptoms. This temporary improvement is offset by the fact that, overall, the patient's condition is worsened by the offending food. It would be expected that if the food is withdrawn from the patient's diet, a considerable improvement will ensure. This does eventually occur, but in the early stages of withdrawal, the patient frequently complains of an increase in symptoms and must be encouraged to persevere until relief is noted (generally after 4 to 7 days). An offending food can be strongly suspected when the patient's immediate reaction to a discussion of food sensitivity is, "Don't take away my chocolate!" (Or coffee, or whatever the crutch may be.)

Nonimmunologic Reactions

In addition to provoking the immunologic reactions already described, food is able to affect the body through a variety of pathways not involving the immune system. These reactions may be all but impossible to distinguish on the basis of symptoms alone from the immunologic reactions already described. Although many chemical mediators may be involved in various adverse food reactions, the most frequent mediator is histamine, which is contained in mast cells throughout the body. Histamine can be released by both immunologic and nonimmunologic reactions. For example, when certain foods (e.g., strawberries and tomatoes) are ingested, they induce the release of histamine without involving the immune system. Other foods, such as aged cheese, contain preformed histamine that is released on inges-

TABLE 14–2. Mechanisms of nonimmunologic food reactions

1. Food intolerance: abnormal, nonimmunologic reaction to ingested food or additive
   Example: lactose intolerance
2. Food poisoning: reaction caused by endotoxins or exotoxins within the food, or released by contaminating microorganisms or parasites
   Example: *Escherichia coli* gastroenteritis
3. Pharmacologic food reaction: adverse reaction to pharmacologic effects of chemicals found in food or additives, or stimulated by them, that is not immunologic in nature
   Examples: direct effect of caffeine (stimulation), red wine (tyramine headache)
   -release of histamine from strawberries, tomatoes, egg whites, tuna, aged cheese
   -effect of additives (monosodium glutamate)

tion. Table 14–2 lists some of the foods that may induce the release of histamine and related substances on ingestion, producing typical food sensitivity reactions in some patients. Thus, food, unlike inhalant allergens, is capable of affecting the body through a wide variety of mechanisms, many of which produce very similar reactions.

In addition to the specific routes of induction of adverse reactions to foods described above, certain enzyme deficiencies may make foods inaccessible to the system, resulting in symptoms that may be virtually indistinguishable from those of food allergy. Lactase deficiency is a well-known example. These are also noted in Table 14–2.[4]

COMPLICATING FACTORS

Cumulative Reactions and Cross-reactivity

Like inhalants, ingestants (foods) contain a variety of substances, any number of which may be sensitizing. Different foods may contain several such antigens in common. As with inhalants, the number of such antigens shared by different foods determines the degree to which these foods will cross-react. In the case of botanical foods (i.e., fruits and vegetables) such cross-reactivity is common, although frequently unrecognized by either patient or physician. For those without extensive botanical knowledge, specific references may be helpful. Appendix 1 contains a cross-reactivity list providing information that is both useful and interesting. For example, how many laypersons would recognize potato and eggplant as close relatives? This cross-reactivity among foods may easily result in an accumulation of similar antigens in the system from several different foods to which the patient is sensitive. The resultant unrecognized increase in the total load of allergens will affect the pattern of cyclic allergy, which you will recall is affected by both dose and frequency of ingestion. Patients may think that they are eating only a limited amount of a particular food, or eating it at infrequent intervals, but if they are in fact eating other foods of the same family, the result may be the same as if large quantities of the primary offending food are eaten regularly. It is the total amount of the allergen in the system at one time, and/or the frequency with which the body is exposed to the allergen, that determines the reaction. Not only must the individual foods be identified to determine the eating habits of the patient, but food families must also be considered.

In nonbotanical foods (e.g., meats), studies of cross-reactivity are limited. In this group of foods, investigation has mainly involved IgE-mediated food allergy, mainly that caused by crustaceans. As previously noted, IgE-mediated food sensitivity is a relative rarity and usually presents no difficulty in diagnosis, as reactions are prompt and frequently severe. Cyclic food responses are more subtle, and hence more difficult to recognize. The non-IgE-mediated antigenic reactions involving meats have not been extensively studied, and hence knowledge of cross-reactivity within this group is limited. When considering cross-reactivity in the nonbotanical food group, it is largely necessary to proceed by analogy to botanical foods, with the knowledge that such analogy is not yet supported by scientific studies, only clinical observations.

A taxonomic classification of botanical foods seems to correlate with allergenic cross-reactivity with considerable accuracy. The more inbred an organism (whether plant or animal), the greater the number of similar antigens it is likely to harbor within its various species. Plants, including food plants, cross-react extensively within genera. It is a reasonable assumption that animals do the same. The earlier the creature separated from the primordial line, the fewer similar antigens are likely to be encountered. Observation and anecdotal experience seem to support this premise, although actual immunologic confirmation would require more ability to characterize non-IgE-mediated food reactions than is currently available. Like plants, animals are usually classified by at least two scientific names, the first of which represents the genus, the second the species. At times, a third term, the subspecies, is added. The working hypothesis for estimating cross-reactivity in nonbotanical foods is that antigens of animals of the same genus will probably cross-react to a large degree, whereas antigens of animals of different genera are less likely to do so. For example, consider chicken and turkey. Many commercial charts of cross-reactivity list as a group simply "bird." This has never been shown to be a uniform group, any more than is "seafood" a single entity. Chicken (*Gallus domesticus*) is the oldest and most widely distributed form of domestic meat known. All chicken is believed to have been derived from the red jungle fowl of India, and despite extensive manipulation of breeding through the centuries, it probably maintains most of the same allergens originally present. Turkey (*Meleagris gallopavo*), on the other hand, is a bird native to the western hemisphere, domesticated only in the last few centuries. Our current knowledge indicates that clinically there is little if any significant cross-reactivity between chicken and turkey. A similar situation exists between beef and bison. The cow (*Bos domesticus*) is presumed to have evolved from the domesticated water buffalo. The American bison (*Bison bison*), on the other hand, is a New World creature whose meat rarely cross-reacts with beef.

On an even more extensive basis, many laypersons have come to believe that they are sensitive to "seafood." Not only multiple genera but multiple phyla exist in the sea, probably more diverse than those on the land. The person suspected of being allergic to "shellfish" is discussing at least two phyla, Crustacea and Mollusca. Although contamination is always a possibility, as when shrimp larvae become lodged in an oyster's filtration system, true cross-reactivity among shellfish is not a problem.

Appendix 5 lists the genera of some of the common staple meat foods in the typical American diet. It must be stressed that this represents only a starting point from which to explore cross-reactivity. However, it has been proved to be a fairly reasonable approach, as opposed to the substitute foods suggested in some of the commercially circulated literature, which suggest that persons allergic to common meats try whale and hippopotamus! Most allergic patients shop in grocery stores where these are unavailable. When cross-reactivity between meats other than those listed is to be considered, a reasonable approach is to use the same principle already applied to the meat sources described: check the scientific name of the animal in the encyclopedia. The first name is normally the genus. If the genus of the meats is the same, there will probably be strong cross-reactivity. If the genera are different, there is less chance that they will cross-react. It must be borne in mind that this is simply a guide. There may at times be some cross-reactivity between different genera, and a person may be sensitive to a variety of meats of different genera. However, consideration of cross-reactivity based on the scientific name of a food provides a useful starting point.

Concomitant Food Reactions

In addition to cross-reactivity between various types of botanical food, cross-reactivity frequently exists between inhaled pollens and ingested foods of the same family. Thus, the ingestion by a patient with active inhalant allergy of a cross-reacting food may produce a greater reaction than expected. This is generally called a *concomitant food reaction*. Such cross-reactivities between inhalants and foods are generally confirmed by RAST inhibition (Fig. 14–1), which is simply a precise technique for confirming the presence of similar or identical antigens in different substances.

The classic example of inhalant and food cross-reactivity is that between grasses and cereal grains (which are in reality grasses). The phenomenon has also been demonstrated between such apparently diverse items as apple (the fruit) and birch (the pollen), as well as ragweed and members of the gourd family (watermelon, canteloupe). A more extensive list of cross-reacting inhalants and foods is found in Appendix 1. The clinical significance of concomitant reactions is that all allergens, although they enter the body by different routes, contribute to the total allergic load. For example, a person mildly sensitive to both apple and birch pollen might have no reaction on eating an apple in the fall, but when birch trees are pollinating, eating the same amount of apple might precipitate a severe reaction. This type of reaction is one more complexity to confuse and confound the allergist and the allergic patient.

Speed of Digestion

Digestive action does not always proceed at the same rate. As a result, foods in the digestive tract are not all uniformly spaced. Even though a food is eaten at the same time each day, if digestion (for one reason or another) is proceeding at different speeds on different days, the food may accumulate in the digestive tract at a given time on one day and be largely absent at that time on another. Food is thus exposed to different quantities of digestive enzymes and absorbed into the circulation in a less predictable manner than is generally imagined. This affects dietary analysis that attempts to identify a cause-and-effect relationship between a food eaten and the symptoms produced, and also complicates treatment by dietary rotation, a technique discussed in the section of this chapter on treatment of food allergy.

Antigen Alteration

As if the above problems were not enough, simply identifying a basic food to which a patient is allergic does not necessarily clarify all the possible ramifications of the situation. With inhalants, the offending substance is delivered to the nasal mucosa in its natural, unaltered state. Although some

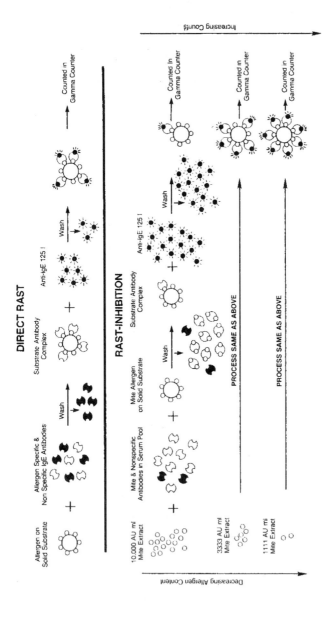

FIGURE 14–1. RAST inhibition is performed as a modification of the radioallergosorbent test (RAST) to determine cross-reactivity between various immunoglobulin E (IgE)-mediated allergens, whether inhalant, food, or both. First, one of the antigens to be tested is serially diluted. The antigen dilutions are then added in measured amounts to a patient's serum known to contain specific IgE for the other antigen to be tested. After this is done, a RAST is run for the second antigen. If the two antigens cross-react, some of the specific IgE will be bound before the serum is exposed to the RAST disk. This will make less unbound IgE available to bind to the RAST disk. The RAST reading will therefore be lower than that seen without exposure to the first antigen. The degree to which the reading drops with each serial dilution is a measure of the cross-reactivity between the two antigens. (From Mason WW, Ward WA. Otolaryngolic Clinics of North America. Philadelphia: W.B. Saunders; 1992:108; with permission.)

foods are usually eaten raw, more commonly foods are processed in some manner before being eaten. This may be by cooking, fermenting, marinating, or any number of methods designed to vary or enhance the palatability of the food. All such procedures are capable of altering the antigens present in the food, and the degree and pattern of such alteration are not predictable. Although some of the antigens of the basic food remain, others are changed, and for this reason the quantity of the basic antigen may be reduced. In additions, new antigens may be added during processing. For example, a patient sensitive to cow's milk would be expected to show some milk sensitivity when eating cheese, but the sensitivity might be less than that displayed when whole cow's milk is ingested. Also, other allergens may have been created by alteration of the antigens of cow's milk during processing into cheese. This same situation may occur when beef or chicken is cooked. This alteration of antigens is one of the factors that has limited the effectiveness of testing for food allergies by using ''pure'' material prepared by reference laboratories. The material used in testing does not truly represent the material to which the patient is actually exposed.

Additives

In addition to the antigen alteration produced by the processing of foods, most foods, even after processing, have various additives applied, either by the person preparing the food or the person consuming the food, before it is eaten. This range of additives, limited only by the tastes of the persons involved, may range from some salt and pepper to spices, flavor enhancers such as monosodium glutamate, lemon, garlic, and a host of other materials. Each carries its own antigens, which may have their own individual effects, or some of the antigens in the additive may be the same as those of the food to which they have been added. In this case, there will be a cumulative effect comparable with that of eating two or more foods in the same family.

A great deal of material has appeared in the literature during the past two decades about the effect of intrinsic or ''invisible'' chemicals present in foods. These include pesticides, antibiotics, and coloring agents. Although such substances may undoubtedly affect some persons, there remains much disagreement as to the degree and nature of their effect. Realistically, attempting to include such substances in an evaluation of food allergy is beyond the scope of the developing allergist, who will encounter enough difficulty in identifying major offenders and trying to provide a significant degree of control by limiting these. A reasonable approach to the problem of intrinsic chemicals is to advise the patient that if, after as much as possible has been done to control food allergy, problems persist when food from a particular source is eaten, that source should be changed. For the patient who is truly this sensitive, organic food sources with no additives are available.

Multiplicity of Target Organs

It has already been stressed that the portal of entry for an allergen has little effect on the site or type of eventual reaction. Although it is true that inhalant allergens primarily affect the respiratory tree, even this is not always the case. Food allergens show no such limitations in their range of action. Before the allergic reaction can occur, the foods must be broken down and digested, and the digested products absorbed into the circulation and carried to the target organ. This much is not difficult to understand, but why allergens circulating throughout the body should affect certain organs and not others is still not understood. Virtually any organ or organ system can serve as a target organ, and the organ is not specific to the food. In other words, cow's milk may produce a rash in one person and asthma in another. The target organ in the first person is the skin, and in the second it is the lungs. The reaction is specific to the patient; if milk causes asthma in one patient, milk will normally continue to cause asthma in the same patient. It will not switch to causing a rash. Of course, there may be more than one target organ from the beginning. Milk, for example, might cause both asthma and diarrhea as soon as the patient becomes sensitized. If this is the case, the symptom pattern may fluctuate in severity over time, varying with the amount of milk consumed and the interval between exposures, but rarely will the pattern change. Symptoms developing in another target organ usually indicate a sensitivity to a different food.

Virtually any organ system in the body may be a target organ for adverse reactions to food. The symptoms depend on the nature of the target organ, not on the type of food, and are not greatly influenced by the type of immunologic or nonimmunologic mechanism causing the reaction. As described in Chapter 3 and reiterated in the portion of this chapter on the nature of food reactions, most such reactions involve the release of histamine or other similar mediators into the tissues of the target organ, which in turn produce tissue edema and inflammation. It can be quite difficult to determine the specific mechanism involved except for the clinical difference between fixed and cyclic reactions. If the target organ is the external carotid artery complex, for example, a migraine headache will result. If the target organ is the intestinal tract, cramping and diarrhea may be expected. The reaction within the tissue at a cellular level is very similar, but the organ is different and hence the symptoms are different.

The "Leaky Gut Syndrome"

Yet another factor may even further complicate the picture of food allergy. Every physician is familiar with the patient who reports being "allergic to everything." Actually, clinical studies on food allergy worldwide have been in agreement that very rarely are patients truly allergic to more than five or six foods. These "universally allergic" patients, however, appear to react adversely to an immense range of foods. Frequently, such reactions have not been a lifelong problem but have developed within a short period of time. This apparent contradiction in patterns, which is not uncommon, can be easily explained.

The mature intestinal tract, functioning properly, is a sophisticated immunologic filter. Food substances are not absorbed from the intestine into the circulation until digestion has broken them down into such small micromolecules that the immune system tends to consider them as building blocks rather than potential offenders. The intestinal tract, however, is easily shocked, and when such shocks occur, the tract becomes much more permeable and absorbs macromolecules of food, which then produce reactions that can mimic true allergy. Several factors can shock the intestinal tract to this degree. They include infection, infancy, and immunologic insult.[4]

Infection is a complex subject, but it is necessary only that the allergist realize that infection can give rise to increased gut permeability.

The infant has not yet developed a mature intestinal tract, and as a result, varying degrees of leakage of macromolecules are common. This is the reason why a small child frequently strongly manifests allergic problems although skin testing and/or RAST indicates little or no response. Skin testing and/or RAST is reliable for IgE-mediated allergy, but major amounts of IgE usually have not developed in infants even if they have the genetic makeup to allow such an abnormality to appear. Prolonged or frequent exposure to allergens is required for significant amounts of specific IgE to develop. As stated elsewhere, it is often of little value to test a child for pollen allergy before the age of 5 or 6 years, and even sensitivity to perennial allergens (e.g., dust, mold, and pet epidermals) is usually minimal before the age of 2 or 3 years. On the other hand, the intestinal tract at birth and shortly thereafter may be "porous." The child with this condition may be expected to demonstrate a wide range of food allergy symptoms, including nasal and eustachian tube congestion. It has been frequently observed that the vast majority of cases of recurrent otitis media appearing before the age of 1 can be controlled simply by eliminating cow's milk from the diet. For the child with major allergy symptoms of any type, analyzing the diet and replacing the major staples (in the infant, usually the formula) with another basic food type will frequently reduce or eliminate the problem. It is reassuring to the parents to note that most such problems will resolve by the age of 6 or 7 years as the intestinal tract matures, provided no permanent damage to the affected target organ occurs in the meantime.

Most pertinent to the present discussion is the effect of true food allergy on the gut. When the gut is exposed to true allergenic offenders, the organ may become shocked, resulting in the apparent development of a multitude of food sensitivities. When the true offenders are identified and removed from the diet, the gut rapidly recovers, and the patient is able to tolerate many or all of the other foods previously considered by the patient to be allergens. To some degree, this leaky gut syndrome is probably related to an untenable increase in the overall total allergic load.

Summary of the Problem of Food Reactions

A person with multiple symptoms, especially if they are not always manifested concurrently, may be suspected of being sensitive to several foods, each causing different symptoms through involvement of different target organs. Although both specific immunologic and nonimmunologic pathways are involved in food hypersensitivity, it is also true that a single food may utilize more than one pathway, and one patient may have more than one type of reaction under way at any one time. Allergenic foods may shock the gut. Foods may act in combination with each other or with inhalants. All these factors explain the virtual impossibility of developing a simple test for food sensitivity. In analyzing the results of the multiple routes and multiple possible reactions, it is necessary to look at the bottom line; determine the specific reactions that have occurred, attempt to identify the cause-and-effect relationship (not an easy task), and maintain a high degree of suspicion for food reactions. Many patients dismissed as hypochondriacs have been cleared of many or all of their symptoms and returned to productivity by successful treatment of food sensitivities.

IDENTIFYING CYCLIC FOOD SENSITIVITIES

It bears repeating that fixed food allergies are easily identified. The reaction is prompt, obvious, and frequently severe. Should any test be needed, an

---

NURSE'S NOTE

There are many types of food reactions. Immediate (Gell and Coombs type I, IgE-mediated) food reactions always carry the potential for anaphylaxis, and foods known to cause them should be avoided indefinitely by the patient. Cyclic food reactions, generally Gell and Coombs type III, may be treated successfully by dietary manipulation. However, this requires careful detective work by the patient and members of the allergy team.

The allergy nurse or assistant is often the person to whom the allergy patient turns for answers, and so this person must be knowledgeable in the area of food families to aid the patient with suspected food allergy. Lists of "hidden sources" of common allergenic foods are available from many antigen suppliers.

When patients are asked to complete a diet diary, it is important that they realize that they will not be "judged" on the results. Otherwise, what is often returned is what patients *think* they *should* be eating, not what they actually consume. If a dietitian is not available in the allergy office, the allergy nurse or assistant is often asked for help in planning a diet that provides adequate nutrients while avoiding offending foods. For example, the patient on a milk-free diet must consider calcium supplementation. Fortunately, it is often possible to obtain this information from commercial sources and books on food allergy.

IgE RAST for the suspected foods will clearly identify the culprit. Identifying food allergens involved in cyclic reactions is more difficult because of their subtlety, tendency to be delayed in presentation, and variation according to the quantity and frequency of ingestion of the causative foods.

When all the factors involved in cyclic food sensitivity are considered, it must appear that any identification of individual offending foods would be a virtual impossibility. It is probably true that if all the contributing factors had to be considered, solving the problem would be impractical, if not impossible. Fortunately, we are helped in this regard by a well-known aspect of allergy known as the *allergic load*. Simply stated, the more offenders present in the system, the worse the problem. This is seen in the priming effect in inhalant allergy and cumulative effects in food sensitivity. Conversely, the more major offenders that can be identified and removed from the system, the better the body's immune system is able to cope with whatever offenders remain. If, therefore, the major offending foods affecting a patient can be identified and removed from the diet, the patient should improve significantly. With control of whatever inhalant allergies are present, still further improvement would be expected. The goal of the allergy team should therefore be to identify as many true major offending elements as possible and to control them.

Although the means does not yet exist to identify all food sensitivities by laboratory tests, on a clinical basis it is generally agreed by experts throughout the world that it is rare for a patient to be significantly sensitive to more than five or six foods. Combinations, additives, and variations in preparation may alter the overall allergen distribution somewhat, but if the basic major offending foods can be identified, dietary manipulation can effectively reduce the patient's total allergic load.

Commercial Tests for Food Allergy

It deserves repetition that other than the IgE RAST for fixed food reactions, no uniformly reliable in vitro test is available for food allergy. Through the years, many tests for food allergy have been offered, beginning with the now extinct cytotoxic test. None has withstood the challenge of reproducibility, even within the same laboratory. Although these tests may have a basic validity, their practicality has been nullified by the inability to obtain the same result twice. In the heyday of such tests, many patients were advised to avoid all the foods giving a positive result on the tests (frequently 20 or more). Unfortunately, a test performed at another laboratory might provide an entirely different list of foods. The end result was condemnation of such tests by the Food and Drug Administration. New tests continue to be promoted, some with little documentation of their validity.

Several screening tests for food sensitivity are currently available; some of these are being promoted commercially and are gaining varying degrees of acceptance. Example are the IgG RAST, the antigen leukocyte antibody test (ALCAT), and the enzyme-linked immunosorbent assay/activated cell test (ELISA/ACT),[3] which are discussed in Chapter 18. Even if such food screening tests are employed, the results provided must be interpreted in the light of clinical confirmation.

The underlying weakness in most in vitro food tests is that they tend to test a single route of reaction, whereas food sensitivity may involve a variety of mechanisms, with all the possible variables already discussed. Thus, the gold standard for the diagnosis of food allergy remains confirmation of the suspected offending food or foods by appropriate in vivo challenge.

Identifying Possible Offenders

The Food Diary

Rather than using the "shotgun" approach inherent in the commercial screening tests, using a food diary can usually provide the same results. People are habit eaters, although many do not realize it. At this point, we can consider only basic foods, without regard to the alterations in antigens and additives discussed above (although there is some benefit in including these, as will be discussed shortly). A typical person will go through the entire gamut of frequently eaten foods in a 14-day period, and foods eaten infrequently enough not to become evident during this period are unlikely to be involved in a cyclic food reaction. The first step, then, is too obtain a diary of foods eaten by the patient during a 14-day period. A patient cannot do this from memory, nor can the patient be depended on to list all commonly eaten foods broken down into types (e.g., corn, wheat, milk). Most laypersons do not know the basic ingredients of food dishes, but simply recognize the dish itself. The best way to obtain such a diary is to provide the patient with a 14-day diary form such as that shown in Appendix 3. This form can be personalized with the office letterhead and may also contain the patient's name, dates covered, and any other information desired.

The patient still needs instruction in filling out the diary. A complete list of foods must be provided, broken down by basic ingredients. For example, there is no such thing as "salad." There is lettuce, tomato, celery, radishes, and other ingredients. Usually, there is dressing, the type of which should be reported, including the brand if eaten at home. Everything ingested should be reported, including snacks, medications, drinks, and anything else taken by mouth. It is sometimes beneficial to give the patient a list of hidden sources of suspected foods, but this should usually be reserved for the next stage of diagnosis unless a very limited number of allergens are suspected, such as milk sensitivity in a toddler. Trying to be conscientious in filling out the diary and at the same time looking for hidden sources of food may prove too much for the average patient at this point. It is likely that not every food will be identified, such as all the ingredients in a stew, but most of the commonly eaten foods should have a place in the diary.

Many 14-day food diaries provide a place in which to record symptoms. This may be of value, but frequently the patient becomes so concerned with trying to relate symptoms to the foods eaten most recently that a reminder needs to be included that most cyclic food allergies are not immediately manifested after ingestion of the offending food. The patient should concentrate on providing as accurate a record as possible and leave the interpretation to the allergy care provider.

Interpreting the Diary

Once the diary has been completed, it should be returned to the office. If the diary is mailed, advise patients to keep a copy. Few things are more frustrating than to have a carefully completed diary lost in the mail. There is an advantage in having patients either mail the diary to the office or drop it off without seeing the doctor. It may take some time to interpret the results, and patients making an appointment and bringing the diary in with them generally expect immediate instructions on how to proceed. At this point, it is up to the allergy care provider to analyze the diary and determine which items are consumed regularly enough to be the likely source of a cyclic food allergy.

Before analyzing the diary, the person performing the analysis must have a reliable list of hidden sources of common basic foods. Before the food can produce an allergic reaction, it must be digested and absorbed; hence, the form in which the food is eaten is of less importance than the presence and quantity of the basic food itself. Appendix 4 contains lists of hidden forms of most of the common foods that frequently cannot be recognized after they have been incorporated in a prepared form. Such foods include milk, wheat, eggs, yeast, corn, and soy. Such foods as tomato, lettuce, beef, and pork are equally important but are easily recognized. Armed with the list of hidden food sources, the person performing the analysis should mark the diary each time the food appears. Probably the easiest way to do this is to acquire a number of highlighters and have each color represent a particular food or food family. This is a time when a knowledge of cross-reactivity becomes important. With the list of hidden sources of common foods and the lists of food families found in Appendix 1 and Appendix 5, preparing a chart in which each hidden food and each food family are represented by a high-lighted color is fairly straight forward. The appropriate color is then used to highlight each food, hidden or not, and each food family as it appears in the diary. The result is a kaleidoscope of color covering the diary sheet.

A certain amount of common sense needs to be applied to this stage of analysis. In going over the hidden sources of major foods, it is not difficult to determine that although the food in question may be present, the amount may be very small. Because the effects of cyclic foods vary with dose and frequency of consumption, it may not be necessary to highlight a food when only tiny amounts are involved.

The usual result of a diary analysis is that an immediate glance shows a major predominance of a very few colors. This clearly indicates the major foods that need to be considered as potential allergens. Rarely will more than five or six foods be involved, and usually fewer. Among these foods are the most likely allergenic offenders. An appointment may now be made for the patient to prepare for the next stage of testing.

If one of the in vitro screening tests had been used, it would have brought things only to this stage. Even if a screening test result is positive, indicating some element of immunologic activity, the range of possible target organs makes it impossible to relate the findings to the patient's symptoms accurately. In addition, about a third of the body appears to be allergenically "silent." Even if immunologic events are occurring, no symptoms result.[4] There is no need to pursue food studies in the absence of symptoms, as eliminating foods cannot relieve symptoms that do not exist.

Preparing the Patient for Challenge

At this stage, the number of potential offending foods has been reduced to a few that can be investigated individually. It is now time to bring the patient in for another appointment, present the results of the dietary analysis, and proceed with withdrawal, followed by challenge with the probable offenders and evaluation of the symptoms produced.

It is frequently a good idea at this visit to show the patient the highlighted diary. As noted, many patients do not realize that they are in fact habit eaters, consuming the same foods or food families on a highly regular basis. The highlighted diary makes the pattern immediately evident and encourages the patient to proceed diligently with the challenge.

At this point, the question is frequently raised of how many foods should be considered for challenge food testing. The factor of allergic load needs to be considered here. Frequently, in analyzing a diet diary, only two or three foods stand out. If these prove to be major offenders, it is frequently possible to obtain good results by controlling only these. In any case, this is a good place to start. More challenges can be made later if needed, based on the same diary.

The Oral Food Challenge

All schools of approach to the diagnosis of food allergy agree that the "gold standard" in food testing is elimination and challenge. What is not always agreed on is the duration of the elimination portion of the study and the nature of the challenge. The authors agree with the concept based on the clinical observations of Rinkel and others more than three decades ago that an ideal period of elimination is 4 days, with a strong challenge on the fifth day. At the time that Rinkel made this observation, no immunologic data were available to support his recommendation, which was made on a clinical basis. The actual format of withdrawal and challenge was established before the principle could be studied and has continued to prove clinically effective.

With the better knowledge of the functions of the immune system available today, a reasonable explanation, which fits the clinical picture, has been proposed for the time frame described. It is generally agreed that most delayed or cyclic food reactions are the result of a Gell and Coombs type III reaction, in which immune complexes (large molecular structures formed from a combination of an antigen and antibody in the blood) attach to the walls of the small vessels in a target organ, damaging the walls and producing a leakage of fluid and inflammatory substances into the tissues of the target organ. Because both antigen and antibody are needed to form immune complexes, either a high level of antigen with less antibody or a high level of antibody with less antigen results in the formation of fewer immune complexes than does a more or less balanced number of each. When the food in question is withdrawn totally from the system, the antigen available is progressively metabolized and leaves the circulation, leaving unattached antibody present in excess. This situation peaks at about the fourth day. When the food in question is abruptly added during the challenge, if the food is in fact allergenic and antibodies to it are present in the system, a large number of immune complexes will be formed rapidly and will affect the target organ, producing a strong onset of symptoms. If the challenge is delayed for several more days, the number of antibodies will gradually diminish, so that fewer are available to form immune complexes. After about 10 days, producing symptoms by challenge becomes difficult. Thus, a challenge should ideally be performed after not fewer than 4 nor more than 7 days of avoidance of the food being tested.

The testing consists of two parts: elimination and challenge.

Elimination

To perform the oral challenge test properly, care must be taken to eliminate the food to be tested from the body as completely as possible. Any food still in the system will provide antigens, which will reduce the marked imbalance between antigen and antibody that is responsible for the challenge reaction. At this point, the patient should be supplied with a list of all the hidden sources of the food to be tested, advised to eliminate all of them, and (to ensure compliance) to read all labels on commercially prepared food. It is also necessary that the patient be aware of terms used in packaging that may not be recognized. Casein and whey, for example, are derived from milk and contain milk antigens. Because only one food will be subjected to oral challenge at a time, it is not necessary at this point that the patient know hidden sources of other foods. This will come later, when these are to be challenged. If it is necessary to identify the hidden sources of only one food at a time, the demand on the patient is considerably less. It is also wise to remind the patient at this time that total elimination is not a permanent requirement but is necessary only for the duration of the test. Such reassurance frequently prevents patients from balking at any possible future demands. Of course, all patients would prefer to have the physician be responsible for all the testing, without any participation or effort required on their part. Unfortunately, this is not possible.

How complete must the elimination be before challenge? Despite all attempts at total elimination, it is still possible for some food from an unrecognized source to slip into the diet. This does not negate the test results, but it does attenuate the response in proportion to the amount of the food consumed. The test can still be completed; it is simply necessary to watch more closely for symptoms.

During the withdrawal portion of testing, patients will often complain of feeling worse for the first day or two, as their body continues to "crave" the food to which they have become "addicted." The chronic ingestion of the offending food has allowed them to achieve something of a balance between antigen and antibody, which they maintain by continually eating the food. This balance between antigen and antibody is upset when the antigen is withdrawn. However, by the fourth day, an improvement in existing symptoms and the patient's sense of well-being generally indicates that the food being withdrawn is probably a true offender.

Challenge

The food to be challenged, and only this food, is to be eaten in quantity on the fifth day. In the traditional approach, the food to be challenged is eaten in its purest form, prepared by boiling. For example, if eggs have been eliminated for 4 days and oral challenge is to be on the fifth day, two eggs would be eaten for breakfast, boiled and with no additives, not even salt or pepper. For the purist, the eggs should be boiled in spring water, and nothing else should be taken by mouth during the challenge period but spring water.

If eggs are in fact an offender, all the patient's symptoms should appear, generally at an exaggerated level. One of the benefits of the oral challenge is that the symptoms precipitated are normally those produced by the food, but to an enhanced degree. This both serves to convince the patient that the food tested is indeed the offender, and allows the physician to see what the symptoms actually are. It is wise to keep a broad outlook at this point. Remember, the number of possible target organs is virtually unlimited, and it is not unusual for an oral food challenge to precipitate totally unexpected symptoms. A person having symptoms of an allergic cough, for example, might not cough on challenge but exhibit a generalized urticaria. This is not a failure of the test, but rather indicates that the physician was unable to connect the food being tested with the symptoms it produced. Because there is no way of predicting the target organ, the test may give the patient and physician an insight into the cause of other symptoms. When this occurs, questioning will almost invariably elicit a report that these symptoms previously existed but no apparent link to allergy was suspected.

If the initial challenge at breakfast does not produce a response, the same food should be eaten in the same manner at lunch. If there is still no response, it may be presumed that the food is in fact not an offender and that the patient may eat it with impunity. Other foods are now open to testing, with exactly the same procedure followed for each. For practical purposes, only one basic food can be tested in a week by this method, as it takes a few days for the effects of the challenge to wear off.

Although the oral challenge is the most definitive means of identifying a food offender, it is time-consuming and therefore most practical when only one or two offenders are felt likely to be present.

The traditional approach concentrates on identifying the basic food elements (e.g., corn, wheat, milk), and for this it is quite accurate. However, it does not account for the modifications of allergens produced by cooking or otherwise processing a food, and hence may miss some sensitivities. This has been demonstrated in studies involving the dimethylsulfoxide food test (DIMSOFT),[5] in which freeze-dried food extracts are mixed with dimethylsulfoxide (DMSO), which carries nonwater-soluble food extracts through the skin. This technique is further described in Chapter 18. In obtaining extracts for use in the DIMSOFT, it was found that basic, freeze-dried food in the raw form did not produce the responses that were obtained when food that had been processed for eating was used in the test. For example, roast chicken produced much stronger responses than the commercially available basic chicken extract, which is made from raw chicken. As a modification of the oral challenge test, if the traditional challenge result is negative or equivocal when ''pure'' challenge material is used (e.g., boiled beef), it may prove worth while to perform the challenge with the food in exactly the form in which the patient usually consumes it (i.e., roast beef). In this case, it is wise to take the ingested material from the center of the roast, avoiding the outermost surface of the prepared food, where the greatest effects of additives would be found. This challenge may not be as pure, but it is more in line with normal lifestyle exposure. Of course, as a practical matter, antigen alteration will occur to a degree in the traditional test, as the patient is not expected to perform a challenge with raw eggs or raw chicken. Boiling is expected to alter the basic allergens less than other forms of preparation, but this has never been actually proved. However, roast chicken may be antigenically somewhat different from boiled chicken. This modification cannot be applied in every case because if the patient generally consumes wheat in the form of bread, which contains numerous other ingredients (egg, milk, yeast), the more traditional method of testing (e.g., cream of wheat) is necessary.

Alternatives to the Oral Challenge

The oral challenge as described above is generally considered the gold standard of this approach to food testing. Whatever other screening tests may have been used previously, or if the dietary history has been used alone, the oral challenge should be performed to confirm the findings. Only in this way can the clinical significance of exposure or test results be confirmed.

The oral challenge, however, has its limitations, as described. The primary limitation is the time necessary to complete the study; usually, only one food can be tested for in a week. There are two ways to speed the diagnostic process, although neither is as easy to perform as the oral challenge test. These tests are the elemental diet and the modified fast.

Elemental Diet

Actually, the elemental diet may be an even more definitive test for the presence of food allergy than the oral challenge, but it is far less widely used. Like so many things in medicine (and in life), the most definitive test is also the most difficult to perform. When the result is positive (i.e., demonstrating the presence of food allergy), this test also allows a variety of foods to be tested in short order. The most difficult aspect of the test is to obtain the patient's cooperation for the elimination part, and then to select and administer the test challenges properly after the period of elimination.

It takes 4 to 5 days for a food to be metabolized completely and eliminated from the body. In the oral challenge test, an elimination period of 4 days is selected, as thereafter the level of antibodies begins to decrease significantly. After 5 days of no exposure to foods with any significant potential for sensitization, the patient's system is essentially free of these foods. Whatever symptoms have been induced by food sensitivity should be greatly reduced and, in most cases, gone by this point. If no change has occurred by the end of 5 days, it is generally safe to assume that food allergy is not playing a significant role in symptom production. The question now arises of how to get the patient through the 5-day period with no foods of allergenic potential. In some studies, a pure fast has been undertaken, allowing the patient nothing but spring water. However, when this is done the body undergoes a degree of catabolic metabolism, and it is frequently difficult to determine whether symptom reduction has occurred as a result of this change in the metabolic state or because of the removal of offending foods. A better solution is to use an "elemental diet" during this time. This is a diet consisting of a food so completely degraded antigenically that the immune system does not react to it, although it still provides adequate nutrition. One such food, Tolorex, has been used effectively for this purpose. Originally designed for astronauts to provide nutrition with a minimum of residue, the food was found fortuitously to have essentially no allergenic potential. Because there is a market for nonallergenic foods, more will almost certainly become available with time.

The disadvantage of Tolorex is twofold. The first is boredom; no other food can be consumed for 5 full days. The second is flavor. Although there has been some improvement in flavor over the years, most people depending on Tolorex complain bitterly. If the patient is adequately motivated, a diet restricted to Tolorex and water for a 5-day period will be the most definitive test for the presence or absence of food allergy. If the symptoms clear or show major improvement, the cause is undoubtedly a food sensitivity. If no improvement occurs, further searching for food allergy is likely to be a waste of time and effort. Tolorex is available without prescription through major pharmacies.

Elemental Diet Challenge   Let us assume that the elemental diet elimination period has been completed successfully and that the patient's symptoms have markedly improved. There are still enough antibodies in the circulation after 5 days to produce a strong reaction if an appropriate antigen is consumed. With the traditional oral challenge, only a single food is removed from the diet; with the elemental diet, the body is relieved of all food antigens, and any potential allergen may be used as a challenge. The benefit is the ability to challenge with a succession of foods during a very short period. The caveat is that when a food challenge produces a reaction, the study must be ended, as no further challenges can be performed until all the immune complexes have been cleared and the symptoms produced by the challenge have disappeared. By this time, further challenges will not usually be productive. Thus, the pattern is reversed from that of the single-food challenge, in which the most likely suspect is withdrawn and challenged first.

The elemental diet followed by challenge is particularly useful when a variety of foods all appear to be potential offenders and the dietary history has not provided a suitably small number of candidates to make the oral challenge the approach of choice. When the challenge is performed after the elemental diet fast, the foods to be tested are prepared in the same manner as for the oral challenge, either in their purest form (as in the basic traditional challenge) or in the form most frequently consumed. When the challenge is performed, however, the sequence is different. The goal of the test is to identify foods that are probably not offenders, based on the dietary history, and that will provide a reasonable diet while further investigations are being made. The usual pattern is to challenge with three foods a day: one at breakfast, one at midday, and one at dinner time. With the body depleted of all antigens, a second challenge later in the day is not usually necessary. The following day, challenge with another three foods may be carried out in the same manner. The same sequence may be repeated if necessary for up to 10 days, after which the reaction is usually minimal even if the food is an offender. This sequence would allow 15 foods to be tested by challenge. Remembering that it is quite rare for more than five or six foods to be significant offenders, this program should allow ample range to test as necessary if reasonably careful screening has been done.

Variations on this format are possible. When a rush procedure is necessary, challenge with two to three foods may be performed at each meal. When a reaction results, however, not only must the rest of the testing be discontinued, but each of the foods included in the group causing the reaction must be tested later by oral challenge independently, to determine which one caused the reaction.

It should be borne in mind that this method is so distasteful for many patients that only a few complete the fast. Care must be taken in the challenge sequence, as when an offender has been identified, the study is over, and encouraging a patient to repeat the study to identify other offenders is most unlikely to meet with acceptance.

Modified Fast or Hypoallergenic Diet

As mentioned, the elemental diet is quite definitive, but in only a very limited number of cases, in which the patient is extraordinarily motivated, is it ever carried to completion. The patient may start with enthusiasm only to abandon the Tolorex within a day or two. A variation on the elemental diet that is less reliable, but that is much more likely to be accepted by the patient, involves selecting a diet to be used exclusively for the 5 days of elimination that is as limited as possible, contains no foods or food families in the patient's normal diet, and is prepared without seasoning or additives. This diet is sometimes referred to as "eating all you want of everything you don't like." The method involves a great deal of effort in selecting the diet contents and still may be affected by some unrecognized cross-reactivity, but it often provides an approach more acceptable to the patient than does the elemental diet. Aside from the selection of diet, this modified fast is performed in the same manner as the elemental diet, with challenge after 5 days.

Summary of Dietary Testing

There are any number of publications covering various innovative approaches to the diagnosis of food allergy. This book is designed for the physician just adding allergy to the practice, or for the physician treating inhalant allergy and becoming frustrated with results that are clearly less than optimal. It is not wise for the physician at this stage of development to undertake diagnostic or therapeutic procedures that are questioned by a significant portion of the medical community. In this text, the diagnostic and therapeutic techniques presented involve only dietary manipulation, an approach that has several advantages. First, it is accepted as valid by all elements of the medical community. Second, no special equipment or training is required. Third, as has often been said by the authors, at no time during the testing does cold steel touch quivering flesh. Any physician, regardless of experience or specialty background, who employs this approach will not be open to criticism, and food-allergic patients will obtain relief in direct proportion to their cooperation in the testing and treatment program.

TREATMENT OF FOOD ALLERGY

Before food allergy can be treated, the offending foods, or at least the major offenders, must be identified. Once this has been done by employing the techniques described, treatment may be undertaken. It must be stressed that, in the beginning at least, manipulating the diet to control the major offenders may be quite adequate to relieve the patient's symptoms. The more foods that are placed in the "avoid" category, the more complicated dietary manipulation will be and the more easily the patient may become discouraged. Three axioms may help the physician plan the patient's treatment:

1. Rarely are more than five or six foods significant offenders.

2. The concept of allergic load applies. If enough of the major offenders are removed, the body's normal immunologic resilience will usually be able to control the rest. Remember that cyclic food reactions are dose- and frequency-related, so that minor amounts of allergenic foods remaining in the diet when used in preparation of foodstuffs will not negate the success of the dietary control. The more complete the elimination, the better the control, but a reasonable compromise is acceptable.

3. If removal of the major offenders is not adequate, additional foods may always be added to the "avoid" list later without disturbing the initial approach, and if the patient has improved somewhat, the additional restrictions are more likely to be accepted.

With these axioms in mind, the approaches to dietary manipulation may be considered. These are simple and straightforward, and are based on the identification of foods as offenders by elimination and challenge.

Elimination

In preparation for the oral challenge test, the patient has already been provided with a list of hidden sources of common allergenic foods, which may have been taken from the lists in the appendixes. Some of the foods for which sensitivity has been tested will probably have produced no symptoms during the oral challenge, and these need not be avoided further. Those producing strong reactions during challenge should now be grouped in order of the severity of the reactions produced, or according to their prevalence in the diet. The most important factor is probably the severity of the reactions, as this will have the greatest effect on the patient's comfort. Less important, but still significant, are foods to which the patient showed a definite but less severe reaction on challenge and that are used very heavily in the diet. These may produce a low-grade but persistent and significant effect on the patient's health. The patient should be made aware of this, and if such foods can be excluded from the diet during the elimination period, so much the better. If these foods are too ubiquitous to be totally eliminated, or if the total number of foods under consideration (including both those causing more severe reactions and those causing less severe reactions but frequently consumed) is simply too much to cope with, even some reduction of exposure to these secondary culprits should provide a significant improvement.

The patient has now been provided with a list of both types of offenders (major and secondary), identified by the oral challenge, and the hidden sources of each. It is time for a conference with the patient. Simply sending the patient out with these lists is highly unlikely to produce optimal results. It is expected that the patient will not be seen for some time after starting this diet, so initial support and reassurance are needed. The patient will almost certainly have questions regarding how to proceed, and there are certain things that almost every patient needs to know:

1. The more completely the offending foods are eliminated, the better the results that can be expected. However, cyclic food allergy is dose- and frequency-related, so an occasional lapse in strict compliance with the diet will not compromise the overall result. If there is a major occasion (e.g., a birthday party or a major holiday) when the offending food is eaten, only a slight setback should be expected. It is only when the offending foods are eaten repeatedly that the benefits the patient hopes to achieve will be lost.

2. Complete elimination of the offending foods for an indefinite period is not necessary. Once the immune system has lost a large degree of its sensitivity to these foods, they may be introduced in moderation without compromising the result. This will be discussed in more detail in the section on reintroduction and rotation.

3. Food sensitivity is not the only factor that can affect the patient's health. Because of the normal human desire for immediate and perfect results, patients attempting to follow a diet, who ''sacrifice'' some favorite foods, tend to expect perfect health to follow. It is usually necessary to remind patients that other factors affect the body. Respiratory infections can occur, digestive upsets unrelated to allergenic foods are still possible, and things other than food may cause headaches. In addition, the majority of food-sensitive patients also have some inhalant allergies, which are affected by climate changes, exposures, and blooming seasons. Before condemning the diet and discarding the dietary restrictions, the patient should consider extraneous factors as the cause of problems. Dietary control is a long-term adjustment, and other conditions will develop both during and after the elimination period. It is the long-term result that must be considered, and patience is necessary.

Reintroduction and Rotation

Reintroduction

The length of time necessary for strict dietary elimination varies from patient to patient. In some cases, a 3-month period is adequate. If the offending foods are reintroduced in less time, a fairly rapid return of symptoms usually results. A 6-month period of elimination is better than 3 months, as this both allows the immune system to lose more of its sensitivity and gives the patient time to become accustomed to a different diet. For some patients, a full year of elimination is necessary. If an offending food cannot be reintroduced after 12 months' omission without a return of symptoms, this signals that the food allergy is "fixed." Fortunately, this is rare.

It is worth noting that the longer and more carefully the elimination diet has been observed in the initial stages, the more the patient is able to "cheat" on the diet as time progresses without having symptoms recur. It may not be wise to advise the patient of this, as it may tend to encourage poorer observation of the diet from the beginning, but the physician should be aware of it because it will aid in evaluating results.

At the end of the elimination period, the patient should schedule another appointment, to evaluate the results of the elimination diet and program the next stage in food allergy control. If the food sensitivities have been properly diagnosed and the patient has been reasonably faithful in following the diet, a major improvement in symptoms should have resulted. Sometimes, it is necessary to go over the symptoms that were present before the diet was started one by one to make the patient aware of exactly how much improvement has occurred. During a period of 6 months, it is easy to forget how pronounced the conditions were that brought about the request for help. Many patients, however, will already be well aware of a major improvement in their overall condition and be quite satisfied with the result of the diet.

Rotation

One of the reasons that cyclic food allergy has been given that designation is that many patients, when released from the original elimination diet, tend to assume that sensitization to the foods eliminated is no longer in effect, so they resume eating all such foods without restriction. The result is a gradual re-establishment of the original sensitivities. The tendency to such sensitization is genetic, and with the same exposure the sensitization will recur and bring the patient full cycle, with all the original problems that brought them to the physician initially. To maintain a good result, the intake of offending foods must be rotated in the diet. When one of the offending foods is eaten only once or twice a week, the immune system will not become sensitive enough to produce problems. It is, of course, necessary to consider the family of the food involved, and not eat foods containing the same antigens as an alternative to the food being rotated. Although it is better to eat the food being reintroduced in larger quantities once a week than in smaller quantities more frequently, it is also only common sense to keep the amount relatively small, if possible. Both dose and frequency relationships are involved in sensitization. If a large number of foods are involved, it is at times necessary to establish a calendar pattern showing which foods may be eaten on certain days. (''If it's Sunday, it must be chicken.'') This is an unpopular restriction, however, and is rarely necessary.

It has been the experience of the senior author that a certain reaction on the part of the patient is remarkably common. When the diet has brought good results and the subject of reintroducing the food on a rotary basis is broached, the following scenario occurs: ''Thank you, doctor. I really feel good now. I'm glad to know that I can introduce the foods again, as long as I rotate them. I don't think I will, though. I've gotten used to doing without them now, and I don't even like them very much any more. If I don't put them back in the diet deliberately, when I see them when dining out or at a friend's, I can eat them without worrying, as I know I won't get them again the next day or the day after.'' This system works extremely well for many patients.

It is advisable to check the patient again in another 6 months, primarily to observe progress and keep posted on further developments. Most patients will continue to do well with whichever approach to rotation is elected. Again, a common scenario is as follows: ''I'm still doing fine and keeping the diet under control. A few months ago, however, I noticed that my old symptoms were coming back. I looked over what I had been eating, and said to myself, 'Aha! You've been cheating! You're eating the food you're supposed to rotate every day!' I cut back to the rotation, and all the symptoms went away.'' When the initial constant level of antibodies has been reduced, it appears that the masking effect has been eliminated and an offending food produces symptoms rather promptly, allowing the patient to recognize a cause-and-effect relationship. In addition, a prolonged period of elimination is unnecessary unless the previous constant level of antigen and antibody has been re-established.

It is unlikely that those patients sensitive to foods will ever be able to eat with impunity whatever they wish in any quantity. It is quite possible, however, for them to establish a level of control that is not difficult to maintain, and that provides them with a major improvement in quality of life.

COMMENTARY ON FOOD REACTIONS

There are several other approaches to the diagnosis and treatment of food allergies. Some are discussed in the last chapter of the book. Others have been detailed elsewhere.[6,7] This text, however, is designed as a guide to the novice allergist. Only elimination and rotation of foods is uniformly accepted as a safe and effective means of controlling food allergies, and therefore only this approach is presented here. It is usually wise for the physician expanding or upgrading a portion of the practice to stay with the most conservative and established approaches, keeping safety strongly in mind. As a reminder here, the reintroduction and rotation of offending foods applies only to cyclic food allergy. With fixed (IgE-mediated) food allergies, the food should be eliminated from the diet completely and permanently. Food allergy is a major part of the overall allergic picture; the true extent is not known because of difficulties in identifying all the factors present. Treating inhalant allergy is a fine place for the novice to begin. However, for the dedicated, it will not be long before it becomes evident that some patients do not respond well to treatment of only inhalant allergies. At this point, the management of food allergy should be the first consideration.

REFERENCES

1. Bahna S. The dilemma of pathogenesis and diagnosis of food allergy. Immunol Allergy Clin North Am 1987;7:299–312.
2. King HC. Food allergy. Curr Opin Otolaryngol Head Neck Surg 1994;2:137–140.
3. Breneman JC, Sweeny M, Robert R. Immunology of delayed type food allergy. Immunol Allergy Pract 1994;13:6.
4. King HC. Exploring the maze of adverse reactions to foods. Ear Nose Throat J 1994;73: 237–241.
5. Breneman JC. Basics of Food Allergy. 2nd ed. Springfield, IL: Charles C Thomas Publishers; 1984.
6. King WP, Motes JM. The intracutaneous progressive dilution multi-food test. Otolaryngol Head Neck Surg 1991;104:235–238.
7. King HC, King WP. Alternatives in diagnosis and treatment of food allergies. Otolaryngol Clin N Amer 1997 (in press).

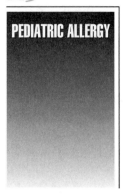

15

PEDIATRIC ALLERGY

Allergy is directly or indirectly involved in up to half the problems encountered in the office practice of otolaryngology. This is true whether the patient population under consideration is composed primarily of adults or children. It has been (very conservatively) estimated that allergic rhinitis occurs in about 10% of children and 20% of adults.[1]However, allergy is probably more commonly present in children than current figures indicate, as in this age group it more frequently takes the form of food hypersensitivity, a disorder that is often overlooked or misdiagnosed. Thus, it is necessary that the pediatric otolaryngologist recognize the many manifestations of allergy affecting children. Although much of the material in this chapter has been presented elsewhere in this text, it is repeated here to provide, a single reference source regarding allergy as it affects the ear, nose, and throat in children.

SIGNS AND SYMPTOMS OF ALLERGY IN CHILDREN

Allergy may affect every organ system and region within the province of the otolaryngologist. However, in children the physician must more carefully look for signs, as verbalization of corresponding symptoms may be lacking because of patient age or (unfortunately) lack of parental attention to these problems.

Head

It is now well accepted that the typical "adenoid facies," characterized by mouth breathing, a retrognathic jaw, and a high palatal arch, may be the result of nasal airway obstruction as well as a hypertrophic adenoid mass. In addition to these features, the child with allergy will often demonstrate facial grimacing and wrinkling of the nose, and a gesture referred to as the "allergic salute": lifting the tip of the nose with an upward sweep of the palm. These gestures result from intense itching of the mucous membranes of the nose, and in many instances, the child soon discovers that a beneficial effect of the actions is to lift the nasal tip and briefly improve the airway. Repetition of the allergic salute for a period of years usually results in a permanent creasing of the skin above the nasal tip, and this "supratip crease" is another aid to the diagnosis of allergy in a child.

Other facial stigmata of allergy appear in the region of the eyes. The most characteristic finding is infraorbital puffiness and discoloration, often referred to as an "allergic shiner." This condition occurs because chronic nasal congestion results in stasis of the venous drainage from the periorbital region. Venous stasis is also postulated to be the cause of "Dennie's sign": lines that radiate downward from the inner corner of the eye in the area of the lower lid, attributed to spasm of the unstriated muscle of Muller resulting from poor oxygenation. Allergic children also frequently have long, silky eyelashes, although the cause for this phenomenon remains obscure.

Finally, some children manifest a characteristic "sad-eyed" look, often combined with tearing and profuse rhinorrhea. In severe instances, this results in chronic excoriation of the soft tissue between the anterior nares and upper lip (Fig. 15–1).

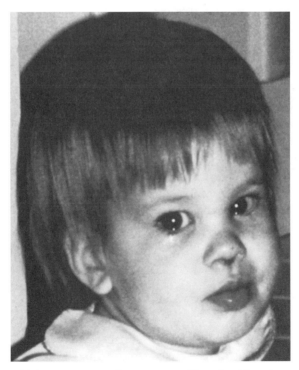

FIGURE 15–1. Child with severe allergy to corn. Note the rhinorrhea, nasal crusting, and teary-eyed appearance.

Eyes

Although the eyes are not truly the province of the otolaryngologist, the astute clinician will observe the patient's eyes, not only for the signs described above but also for conjunctival or scleral injection, often indicative of the chronic rubbing that results from pruritis in these areas.

Ears

The skin of the allergic child is often dry, scaly, or excoriated, and this condition can involve the skin of the concha and external canal. Although controversy continues regarding the role of allergy in recurrent otitis media or chronic middle ear effusion, studies indicate that this factor cannot be ignored. McMahan et al[2] found that of 119 children undergoing tube insertion for otitis media with effusion, 93% had positive results on radioallergosorbent testing (RAST) for inhalants, foods, or both. Renfro[3] found that skin test results were positive in all of a study group of children receiving a set of tubes for the second time or more.

Nose

The nasal membranes (like all mucosa of the upper aerodigestive tract) are afflicted with intense pruritis during an allergic flare, giving rise to the allergic salute, supratip crease, and other signs already described. Other characteristic nasal manifestations of allergy are sneezing, discharge of clear mucus, and congestion. At one time, the presence of nasal polyps was felt to be a definite indication of the presence of allergy. This is not always the case, although an estimated 25 to 30% of patients with polyps are allergic.

The presence of nasal mucosal edema, combined with hypersecretion, often results in stasis within the sinuses. Thus, allergic children frequently have sinusitis; this is slower to resolve and recurs more rapidly than in nonallergic children.

Pharynx

Signs of allergy may include prominent pharyngeal lymphoid follicles, producing a "cobblestone" appearance, often with prominent lateral bands. Hypertrophic adenoids and tonsils have also been attributed to uncontrolled allergy, with resultant chronic postnasal drainage.[4] Similar hypertrophy of lingual tonsillar tissue may result in a sensation of having a "lump in the throat," chronic throat clearing, or even dysphagia.

Although recurrent episodes of pharyngitis cannot be directly attributed to the presence of allergy, there is little doubt that chronic mouth breathing (with resultant drying of the mucous membranes and loss of the cleansing function of the nasal mucosa) and postnasal drainage provide a fertile field for the microorganisms to which children are frequently exposed.

Larynx

Recurrent or chronic hoarseness may suggest the presence of allergy and may be related to chronic throat clearing or episodes of allergic edema of the vocal folds.

FAMILY HISTORY AND ENVIRONMENTAL EXPOSURE

There is little doubt that a predisposition to the development of allergy is an inherited characteristic. The presence of atopy in parents and siblings should alert the physician to possible allergy in the patient. Although exact figures vary, it is generally accepted that a child with one allergic parent has roughly one chance in three of being allergic, whereas if both parents are allergic, the chance increases to more than two in three.

For clinical allergy to develop, repeated exposures to the allergens must occur, so that the formation of antigen-specific IgE is eventually triggered. Most allergy in children below the age of 2 years is caused by food hypersensitivity. Inhalant allergy becomes a significant factor after this age, and the earliest incriminated antigens are those to which the child is exposed: dust mite, mold, and animal danders. By about the age of 6, pollens are also significant offenders. Although in adults it is often necessary to employ a number of antigens when testing for inhalant allergy, the number may be minimized in children through a judicious history that focuses on exposure and circumstances under which symptoms are noted.

ADJUNCTIVE TESTS

An increase in the eosinophil fraction of leukocytes in a differential count should suggest the presence of allergy (although other disease states, such as infection with intestinal parasites, may also cause eosinophilia). More specific is the finding of eosinophils in an eosin-methylene blue-stained smear of nasal secretions. The exact details of specimen collection, staining, and interpretation are beyond the scope of this work and are described elsewhere.[5] Although the finding of eosinophils (indicating allergy) or neutrophils (indicating an infectious component) in nasal secretions constitutes a respected means of confirming a clinical diagnosis, this test is not entirely accurate. For example, long-term topical application of corticosteroids to the nasal mucosa has been shown to diminish the number of nasal eosinophils.[6] In addition, sampling techniques are highly variable (from having the patient blow the nose into waxed paper to the use of a plastic blunt curette to obtain nasal scrapings), and the experience of the person preparing and examining the slides significantly impact the accuracy of the test results.

Another adjunctive test that has traditionally been employed in the diagnosis of allergic rhinosinusitis is examination of sinus radiographs. Unfortunately, it is now accepted that conventional sinus x-ray films are of little benefit in confirming disease in the ethmoid sinuses, and that computerized tomography (CT scans) of the sinuses is required for accurate diagnosis. To investigate antral disease, either an open-mouth, upright Waters view of the sinuses or the use of A-mode ultrasound scans may be helpful, as may be transillumination.[7]

TREATMENT BASED ON A PRESUMPTIVE DIAGNOSIS OF ALLERGY

The diagnosis of upper respiratory inhalant allergy is made by history. Physical examination confirms the manifestations. After these steps, specific testing may be carried out to determine the offending antigens with certainty. However, a positive allergy test result without historical verification of symptoms likely produced by that antigen does not establish a diagnosis of ''allergy'' or justify treatment.

It is important for the clinician to realize that effective clinical management may be instituted based solely on a presumptive diagnosis of allergy made through history and physical examination alone. Thus, it is unnecessary to await the results of testing to afford some degree of relief to the child (and parents). In some instances, these measures are sufficiently successful to warrant deferring specific allergy testing.

Environmental Control

Although a great deal of upper respiratory allergy in very young children (especially below the age of 2 years) arises from food hypersensitivity, inhal-

TABLE 15–1. Measures to minimize dust mite exposure in children

1. Eliminate mite reservoirs.
   A. Encase mattress and pillows with barrier material.
   B. Wash all bedding weekly in hot water (135 F).
   C. Tumble stuffed animals in dryer weekly on hot cycle.
   D. Store stuffed animals in "hammock" over bed.
   E. Eliminate or minimize carpets and draperies in bedroom.
2. Utilize filtration devices and minimize visible dust.
   A. Use electrostatic or high-efficiency particulate arresting (HEPA) filters.
   B. Clean filters regularly or (if using conventional filters) change monthly.
   C. Dust regularly (patient should not do dusting), using treated cloth to avoid spreading dust.
3. Reduce indoor humidity (<50%).
   A. Install air conditioner, dehumidifier.
   B. Eliminate or minimize houseplants.
   C. Ventilate home.
4. Use acaricides (e.g., benzyl benzoate) and antigen-denaturing agents (e.g., tannic acid).

ant allergy in infants and young children in most cases is sensitization that develops to allergens found in the home environment, to which they are most frequently exposed: dust mite, molds, and animal danders.

Dust mite is an acarid that thrives in a warm, moist environment and feeds on human skin scales. Its antigen is found in the dung balls deposited by the organisms. The most common sites for dust mite exposure in children are stuffed animals and toys, bedding, upholstered furniture, and rugs. A number of measures are available for diminishing dust mite exposure (Table 15–1), and parents should be urged to employ them as much as possible.[8] Because this antigen is so commonly involved, dust mite avoidance measures are merited on an empiric basis in the management of children suspected of upper respiratory inhalant allergy, even before specific testing has been performed.

Molds are a frequent indoor antigen. Their growth requirements are similar to those for dust mite, and control of relative humidity in the home will be helpful. It is often problematic to keep the indoor relative humidity above 40% (to combat the harmful effects of dry air on respiratory mucosa), yet below 50% (to minimize dust mite and mold growth). The purchase of a hygrometer or the use of a central humidifier with a humidistat is recommended. In addition to humidity control and avoidance of reservoirs such as houseplants, mold elimination should focus on treating visibly moldy surfaces. Commercially prepared "mildew sprays" are available. Also, a solution of household bleach (one part of bleach in nine parts of water) sprayed or wiped onto affected surfaces is an effective treatment for mold and mildew.

Animal danders are common sources of allergy in children, and the cat is by far the most frequent and serious offender. It appears that the allergen associated with cats is produced by the sebaceous glands in the cat skin (not just the salivary glands, as once thought). The allergen becomes airborne when skin scales are shed, and because the particles are quite small (2 to 4 μm), they remain airborne for prolonged periods. Even removing the cat (a suggestion that is usually met with significant resistance) does not solve the problem, as dander may continue to be present in the environment for 3 to 4 months afterward. Nevertheless, a number of measures may be instituted that will alleviate some of the symptoms suffered by children allergic to their beloved cat[7] (Table 15–2).

Pharmacotherapy

In addition to avoidance of known provoking factors, the treatment of suspected allergic rhinitis in children will involve the administration of appropriate pharmacotherapeutic agents. Although these should be administered in an appropriate stepwise fashion, in the same manner as in the treatment of adults,[9] certain factors unique to the treatment of children must be considered.

Antihistamines

Considerable effort has been expended within the past decade on the development of new, nonsedating H_1-receptor antagonists. Not all members of this

---

TABLE 15–2. Measures to minimize cat dander exposure in children

1. Limit exposure to the cat.
    A. Remove (when possible), or
    B. Eliminate from indoor access, or
    C. Eliminate from bedrooms.
2. Limit reservoirs (carpets, draperies, upholstered furniture).
    A. Eliminate carpets and draperies, or
    B. Frequently clean reservoirs, using HEPA vacuum, and
    C. Use efficient air filtration system (HEPA, electrostatic).
3. Minimize shed antigen and its effect.
    A. Wash the cat weekly.*
    B. Administer acepromazine to cat.*
    C. Apply Allerpet to cat.*
    D. Apply tannic acid to carpet (to neutralize antigen).

* Efficacy of these measures has been questioned.[24]

TABLE 15–3. Dosages of selected antihistamines for pediatric use*

Generic name	Patient age	Pediatric dosage	Adult dosage
First-generation antihistamines			
Brompheniramine	2–6 years old	1 mg q 4–6 h	8–12 mg b.i.d.
	6–12 years old	2 mg q 4–6 h	
Chlorpheniramine	6–12 years old	2 mg up to q.i.d.	8–12 mg b.i.d.
Clemastine	6–12 years old	0.67–1.34 mg b.i.d.	2.68 mg up to t.i.d.
Diphenhydramine	<6 years old	6.12–12.5 mg q 4–6 h	25–50 mg q.i.d.
	6–12 years old	12.5–25 mg q 4–6 h	
Second- and third-generation antihistamines			
Cetirizine	2–6 years old	5 mg once daily	10 mg once daily
	6–11 years old	10 mg once daily	
Loratadine	2–9 years old	5 mg once daily	10 mg once daily
Astemizole†	2–6 years old	0.2 mg/kg/once daily	10 mg once daily
	6–12 years old	10 mg once daily	
Fexofenadine†	3–6 years old	15 mg b.i.d.	60 mg b.i.d.
	6–12 years old	30 mg b.i.d.	

* Suggested dosages based on USP[11] and industry sources. However, latest prescribing information should be consulted for most current information.

† Pediatric use not approved in United States.

class currently in use in the United States are approved for pediatric use, although research continues to develop acceptable and safe formulations for the treatment of children.[10] In prescribing antihistamines, the physician must remember that newborns and premature infants are especially susceptible to the antimuscarinic effects of these drugs, and that children of any age may exhibit paradoxical excitement, rather than sedation, as a result of such treatment. Table 15–3 lists typical antihistamines, both first-generation and newer preparations, with suggested current pediatric dosages.[11] Topical antihistamines, such as azelastine and levocabastine, are now available, but at this writing their pediatric dosage has not been established.

Decongestants

Sympathomimetic drugs to relieve nasal congestion may be administered topically or systematically. Topical nasal application of a decongestant may result in rebound rhinitis if continued for longer than 4 to 7 days. In addition, the stimulatory side effects of these drugs may be unacceptable to the parents, especially if they are administered in a regimen that includes nighttime dosing. The systemic decongestant most commonly employed in the treatment of children is pseudoephedrine, at a dose of 15 to 30 mg three times daily.

Cromolyn

The topical application of cromolyn to the nasal mucosa before an anticipated allergen exposure has been shown to be effective in preventing the development of an allergic reaction.[12] In addition to prophylactic administration, its regular use by patients with immunoglobin E (IgE)-mediated allergic rhinitis will often provide symptom control. The primary advantage of cromolyn, in addition to its specificity, is that it does not produce significant side effects, either local or systemic. The major cautions associated with the use of cromolyn are that it must come in adequate contact with nasal mucosa, that it is ineffective in the treatment of polyps and nonallergic rhinitis, and that some patients with severe allergic rhinitis do not obtain satisfactory results with cromolyn (requiring topical corticosteroids instead).[13] Cromolyn, which is now available without a prescription, has been approved in the United States for administration to adults and children age 5 years and over, at a dosage of one spray in each nostril up to six times daily.[14]

Topical Corticosteroids

Intranasally administered corticosteroids are extremely effective in the symptomatic management of both seasonal and perennial allergic rhinitis, as well as many nonallergic rhinitides. The primary effect of glucocorticoids on the allergic event is blunting of the late-phase reaction, although prolonged pretreatment with a topical form will also lessen the severity of acute-phase reactions. Because of their potential side effects, both local and systemic, these preparations should be utilized only after a failure of more conservative measures.[15] This is especially true when treating children. The potential adverse effects associated with nasal corticosteroids are discussed in detail in Chapter 8. In children, one important consideration is potential inhibition of the growth of long bones. This is most often discussed in association with inhaled corticosteroids (administered for asthma), and it has less convincingly been shown to be a consequence of nasal corticosteroid use. Nevertheless, caution is advised.

Proper use of topical nasal steroids requires adequate mucosal contact, instruction of the patient (and parents) in the proper mode and schedule of administration, and constant monitoring for undesirable effects, which may be either local or systemic. The potential for the development of systemic effects after topical administration is explained by absorption from the nasal mucosa, and from the gastrointestinal tract when these preparations are swallowed. Fortunately, many of the nasal corticosteroids undergo significant first-pass liver metabolism into inactive or less active forms. However, the degree of this degradation varies with the corticosteroid in question. Newer

TABLE 15–4. Topical nasal corticosteroids*

Preparation	Spray, μg	Age, y	Sprays per nostril. frequency
Beclomethasone	42	6–12 y/o	1 t.i.d
		12 y/o	1 b.i.d to q.i.d
Beclomethasone AQ	42	6–12 y/o	1–2 b.i.d
		12 y/o	2 b.i.d
Beclomethasone AQ	84	6 y/o	1–2 once daily
Flunisolide	25	6–14 y/o	1 t.i.d or 2 b.i.d
		15 y/o	2 b.i.d
Triamcinolone	55	6–11 y/o	1 once daily
		12 y/o	2 once daily
Triamcinolone AQ	55	6–11 y/o	1 once daily
		12 y/o	2 once daily
Budesonide	32	6 y/o	2 b.i.d or 4 once daily
Fluticasone	50	6–11 y/o	1 once daily
		12 y/o	2 once daily
Mometasone	25	12 y/o	2 once daily

AQ, aqueous form.
* Suggested dosages based on USP[16] and industry sources. However, latest prescribing information should be consulted for most current information.

corticosteroid nasal sprays continue to be introduced, and most of these have an improved margin of safety between the maximum recommended dose and that at which a systemic effect may be noted. Table 15–4 lists the most common topical nasal corticosteroids. Most topical nasal corticosteroids are now approved for use in children. The dosage for such use varies with each product, and the physician should carefully scrutinize the product literature and other sources before prescribing.[16]

Anticholinergics

Topical anticholinergics are sometimes utilized to control profuse rhinorrhea caused by both allergic and nonallergic rhinitis.[17] However, the use of these agents is rarely necessary in children. When they are indicated, 0.03% ipratropium hydrobromide (Atrovent Nasal) may be administered to children ages 12 years and older in dosages of two sprays in each nostril three times daily to control rhinorrhea. If this treatment is to be effective, results will be seen in a week or less. There is little to recommend the use of systemic anticholinergics for this same purpose, for either adults or children.

ESTABLISHING THE DIAGNOSIS OF ALLERGY

Although treatment may be administered based on the presumptive diagnosis of inhalant allergy, proof of the presence of IgE specific to various allergens

TABLE 15–5. Advantages and disadvantages of in vitro testing

Advantages
  Not affected by skin reactivity
  Not affected by drugs
  No risk for systemic reaction
  Only one needle stick required
  More specific than skin tests
Disadvantages
  Equipment and trained personnel required
  Not all antigens available
  Lack of correspondence between antigen strength in treatment concentrate and in
    vitro level (because of standardization differences)
  Delay in availability of results
  Less sensitive than skin tests

is necessary to recommend more appropriate environmental control and administer definitive immunotherapy.

For more than a century, the benchmark of inhalant allergy testing has been skin testing of one type or another. Currently, the methods used are a combination of prick testing and intradermal testing, or intradermal testing with a series of progressively more concentrated antigens (skin endpoint titration, or SET). Either method is acceptable, although SET also determines a safe starting point for immunotherapy.[18] Skin testing on cooperative children can generally be carried out as an office procedure. However, it has been shown that SET performed under general anesthesia at the same time as other procedures (e.g., adenotonsillectomy, pressure-equalization tube insertion) is safe and accurate.[19] The details of skin testing are presented in Chapter 6.

In vitro allergy testing presents both advantages and disadvantages in comparison with skin testing (Table 15–5). These tests may be quantitative (radioallergosorbent testing, or RAST; enzyme-linked immunosorbent assay, or ELISA), semiquantitative (dipstick tests), or qualitative (''yes-no'' assays for multiple antigens). Only quantitative in vitro tests may be used as the basis for immunotherapy, and the treatment vial formulated from such results must be checked on the skin (''vial test'') before immunotherapy is begun.[20] In vitro tests are also discussed in depth in Chapter 6.

DEFINITIVE MANAGEMENT OF UPPER RESPIRATORY ALLERGY

As already mentioned, allergy testing allows ''fine tuning'' of environmental control, based on the certain knowledge that specific antigens are triggering

NURSE'S NOTE

If the allergic child must undergo a general anesthetic (e.g., for tonsillectomy, adenoidectomy, and/or tube insertion), allergy testing may be accomplished more easily. At this time, it is easy to obtain a blood sample for RAST determinations. Skin testing can also be performed under anesthesia, and if carried out efficiently, it should not prolong the anesthetic time. Unless a phenothiazine preparation has been utilized as part of premedication or given during the procedure, general anesthesia should not affect skin test responses. However, skin testing under anesthesia requires careful preplanning.

1. The person most experienced in skin testing should perform the tests.

2. A preoperative conference between the physician and the person doing the testing should take place to determine the antigens to be tested and minimize the number of tests that must be applied. This involves a knowledge of cross-reactivity and of the index antigens for the area, and a careful analysis of the patient's history to avoid testing for unnecessary antigens. In addition, an experienced tester may utilize vertical testing, as described more fully in Chapter 6.

3. The patient should be observed carefully in the recovery room for any late-phase reactions and the results recorded. In addition, continued postoperative observation for a masked systemic reaction is necessary, although careful attention to skin whealing responses during the testing should make this highly unlikely.

If skin testing must be done with the patient in an awake state, we have found that pretesting application of EMLA Cream (2.5% lidocaine, 2.5% prilocaine) to the test site will minimize discomfort without affecting skin reactivity.[21] This cream should be applied to the test site in a thick layer 90 minutes before the start of testing and the area covered with an occlusive dressing. A dressing is provided with 5-g tubes of EMLA Cream, or a plastic wrap may be used. For testing, the wrap is removed, the remaining cream is wiped away, and skin tests are applied as usual, including controls.

allergic responses. It should be emphasized that the avoidance of an inciting allergen remains the best treatment for allergy.

More important is the use of information gained through allergy testing to administer immunotherapy, which is the only available treatment for allergy producing long-lasting effects proved to persist for years after the conclusion of a course of therapy.[22] Suitable candidates for immunotherapy are persons with proven IgE-mediated atopy for allergens that are unavoidable or that produce symptoms unresponsive to more conservative measures; they include patients with symptoms spanning multiple seasons or single-season allergy that is consistently severe, as well as those for whom pharmacotherapy gives imperfect relief or interferes with quality of life. The final consideration in determining suitable candidates for immunotherapy is whether the patient and/or parents are motivated, cooperative, and likely to follow through with a 3- to 5-year course of injections.

A frequently asked question is, "At what age would you give immunotherapy?" No hard and fast rule exists, and most otolaryngic allergists would administer immunotherapy to children above the age of 2 years if necessary. However, most inhalant allergy in children below the age of about 5 is caused to a great degree by perennial antigens, such as animal danders and dust mite. The best management in these situations is avoidance and environmental control. Above this age, pollens become more problematic and immunotherapy may often be necessary. In any instance, the willingness and ability of both the child and parents to cooperate in a program of immunotherapy must be taken into account before such a regimen is begun. If the parents can be enlisted as active participants in the treatment program, the success of immunotherapy is greatly enhanced.

Dose advancement in children proceeds in a similar fashion to that used in adults. Children frequently exhibit local reactions that are more pronounced than those seen in adults, and they should always be observed for a full 20 minutes after injections. This may require more cautious dose advancement. Continued local reactions should suggest inquiries about the concomitant ingestion of cross-reacting foods (e.g., cereal grains in grass-allergic patients), which affects the patient's overall sensitivity. Also, continued local reactions without a change in antigen exposure should suggest the presence of hidden infection.

NURSE'S NOTE

Children tend to be more labile in their reactivity to immunotherapy than are adults, and they should be observed carefully for reactions after injections. Dose advancement may have to proceed more slowly than desired but is usually possible with good control of symptoms.

Even small children will cooperate during injections when they begin to feel better. Cooperation from the child is often not as difficult to obtain as from parents. A greater challenge is to get busy parents to interrupt their schedules to bring a child in for repeated injections.

Further details on immunotherapy are presented in Chapter 9.

MANAGEMENT OF FOOD ALLERGY IN CHILDREN

Food allergy is an often-neglected problem in the allergic child, partially because there is no general agreement among physicians as to what constitutes true "food allergy." Almost everyone will accept as allergic immediate, IgE-mediated food reactions, in which anaphylactic-type reactions (e.g., rhinorrhea, angioedema) follow within 10 to 20 minutes ingestion of the offending food. Fortunately or unfortunately, these probably constitute only 10% or so of food reactions. Numerous other symptoms may be produced by delayed hypersensitivity, involving Gell and Coombs type III (IgG-mediated) reactions.

Initial Approach to Food Allergy in Children

The first recommended measure in dealing with suspected food allergy in children is the elimination of all "junk food" from the diet for the period of a week. Generally, this measure will greatly reduce the child's intake of corn (found in corn syrup in soft drinks, corn chips, corn oil used in frying, and other foods), milk (as milk, ice cream), and soy (added to numerous products).

In addition to this initial measure, a diet diary should be kept for a period of 1 to 2 weeks. This may be done in numerous ways, from listing how often the child ingests certain foods to simply writing down everything taken into the child's mouth. It is important to assure the patient (and parents) that they will not be censured for what they report, and that this diary is simply a diagnostic tool. Otherwise, the diary returned may bear little or no resemblance to the actual diet consumed.

Analyzing a diet diary for potential food allergy involves looking for foods eaten frequently (on a daily basis) and often "craved." The major offenders, both in children and adults, are corn, wheat, milk, soy, and egg. Occasionally, items such as chocolate or tea will require investigation.

Testing for Food Allergy

In vitro testing is a simple and accurate way to test for inhalant allergies. Unfortunately, in vitro testing for food allergy is helpful only in establishing IgE-mediated food allergy. Because such allergy is characterized by symptoms that rapidly follow food ingestion (e.g., angioedema after eating shrimp), it rarely presents a diagnostic problem. Although skin testing for foods has been shown to be effective when properly performed, the average practitioner has no desire to go this far in an allergy practice. However, it is possible to carry out evaluation and treatment of food sensitivity adequately by methods that do not involve skin tests or injections. Other methods for food allergy testing are discussed in Chapters 14 and 18.

Testing for Food Allergy by Dietary Manipulation

For the average clinician, the best (and most accurate) means of diagnosing a food allergy remains the simple (but difficult) process of having the patient omit the potential offender from the diet (observing for improvement in symptoms), then ingest it under controlled circumstances (observing for the development of symptoms). This may be done in one of two ways: the single-food withdrawal and oral challenge feeding test (OCFT), or the elimination diet with add-back challenge.

Single-Food Withdrawal and OCFT

When one or only a few food groups are suspected of causing allergic symptoms, this test is the most effective means of proving such a relationship, both to the clinician and to the patient and family. The suspected food, in all its forms, is omitted from the diet for from 4 to 7 days. An improvement in symptoms after omission is the first indication that the tested food may be the source of allergic problems. This is confirmed by a ''challenge'' refeeding.

The challenge feeding consists of ingestion of the test food, in the purest possible form, followed by observation for the development of symptoms. It is noteworthy that symptoms produced by the OCFT may take the form of headache, rhinorrhea, nasal congestion, or even abdominal distress. If symptoms are not produced with the initial feeding, it is advisable to administer more of the test food after 3 hours. If no symptoms result, the food may be considered safe for addition back to the diet.

Basic Elimination Diet with Add-Back Challenge

In the OCFT, each food under consideration is tested individually. If there is no clear history to suggest offending foods, or if a multitude of foods are to be tested, it may be necessary to place the patient on a diet free of all the foods in question for about a week, then challenge daily with different foods. Foods that do not provoke a reaction may be added back to the diet. This is a more difficult test to carry out than the OCFT, both in formulating a basic diet and interpreting the results of the challenges. For further information on both the OCFT and basic elimination diet with add-back challenge, the interested clinician may consult Chapter 14.

Treatment of Food Allergy

Controversy exists regarding the benefit of immunotherapy for food allergy, as well as the form such treatment should take (e.g., injections, sublingual drops). For the clinician wishing to initiate treatment based on the results of an OCFT, dietary manipulation is the preferred initial means for such management.

The first step in treating food allergy is the elimination of the proven allergenic food from the diet. This may be extremely difficult, especially when dealing with such ubiquitous foods as corn, wheat, milk, egg, and soy (which are, unfortunately, the major food offenders). However, such elimination during a period of about 12 weeks may result in the development of sufficient tolerance to allow reintroduction of the food into the diet on a limited basis. If attempts to reintroduce an allergenic food result in reactions, further avoidance must be counseled. If after a total of 2 years' avoidance symptoms still follow the ingestion of the food, the allergy must be considered fixed and the food avoided indefinitely.

The second dietary measure employed is the institution of a rotary, diversified diet. The rationale for this diet is avoidance of repeated ingestion of any given food or food family. Specific foods (in all forms) are eaten no more often than twice weekly, and the diet is "rotated" to include a large variety of foods. This not only prevents a buildup of immune complexes by repeated ingestion of offending foods, but also minimizes the development of new food sensitivities through daily exposure.[23]

CONCLUSION

Allergy in children is not an uncommon occurrence, and it frequently is manifested in disorders of the ears, nose, and throat. The otolaryngologist who chooses to ignore the possibility of a contributory allergic component may achieve inadequate results with medical management and surgical intervention that would otherwise be effective. Despite the oft-voiced hope that children will "outgrow their allergy," it appears that this occurs in fewer than 10% of cases. Modern otolaryngologists who treat children must be conversant with the manifestations and appropriate treatment of allergy to offer the best care to their patients.

REFERENCES

1. Smith JM. The epidemiology of allergic rhinitis. In: Settipane GA, ed. Rhinitis. Providence, RI: New England and Regional Allergy Proceedings; 1984:86–91.
2. McMahan JT, Calenoff E, Croft DJ, et al. Chronic otitis media with effusion and allergy: modified RAST analysis of 119 cases. Otolaryngol Head Neck Surg 1981;89:427–431.
3. Renfro B. Pediatric otolaryngic allergy. Otolaryngol Clin North Am 1992;25:181–196.
4. Krause HF. Diagnostic patterns of otolaryngic allergy: symptoms. In: Krause HF, ed. Otolaryngic Allergy and Immunology. Philadelphia: WB Saunders; 1989:51–65.
5. Jalowayski AA, Zeiger RS. A Practical Guide for the Examination of Nasal Cytology in the Diagnosis of Nasal Disorders. Richmond, VA: AH Robins Co; 1981.
6. Driscoll PV, Naclerio RM, Baroody FM. Intranasal corticosteroids reduce eosinophils in nasal secretions but not in the submucosa after allergen challenge. J Allergy Clin Immunol 1994;93:216 (abst).
7. Mabry RL. Office Diagnosis of Sinus Disorders: the Role of Ultrasound Scanning, Laryngoscope 1984;94:1042–1044.
8. Squillace SP. Environmental control. Otolaryngol Head Neck Surg 1992;107:831–834.
9. Mabry RL. Overview: the allergic reaction and site-based therapy. Otolaryngol Head Neck Surg 1992;107:828–830.
10. Simons FER. Allergic rhinitis: recent advances. Pediatr Clin North Am 1988;35:1053–1073.
11. Antihistamines (systemic). Drug Information for the Health Care Professional. 17th ed. Rockville, MD: US Pharmacopeial Convention; 1997:318–337.
12. Schwartz HJ. Cromolyn sodium and its effect on nasal disease. Am J Rhinol 1988;2:129–133.
13. Mabry RL. Uses and misuses of intranasal corticosteroids and cromolyn. Am J Rhinol 1991;5:121–124.
14. Cromolyn (nasal). Drug Information for the Health Care Professional. 17th ed. Rockville, MD: US Pharmacopeial Convention; 1997:1084–1086.
15. Mabry RL. Corticosteroids in the management of upper respiratory allergy: the emerging role of steroid nasal sprays. Otolaryngol Head Neck Surg 1992;107:855–860.
16. Corticosteroids (nasal). Drug Information for the Health Care Professional. 17th ed. Rockville, MD: US Pharmacopeial Convention; 1997:925–930.
17. Mabry RL. Topical pharmacotherapy for allergic rhinitis: new agents. South Med J 1992;85:149–154.
18. AMA Council on Scientific Affairs, Panel on Allergy. In vivo diagnostic testing and immunotherapy for allergy. JAMA 1983;258:363–367.
19. Renfro B. Pediatric otolaryngic allergy. Otolaryngol Clin North Am 1992;25:181–196.
20. Mabry, RL. Blending skin endpoint titration and in vitro methods in clinical practice. Otolaryngol Clin North Am 1992;25:61–70.
21. Shapiro GG, Soler JS, Cierman CW, et al. Effect of EMLA on allergy skin tests. J Allergy Clin Immunol 1994;93:280 (abst).
22. Gordon BR. Immunotherapy: rationale and mechanisms. Otolaryngol Head Neck Surg 1992;107:861–865.
23. King WP. Food hypersensitivity in otolaryngology. Otolaryngol Clin North Am 1992;25:163–179.
24. Klucka CV, Ownby DR, Green J, Zoratti EM. Cat washings. Allerpet or acepromazine does not diminish Fel D 1 shedding. J Allergy Clin Immunol 1994;93:180.

Although the complaint "Doctor, I have sinus" is commonly heard by the otolaryngologist, the exact meaning of "sinus" to a patient remains a highly individual matter. Some of these patients have primary complaints that represent allergy. Others have infection, vasomotor rhinitis, or even migraine headaches. Therefore, the most important initial step is to establish the exact symptoms, that are troubling the patient, the chronology of the illness, and (if applicable) the response to various previous therapeutic attempts. In other words, the presence or absence of active sinus disease must be determined by a history, physical examination, and appropriate ancillary tests (endoscopy, radiographic studies). This chapter assumes that all this has been done, and that the patient indeed does suffer from some form of sinusitis. In such instances, there is often a distinct relationship between such sinus problems and allergy, and it behooves physicians engaging to treat these patients to understand and address this relationship. To do so ensures better results, and to ignore such a concordance increases the chance of a poor therapeutic outcome or a rapid recurrence of symptoms.

ROLE OF THE OSTIOMEATAL COMPLEX

The concept of the ostiomeatal complex (OMC) as the key to sinus disease is generally attributed to the work of Messerklinger.[1] However, even earlier, Proctor[2] underscored the importance of the ethmoids and infundibulum as the key structures in producing disease in other sinuses. The OMC is located in the middle meatus and represents the region into which empty the maxillary, anterior ethmoid, and frontal sinuses. It is bounded by the ethmoid bulla, the uncinate process, and the middle turbinate (Fig. 16–1). Although anatomic abnormalities may result in OMC blockage, by far the most frequent cause of such obstruction is mucosal edema. Edema may be caused by infection, allergy, or various nonatopic triggers (Table 16–1).

RELATIONSHIP OF ALLERGY AND SINUSITIS

There has been gradual acceptance that allergy may be a significant contributor to sinus disease. In 1995, Slavin[3] reviewed the concordance of allergy

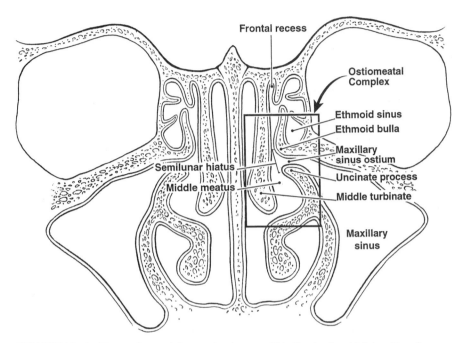

FIGURE 16–1. The ostiomeatal complex (*area within the box*), which is of key importance in the prevention and management of sinus disease.

and sinus disease (as high as 75% in some series) and indicated that this finding, significantly more frequent than the prevalence of allergy in the general population, "supports the impression that allergy is an important associated and probably predisposing factor in sinusitis." In one study, patients with acute sinusitis showed a significantly higher number of positive results on allergy skin tests in comparison with control groups.[4] In children, a high correlation between allergy and sinus disease has also been demonstrated.[5,6] Such studies have made it clear that it is no longer necessary to defend the practice of investigating and treating allergy in every patient with sinus disease. Rather, to omit such a consideration would appear to be questionable.

Allergy may affect the sinuses in three ways: by the direct effect of the allergic event, by enhancing reactivity (or priming), and by contributing to the formation of polyps.

Direct Effects of the Allergic Reaction on Sinuses

An acute Gell and Coombs type I, immunoglobulin E (IgE)-mediated allergic event results in the release by tissue mast cells and basophils of both pre-

TABLE 16–1. Factors contributing to ostiomeatal complex obstruction

I. Anatomic abnormalities
  A. Septal deviation
  B. Mass lesions
    1. Polyp
    2. Foreign body
    3. Tumor
  C. Abnormalities of middle turbinate
    1. Paradoxical middle turbinate
    2. Concha bullosum
  D. Abnormalities of lateral nasal wall
    1. Enlarged uncinate process
    2. Enlarged extramural ethmoid cells
II. Mucosal edema
  A. Infection
  B. Allergy
  C. Medicamentous rhinitis
  D. Hormonal aberrations
  E. Vasomotor rhinitis
    1. Stress, temperature change, eating
    2. Cigarette smoke, air pollution, chemical exposure

From Mabry RL. Medical management of sinusitis. In: Rice DH, Schaefer SD, (eds.). Endoscopic Paranasal Sinus Surgery. 2nd ed. New York: Raven Press; 1992:95–104; with permission.

formed and newly formed mediators of inflammation. These include inflammatory agents (e.g., histamine, platelet activating factor, tryptase, kinins), spasmogens and mucous secretagogues (e.g., prostaglandins, leukotrienes), and cellular attractants (neutrophil and eosinophil chemotactic factors). This process results is an acute reaction characterized by mucosal edema, mucous secretion, and vasodilation with increased vascular permeability. A late stage, marked by cellular influx, maintains many of these circumstances. As a consequence of such a reaction in the nasal mucosa, obstruction of the ostiomeatal complex may occur. The increased production of mucus by the sinus mucosa is trapped within the various sinus cavities, resulting in stagnation. These thick secretions form a medium for the aerobic and/or anaerobic growth of pathogens, setting the stage for secondary infection or perpetuating existing infection. Thus, in patients with borderline competence of the ostiomeatal complex, allergic reactions and the edema and hypersecretion that accompany them may tip the balance from adequate function to disease.

Allergy and Altered Responsiveness (Priming)

In 1968, Connell[7] reported his observations that in pollen-allergic patients, more nasal symptoms (especially obstruction) were produced by the same amount of pollen exposure at the end of a pollen season than at its beginning. He called this phenomenon *priming*. He found it to be related to the degree of allergen exposure (i.e., threshold lowered more by larger allergen challenges). It was specific to the challenged mucosa, so that if only the lower airway was challenged, no priming was exhibited by the nasal mucosa. Connell also found that the affected mucosa demonstrated heightened sensitivity to challenges by other stimuli. The phenomenon was reversible, ceasing after allergen challenges were discontinued.

The mechanism of priming has been clarified by further studies.[8] It appears to result from the release of additional mediators, such as histamine, toxoid-antitoxoid mixture esterase (TAME), and prostaglandin D_2, caused by an increased influx of inflammatory cells.

It has been shown that priming can affect eustachian tube function.[9] The parallel between the eustachian tube and the OMC is readily apparent. Thus, it certainly seems logical that repeated allergic challenges and untreated allergic reactions could adversely affect the function of the narrow channel through which the key sinuses ventilate and drain. It follows that appropriate management of allergy, including the prevention of the allergic reaction whenever possible, should be part of the management of sinusitis.

Allergy and Polyps

In the early days of our specialty, polyps were classified as being of "allergic" or "inflammatory" origin, based on the presence or absence of eosinophils within their stroma. Likewise, the view formerly espoused that all polyps have an allergic origin has given way to the opinion voiced by Slavin[10] that allergy occurs infrequently and independently in patients with nasal polyps, and that "the routine allergic evaluation of patients with nasal polyps should be discouraged in the name of health care cost containment."

Recently reported observations[11] indicate that polyp development begins as epithelial rupture (caused by edema). Tissue prolapse, the development of a vascular stalk, and epithelialization of the prolapsed tissue follow, resulting in the formation of a full-blown polyp. The cause of rupture can be trauma, infection,[12] allergy,[13] or a combination of factors.

The fact remains that allergy may be a cause (possibly a very significant one) of sinonasal polyps. The review by Slavin that led him to the conclusion that allergy is not a significant factor in polyp development included allergy testing primarily by prick/puncture methods. Although prick testing is generally adequate to diagnose significant degrees of sensitivity to inhalant antigens, negative prick test results must followed by intradermal tests (which are much more sensitive) before the true absence of atopic skin reactivity can be confirmed. In addition, the material reviewed by Slavin did not include investigation for food allergy, which may influence polyp development. Thus, his evaluation of a possible effect on polyps may have significantly underestimated the incidence of allergy in the populations considered.

An interesting phenomenon is the presence of allergen-specific IgE in the nasal mucosa and/or polyps of patients with no systemic evidence of allergy.[14] This suggests that in some patients local allergy may play a role in sinonasal polyposis.

Certainly, experienced rhinologists who deal with allergy have made the clinical observation (unfortunately, unconfirmed thus far by scientific studies) that in patients in whom allergy and polyps coexist, appropriate management of the allergy significantly lessens the likelihood of polyp recurrence. Therefore, as a practical matter, all patients with rhinosinusitis and nasal polyposis should have some sort of allergy workup. This may be as simple as a thorough history with attention to indicators of allergy, or as complex as complete evaluation for inhalant and food sensitivity.

PHARMACOTHERAPY FOR ALLERGY IN THE PATIENT WITH SINUSITIS

Some consideration must be given to the effect of concomitant allergy and sinus disease when various medications are considered in these patients.

Antihistamines

For years, it was thought that antihistamines should not be administered to patients with sinusitis, lest these compounds thicken nasal secretions, thereby contributing to stagnation of secretions and crust formation with obstruction. For similar reasons, the use of antihistamines in asthmatic patients was questioned. This idea remains valid in regard to the administration of conventional, first-generation (sedating) antihistamines, which have significant anticholinergic, side effects. However, the second- and third-generation preparations, such as loratadine, cetirizine, and fexofenadine, are essentially free of this side effect and may safely (and effectively) be used to provide symptomatic relief in patients with allergy and sinus disease and/or asthma.[15]

Patients with sinusitis often require antibiotic therapy. It has been shown that the administration of either of the antihistamines terfenadine and astemizole concurrently with either of the macrolide antibiotics erythromycin and troleandomycin, which are also metabolized by the P-450 cytochrome oxidase system, may result in cardiac arrhythmias, such as torsades de pointes, in a very small percentage of patients.[16] This warning has not been extended to some of the newer macrolides, such as clarithromycin and azithromycin. Other compounds, most notably systemic antifungals, may also produce arrhythmias when given with terfenadine or astemizole. Fortunately, this is not a problem with the newer antihistamines.

Decongestants

Patients with both allergy and sinusitis experience nasal obstruction as a result of the disease process. Because both problems tend to be chronic, these patients are more prone than others to become dependent on topical nasal decongestants, producing a "rebound rhinitis." This may occur in as little as 5 to 7 days. One study (using normal volunteers, not patients with rhinitis) has suggested that restricted usage of a long-acting preparation (e.g., oxymetazoline) for even longer periods may not produce a rebound phenomenon.[17] Nevertheless, until further work confirms this, it is best to utilize systemic decongestants, rather than topical preparations, in patients with allergy and/or sinus disease.

Mucolytics

Although the clinical studies available to support the use of mucolytics sinusitis,[18] most physicians (based on clinical experience) routinely employ them (e.g., guafenesin) to thin secretions that have become thick and tenacious, thereby aiding sinus drainage and evacuation of secretions. However, patients with associated allergy may often complain that these drugs are "making their allergy worse," as the end result that they perceive is an increase in thin nasal secretions. A word of forewarning is generally sufficient to result in patient acceptance of this treatment, when needed.

Mast Cell Stabilizers

The prototype of this category of drugs, cromolyn, is an excellent preventive agent in the treatment of allergic rhinitis. Appropriate use of cromolyn before an anticipated allergy exposure may prevent a priming phenomenon caused by repeated allergic events. In a few fortunate patients with allergy and recurrent sinusitis who have borderline obstruction of the ostiomeatal complex, preventing the direct effects of the allergic reaction already described by the regular use of a mast cell stabilizer may permit adequate sinus ventilation and drainage, thereby avoiding the need for surgical intervention.

It should be pointed out that cromolyn is not effective in the treatment of polyps, nor does it have a primary anti-inflammatory effect (such as is exhibited by corticosteroids). As pointed out below, if patients are placed on nasal corticosteroids, the use of cromolyn becomes redundant.

Finally, in our experience we have noted that patients using cromolyn in the face of active nasal and sinus infection often complain that it produces a nasal burning. This should cause the clinician to suspect infection strongly and treat it appropriately.

Corticosteroids

These potent anti-inflammatory drugs are frequently effective in treating rhinosinusitis from a variety of causes, not just allergy. As pointed out in the chapter on pharmacotherapy, appropriate instruction of the patient regarding the proper use of corticosteroids is required, as well as monitoring to ascertain the need for their continued use and to watch for undesirable topical or systemic effects.

At least theoretically, corticosteroids inhibit the body's natural defense against infection through their effect on the inflammatory response. It is prudent to interrupt a course of topical corticosteroid treatment if an active infection supervenes until it has been controlled by antibiotic therapy.

IMMUNOTHERAPY IN THE PATIENT WITH SINUSITIS

Because of the concordance between allergy and sinusitis, many patients with sinus disease are candidates for immunotherapy. When the appropriate treatment of the sinus disease fails to produce adequate resolution and surgery is indicated, the question that constantly arises is whether these injections should be begun before surgery or afterward. Ideally, allergy therapy should be instituted 6 to 12 weeks before surgical intervention is employed. This is not to make the surgery unnecessary (although, happily, that is sometimes the result). Rather, addressing allergy before surgery and continuing the therapy after surgery provides the greatest likelihood of a desirable long-term result.[19]

If the need for surgical intervention is pressing, immunotherapy may be begun after surgery. However, these patients should be urged to start allergen avoidance and environmental control measures at the earliest possible moment. Likewise, appropriate pharmacotherapy should be instituted. If surgery must precede immunotherapy, it is best to wait for about 4 weeks to do any skin testing or begin allergy injections, to allow the immune system to normalize after the stress of surgery.

It is important, when immunotherapy is begun in patients with both allergy and sinus disease, to be certain that all parties concerned understand the indicators of success. Some of these patients may not have "typical" allergic symptoms of rhinorrhea, sneezing, and pruritis. However, if they understand that their allergy treatment is aimed at preventing episodes of hypersecretion and mucosal edema, they will be able to appreciate the benefits of fewer "sinus"-type symptoms.

NURSE'S NOTE

Allergy nurses and assistants should be alert to the situation in which a patient, for no apparent reason, begins to have significant local reactions after allergy injections. If these patients have experienced no increased antigen exposure or had no change in their dosage, the possibility of a complicating infection should be strongly considered. Most patients receiving allergy injections tend to blame all their nasal symptoms on allergy and never consider that infections may produce similar problems. It is helpful to encourage these patients to see the physician to check this possibility, and to assess the reason for their local reactions.

Patients on immunotherapy in whom an active infection develops involving the nose and sinus frequently demonstrate increased (and often unacceptable) local reactions at their injection sites, with no change in antigen dose or allergen exposure. This may call for a brief dose adjustment or even the omission of injections for a week or so, and it should also trigger a search for and appropriate treatment of the infection. Rarely will these episodes significantly alter the overall course of immunotherapy. However, the allergy nurse or assistant should be constantly alert for situations in which large local reactions occur for no apparent reason (such as an increased exposure to allergens or a change in dose). When this occurs, the possibility of an infection should be entertained, and the patient should be seen by the physician if necessary for further evaluation.

SURGERY IN THE ALLERGIC PATIENT

A question often raised in the past was whether nasal and sinus surgery in allergic patients should be deferred to avoid operating during times of peak exposure to antigens causing allergic reactions. This no longer represents a major problem, as measures are now available to provide control of nasal allergic symptoms that might otherwise be accentuated by surgical intervention. Nevertheless, every effort should be made, both before and after surgery, to minimize the patient's allergic symptoms through environmental control, appropriate pharmacotherapy, and immunotherapy. If possible, immunotherapy should be instituted 6 to 12 weeks before surgery, as it is often possible to see positive results in even this short a time. Of course, all these measures should also be continued for as long as necessary after surgery.

A helpful measure is the use of intraturbinal corticosteroid injection at the conclusion of nasal and sinus procedures in patients with allergy. This minimizes reactive edema and allergic problems during the immediate postoperative period. The injection is effective within hours and the effects last 4 to 6 weeks, so that the use of intranasal corticosteroids is unnecessary within the first week or two after surgery (when the nasal mucosa is often hyperreactive to stimuli such as sprays). Details of the proper use of this procedure are found in Chapter 8; they should be kept firmly in mind to avoid the potential complication of retinal vasospasm or embolization, which has been reported in rare instances.[20]

Some patients with allergic rhinitis also have asthma and may be receiving systemic corticosteroids at the time of needed nasal and sinus surgery. Exogenous administration of a glucocorticoid may result in adrenal suppression through the hypothalamic-pituitary axis (HPA) feedback mechanism. This will vary with dose and duration of administration. For example, administration of 20 to 30 mg of prednisone (or the equivalent dose of another corticosteroid) for as little as 5 to 7 days may produce adrenal insufficiency, with recovery in about a week after the drug is discontinued. Lower doses administered for 30 days may produce significant adrenal suppression, which requires longer for recovery.[21] When patients have received systemic corticosteroids before surgery, it is advisable to keep in mind the possibility of adrenal suppression, which may be manifested by an addisonian crisis during the stress of surgery. Supplementation with exogenous corticosteroids is generally advisable in these situations. If this is the case, the anesthesiologist is usually able to offer specific suggestions regarding dosing and duration of such supplementation.

GOALS OF ALLERGY THERAPY IN SINUSITIS

The goals of allergy therapy in patients with sinusitis are outlined in Table 16–2. Environmental control should be practiced by all patients with rhinos-

TABLE 16–2. Goals of allergy therapy in sinus disease

I. Teach environmental control.
  A. Specific antigenic triggers
  B. Nonspecific triggers
    1. Smoke
    2. Chemicals
II. Instruct in proper use of medication.
  A. Antihistamines
  B. Decongestants
  C. Cromolyn
  D. Corticosteroids
III. Administer immunotherapy when indicated.
IV. Consider allergy in all cases.

inusitis. In those with allergy, this obviously entails avoiding allergenic triggers insofar as possible. However, nonspecific irritants such as tobacco smoke and chemicals should be avoided by all patients. Education in this regard often falls to the nurse or allergy assistant, but physicians should participate by constantly reminding patients of this important facet of care.

NURSE'S NOTE

Patients on allergy injections may either neglect to take their medications (feeling that the injections should take care of the problem) or take them improperly. It generally falls to the allergy nurse or assistant to inquire continually if patients are using the medications that have been prescribed, and if they are using them properly. Intranasal cromolyn should be used before an anticipated allergy exposure. Antihistamines should be taken to control ''wet'' symptoms, whereas decongestants relieve nasal obstruction. (Unfortunately, many patients don't understand the difference.) Topical nasal steroids should be used regularly, not just ''when I think I need them,'' and the proper technique of use will not only make them more effective but will prevent local side effects, such as nasal irritation. Antibiotics given for infection should be taken for the full course prescribed. Patients with sinusitis may need to be reminded of the benefits and proper technique of nasal irrigation.

Printed material about the proper use of medications is available from the American Academy of Otolaryngology-Head and Neck Surgery (One Prince St, Alexandria, VA 22314) or the U.S. Pharmacopeial Convention (12601 Twinbrook Pkwy, Rockville, MD 20852), as well as from many drug companies.

Patients with rhinosinusitis are almost universally provided with one or more medications to use for symptom control. Unfortunately, the directions for proper use of these agents are often misunderstood or forgotten. Therefore, it is important to determine at every visit whether patients are using the medications provided, and to what extent they are necessary. Furthermore, inquiry should be made as to how they are using them. For example, it has been shown quite well that nasal corticosteroids must be used on a regular basis, not "as needed," for maximum effectiveness.[22] Nevertheless, patients are constantly encountered who employ corticosteroid nasal sprays in single doses every day or two, "when they feel they need them." Patients must be educated and constantly reminded that 2 to 5 days of regular use are required for nasal steroid sprays to be effective, and especially for them to provide protection from the acute-phase (rather than the late-phase) allergic reaction. Similar misunderstandings are often encountered in dealing with patients' perception of the proper use of antihistamines and decongestants. Much of this instruction in the proper and continuing use of their medications falls to the allergy nurse or assistant and is a major contribution to patients' ongoing care.

The indications for allergy immunotherapy are detailed elsewhere in this text. Not all patients with allergic rhinosinusitis require this form of therapy, but there are many situations in which it can be of benefit. Unfortunately, for patients to be considered for immunotherapy, the treating physician must think of it first. Physicians who are appropriately trained in both the medical and surgical management of rhinosinusitis, including the provision of immunotherapy when indicated, can offer the most comprehensive care to their patients.

In summary, it is important for the physician dealing with patients who have sinus disease to include allergy in the total consideration of diagnosis and treatment.

REFERENCES

1. Messerk linger W. Uber die drainage der menshichen nasennebenhohler unter normalen ausfuhrungssystem. Monatsschr Ohrenheilkd 1967;101:313–326.
2. Proctor DF. The nose, paranasal sinuses and pharynx. In: Walters W, (ed.). Lewis-Walters Practice of Surgery. Hagerstown, MD: WF Prior; 1966:1–37 (vol 4).
3. Slavin RG. Infectious sinusitis: when usual treatment fails. Presented at the Annual Meeting of the American College of Asthma, Allergy and Immunology, Dallas, Texas, November 13, 1995.
4. Savolainen S. Allergy in patients with acute maxillary sinusitis. Allergy 1989;44: 116–122.
5. Rachelefsky G, Siegel SC, Katz RM, et al. Chronic sinusitis in children. J Allergy Clin Immunol 1991;87:219 (abst).

 6. Shapiro G, Virant F, Furukawa CT, et al. Immunologic defects in patients with refractory sinusitis. Pediatrics 1991;87:311–316.
 7. Connell JT. Quantitative intranasal pollen challenge. J Allergy 1968;41:123–139.
 8. Wachs M, Proud D, Lichtenstein LM, Kagey-Sobotka A, Norman PS, Naclerio RM. Observations on the pathogenesis of nasal priming. J Allergy Clin Immunol 1989;84: 492–501.
 9. Skoner D, Doyle W, Boehm S, Fireman P. Priming of the nose and eustachian tube during natural pollen exposure. Am J Rhinol 1989;3:53–57.
10. Slavin RG. Allergy is not a significant cause of nasal polyps. Arch Otolaryngol Head Neck Surg 1992;118:771.
11. Tos M. The pathogenetic theories in formation of nasal polyps. Am J Rhinol 1990;4: 51–56.
12. Norlander T, Fukami M, Westrin KM, Stierna P, Carlsoo B. Formation of mucosal polyps in the nasal and maxillary sinus cavities by infection. Otolaryngol Head Neck Surg 1993; 109:522–529.
13. Bernstein JM, Gorfien J, Noble B. Role of allergy in nasal polyposis: a review. Otolaryngol Head Neck Surg 1995;113:724–732.
14. Shatkin JS, Delsupsehe KG, Thisted RA, Corey JP. Mucosal allergy in the absence of systemic allergy in nasal polyposis and rhinitis: a meta-analysis. Otolaryngol Head Neck Surg 1994;111:553–556.
15. Busse WW. Role of antihistamines in allergic disease. Ann Allergy 1994;72:371–375.
16. Honig P, Baraniuk JN. Adverse effects of H_1-receptor antagonists in the cardiovascular system. In: Simons FER, ed. Histamine and H_1-Receptor Antagonists in Allergic Disease. New York: Marcel Dekker; 1996:383–412.
17. Yoo JK, Seikaly H, Calhoun K. Extended use of topical nasal decongestants. Laryngoscope 1997;107:40–43.
18. Wawrose SF, Tami TA, Amoils CP. The role of guaifenesin in the treatment of sinonasal disease in patients infected with human immunodeficiency virus (HIV). Laryngoscope 1992;102:1225–1228.
19. Davis WE, Templer JW, Lamear WR, Davis WE Jr. Middle meatus antrostomy: patency rates and risk factors. Otolaryngol Head Neck Surg 1991;104:467–472.
20. Mabry RL. Corticosteroids in otolaryngology: intraturbinal injection. Otolaryngol Head Neck Surg 1983;91:717–720.
21. Corticosteroids-glucocorticoid effects (systemic). Drug Information for the Health Care Professional. 17th ed. Rockville, MD: US Pharmacopeial Convention; 1997:958–966.
22. Juniper EE, Guyat GH, O'Byrne PM, et al. Aqueous beclomethasone dipropionate nasal spray: regular versus "as required" use in the treatment of seasonal allergic rhinitis. J Allergy Clin Immunol 1990;86:380–386.

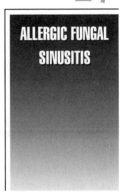

The subject of "fungal sinusitis" has received a great
deal of attention during the past decade or more. No
aspect of this problem has received more recent attention than the entity known as, *allergic fungal sinusitis*
(AFS). Because of its allergic aspects, AFS is important to all rhinologists, especially to those dealing with
allergy.

AFS must be differentiated from other pathophysiologic states in which fungal organisms affect the paranasal sinuses. Included in this group are invasive
fungal sinusitis (typically, but not universally, seen in immunocompromised
patients), mycetomas (noninvasive fungus balls typically found in one maxillary or sphenoid sinus), and saprophytic fungal growth on crusts and purulent
exudate within diseased sinuses.[1] AFS is the only one of these disorders with
an allergic component, which must be understood (and managed) to provide
the greatest likelihood of control in this typically recalcitrant disease.

HISTORICAL BACKGROUND

AFS was originally termed *allergic Aspergillus sinusitis* and was felt to
represent the sinonasal equivalent of allergic bronchopulmonary aspergillosis
(ABPA). The diagnostic criteria for ABPA include bronchial obstruction,
eosinophilia, positive immunologic test results, positive sputum cultures for
Aspergillus, and a history of expectoration of brown plugs (representing
fungal debris).[2] In 1981, Millar et al[3] first termed this entity *allergic aspergillosis of the paranasal sinuses*.

The most definitive early study in this area was that of Katzenstein and
colleagues,[4] who retrospectively reviewed specimens from more than 100
sinus operations, finding seven instances of histologic findings similar to the
mucoid impactions found in the bronchi of patients with ABPA. It was
Allphin et al[5] who finally suggested that many fungi, not just *Aspergillus*
species, were capable of causing this clinical picture, and also suggested the
term now used, *allergic fungal sinusitis* (AFS).

PATHOPHYSIOLOGY

There now is little doubt that AFS is truly an allergic disorder, not a fungal
infection. These patients have been shown to have markedly increased total

levels of immunoglobulin E (IgE) and positive results on allergen-specific IgE assays for both fungal and nonfungal antigens.[6] Results of skin tests for fungal antigens have also been noted to be positive in patients with AFS.[7]

It has been conjectured that AFS occurs in the same manner as ABPA. The process has been described as a vicious cycle in which fungus, trapped in viscid secretions contained in the constricted airway, results in continued exposure to large quantities of antigenic material. The most likely scenario for the development of AFS is that proposed by Manning et al,[8] in which obstruction of the sinus ostia and stasis of secretions may be promoted by allergy and bacterial infection, as well as anatomic abnormalities. When this occurs in patients with a genetic predisposition to atopy, prolonged contact between the sinus mucosa and entrapped fungal elements results in both Gell and Coombs type I (IgE-mediated) and type III (immune complex) reactions. These cause further mucosal edema and polyp formation, plus the formation of an eosinophilic debris termed *allergic mucin*.

CLINICAL DIAGNOSTIC CHARACTERISTICS

As already mentioned, other forms of fungal involvement of the sinuses occur, and these must be differentiated from AFS. Invasive fungal sinusitis, which generally affects immunocompromised patients, is characterized by tissue invasion and necrosis, neither of which is seen in AFS. Mycetomas are large "fungus balls" that are found in one sinus, generally the maxillary or sphenoid, in immunocompetent patients. In these situations, surgical extirpation and marsupialization are curative. It is frequently the case that fungi grow saprophytically in the debris and purulent exudate found in the sinuses of patients with chronic purulent sinusitis. This represents merely a fungal presence, not an infection, and is generally of no clinical significance.

One entity that may present a greater diagnostic challenge has been described by Ferguson,[9] who terms it *allergic mucin sinusitis*. In this situation, the histopathologic picture mimics that of AFS, with the exception of demonstrable fungal forms.

The typical clinical presentation of AFS is chronic pansinusitis with polyposis, often with a history of recurrent problems despite one or more previous sinus operations. If sinus disease is long-standing or severe, bone remodeling may result in proptosis or diplopia. However, other patients may present with simple nasal congestion and purulent sinusitis. These patients are generally young but may range in age from preadolescence to middle age; AFS shows no predilection for either sex. The patients do not show an increased incidence of salicylate sensitivity, and only about one third are asthmatic.

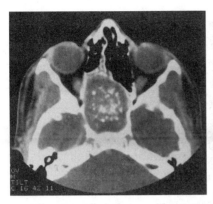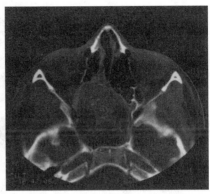

FIGURE 17–1. CT scan of patient with expansile mass of allergic fungal sinusitis involving the sphenoid. Both soft-tissue *(left)* and bone *(right)* windows demonstrate a typical speckled pattern of high attenuation. (From Manning SC, Merkel M, Kriesel K, Vuitch F, Marple B. Computed tomography and magnetic resonance diagnosis of allergic fungal sinusitis. Laryngoscope 1997;107:170–176; with permission.)

Atopy is virtually a universal finding in these patients, who often have allergic rhinitis. Interestingly, many patients with AFS have received immunotherapy previously and have discontinued it because of adverse local or constitutional reactions.

The radiographic findings in AFS are typical.[10] Multiple sinuses are opacified. Long-standing or severe disease may have caused bone remodeling or erosion involving the lamina papyracea, orbital apex, or cribriform plate. Heterogenous densities on computed tomography (CT scans) of patients with AFS (Fig. 17–1) have been described and are theorized to result from high levels of magnesium, manganese, and iron in allergic mucin within the sinuses.[11] Magnetic resonance imaging (MRI) may be useful, especially if erosion is suspected. On T_1-weighted images, allergic mucin is seen as isointense or slightly hypointense masses, which frequently become completely black on T_2-weighted images (Fig. 17–2).

Although the disorder may be suspected based on history, physical examination, and radiographic characteristics, surgical and histopathologic findings are able to provide more definitive diagnostic information. At surgery, in addition to polyps and mucosal hyperplasia, sinuses involved with AFS contain a unique material, allergic mucin (Fig. 17–3). This is a thick, viscous, tenacious material that may vary in color from light tan to brown to green to black. Its consistency is sometimes compared with that of axle grease or peanut butter. It is typically very difficult to remove from the involved sinuses, usually requiring irrigation, suction, and painstaking dissection. The

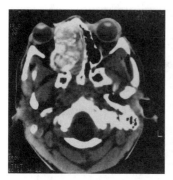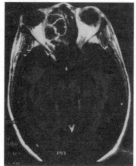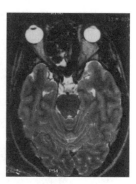

FIGURE 17–2. Patient with allergic fungal sinusitis involving right ethmoid and expanding into orbit. The CT scan *(left)* demonstrates the extent of disease and orbital involvement. The T_1 MRI *(center)* shows low signal in the center of the mass, with a high signal on the periphery. On the T_2 MRI *(right)*, the central area demonstrates a void signal. (From Manning SC, Merkel M, Kriesel K, Vuitch F, Marple B. Computed tomography and magnetic resonance diagnosis of allergic fungal sinusitis. Laryngoscope 1997;107:170–176; with permission.)

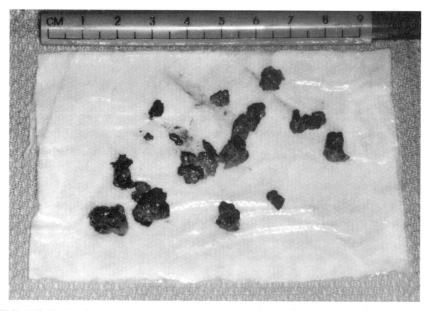

FIGURE 17–3. Allergic mucin removed from a patient with extensive allergic fungal sinusitis. This thick material, often compared in consistency with peanut butter or axle grease, is a hallmark of AFS.

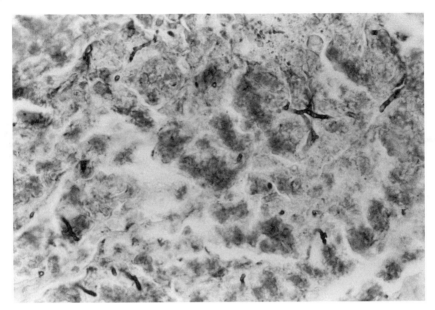

FIGURE 17–4. Histopathology of allergic fungal sinusitis. On a background of sheets of eosinophils, a fungal stain demonstrates noninvasive fungal hyphae. Clumps of degenerating eosinophils form Charcot-Leyden crystals.

accumulation of this material is responsible for the bone remodeling or pressure erosion that characterizes AFS.

Histopathologic examination of allergic mucin reveals an eosinophilic substrate that, when stained appropriately, demonstrates the presence of noninvasive fungal elements (Fig. 17–4). The substrate is composed of sheets of eosinophils (both intact and in varying degrees of degradation) and contains Charcot-Leyden crystals. These elongated eosinophilic bodies represent the product of eosinophil degradation. They are not specific for AFS and may be found in any secretions rich in eosinophils, such as the sputum of asthmatic patients.

DIAGNOSIS

Although during the last decade AFS has been recognized as being less rare than initially thought, its exact incidence remains unclear. This is primarily because no single set of criteria for the establishment of this diagnosis have been universally accepted. Even with the varied standards of diagnosis that currently exist, it is estimated that about 7% of the cases of chronic sinusitis that require surgery involve AFS.[12]

The initial descriptions of allergic *Aspergillus* sinusitis included the common factors of immunocompetence (as opposed to the immune deficiency seen in patients with invasive fungal sinusitis), positive skin test reactions to *Aspergillus* antigen, other positive serologic findings (high levels of fungal-specific antigen and elevated total IgE), and typical histopathologic findings of allergic mucin containing noninvasive fungal forms.

Corey[13] and others have described immunologic characteristics that might suggest preoperatively the presence of AFS. These are derived from those for ABPA, which include peripheral eosinophilia, immediate cutaneous reactivity and the presence of precipitating antigens to *Aspergillus*, elevated total serum IgE, and elevated levels of *Aspergillus*-specific IgE and IgG. Such immunologic information may be highly suggestive of AFS. However, clinical characteristics must also be considered in making this diagnosis.

Numerous authors have set forth their own diagnostic criteria,[14–16] all of which generally include immunocompetence, typical radiographic findings, presence of typical allergic mucin with noninvasive hyphae, and presence of atopy. Among the best-known and most-used are the criteria set forth by Bent and Kuhn.[17] After an analysis of 15 cases of AFS, they found five characteristics common to all (Table 17–1): Gell and Coombs type I hypersensitivity, nasal polyposis, characteristic CT appearance, eosinophilic mucus without fungal invasion, and positive fungal stain of sinus contents removed at surgery. They found that a unilateral predominance, a history of asthma, the presence of Charcot-Leyden crystals, and peripheral eosinophilia

TABLE 17–1. Characteristics of AFS

Gell and Coombs type I hypersensitivity
  Positive skin test results
  Positive in vitro test results
  Strongly positive history
Nasal polyposis
Characteristic findings on CT scan
  Clouding of multiple sinuses
  Areas of increased attenuation, especially on bone windows
  Bone destruction and remodeling variably present
Allergic mucin
  Typical gross appearance
  Eosinophilic material on histopathology
Identifiable fungal forms with appropriate fungal stains
  Noninvasive
  Fungal cultures variably positive

Adapted from Bent JP III, Kuhn FA. Diagnosis of allergic fungal sinusitis. Otolaryngol Head Neck Surg 1994;111:580–588.

were often (but not universally) present in their series. Our experience has been similar to theirs, and we base the diagnosis of AFS on the presence in atopic patients of pansinusitis with polyposis, with typical gross and histologic findings of allergic mucin, including noninvasive hyphae.

It is important to point out that cultures may not be positive for fungi in all patients with AFS. Conversely, the presence of a positive fungal culture does not confirm the diagnosis, as this may simply represent a saprophytic fungal overgrowth in a diseased sinus. Furthermore, it is important that the specimen removed at sinus surgery and submitted for histopathologic examination include the allergic mucin material, not just the polypoid mucosa. In AFS, fungal forms will be found only in the former location, not in the latter.

PRINCIPLES OF TREATMENT

The management of AFS to some degree parallels that recommended for ABPA. In ABPA, the aim of treatment is to break the ''vicious cycle'' of entrapped viscid secretions in the constricted airways serving as the allergic stimulus for a reaction responsible for the formation of more secretions. This has traditionally involved treatment with systemic corticosteroids (administered for their anti-inflammatory effect), plus bronchodilators, expectorants, and other measures aimed at tracheobronchial toilet.[18] The major difference is that in AFS, it is possible to aid in breaking this cycle by physically removing the retained allergic mucin and opening the involved sinuses to make subsequent cleaning possible. Despite surgical intervention, the use of corticosteroids has also been a mainstay of the medical management of AFS. However, recent advances in treatment strategy may change this situation.

Although some early investigators implied that AFS represents merely a more indolent form of fungal infection, without invasion, this view is no longer widely held. Thus, the use of systemic antifungal agents has little or no place in the treatment of AFS. The use of topical antifungal agents in irrigation solutions following surgery has been suggested, but the efficacy of such treatment has yet to be definitely established.[19]

PREOPERATIVE MANAGEMENT

Once a working diagnosis of AFS has been reached, it is almost certain that eventual surgical intervention will be necessary. However, efforts at preoperative preparation will be repaid by better postoperative results. Probably the most important step is the administration of a short burst of systemic corticosteroids before surgery, to decrease the inflammatory response in the sinonasal region and (it is hoped) make surgical extirpation easier. An expeditious means of administering a tapered dose is the use of a tapered-dose package, such as a Medrol Dosepak. A useful variant is to prescribed two such packages, with instructions to the patient to take the first day's pills from pack 1 on day 1, the first day's pills from pack 2 on day 2, and so forth. Topical nasal steroids may also be given, but extensive polyp disease may prevent medication from reaching significantly into the nasal cavity. Administration of antibiotics preoperatively is recommended, as almost all these patients will have some element of purulence in the stagnant secretions within their sinuses. The use of nasal irrigations to cleanse thick mucus preoperatively may be helpful and serves to educate the patients in a modality that most will require after surgery.

Allergy testing should have been done before surgery as part of the workup. Although immunotherapy for fungal antigens should be withheld until after surgery, patients should be counseled preoperatively regarding avoidance measures (for both fungal and nonfungal antigens). In addition, this counseling should be repeated after surgery, during the course of immunotherapy, as the allergy staff comes into continued contact with the patient.

NURSE'S NOTE

The nurse or allergy care giver usually has most of the responsibility for instruction in environmental control. This is especially important in the case of patients with AFS, who must be continually educated in mold-avoidance measures. These include not only minimization of exposure to molds, but also avoidance of foods that are sources of mold and fungi, such as beer, wine, and cheese. Also patients often need assistance in locating commercial sources for materials they need to carry out their environmental control programs.

This instruction in environmental control can begin before surgery or the institution of immunotherapy, but it must be constantly reinforced and updated.

OPERATIVE MANAGEMENT

The surgical techniques employed in patients with AFS are beyond the scope of this text. However, the goals of surgery in these patients are (1) removal of obstructing sinonasal polypoid tissue, (2) removal of all allergic mucin, and (3) wide exteriorization or marsupialization of all involved sinuses. The use of a powered instrument such as a microdebrider

TABLE 17–2. Instructions to patient for nasal irrigation

The Grossan nasal irrigation tip attaches to a WaterPik and is used to irrigate the nose and sinuses with saline solution (salt water). This is especially beneficial after nasal and sinus surgery but may also be helpful for patients with chronic thick nasal secretions.

The Grossan nasal irrigation tip may be purchased at many pharmacies, or directly from Hydro Med Inc,* without a prescription. Although in some circumstances it is necessary to use commercially obtained sterile saline solution for irrigation, in most instances it is possible to prepare your own saline solution by *adding two heaping teaspoons of salt and one teaspoon of baking soda to a quart of boiled water (cooled to room temperature)*.

Attach the irrigator tip to the WaterPik and add saline solution to the device's reservoir. Set the WaterPik between medium and high, so that the stream delivered squirts about four inches. Bending over a sink, place the tip comfortably in one nostril and aim the stream toward the top of the nasal cavity, directing the stream from the front to the back to cover all areas. If you have had turbinate surgery, also direct the stream along the floor of the nose. The water may drain out the back of the nose into the mouth and throat, or it may return from the opposite nostril or around the irrigator tip. Use about half the saline solution on each side.

For most patients, irrigation should be begun about 2 weeks after surgery, unless you are instructed to begin it sooner. Irrigate at least twice daily, although you may irrigate up to four times daily if desired. Continue the irrigations until instructed to discontinue them. They may be useful in the future to cleanse crusts and thick nasal mucus, but if these problems persist, be sure to see the doctor.

* Hydro Med Inc, 4419 Van Nuys Blvd, Suite 310, Sherman Oaks, CA 91403; phone, 800-560-9007; web address, http://www.ent-consult.com.

is extremely helpful in these cases.[20] It is extremely important to remove only the diseased mucosa, as frequently the process of opening the sinuses and removing accumulated allergic mucin, coupled with hygiene and follow-up, will allow otherwise "irreversibly diseased" mucosa to return to normal function. On the other hand, extensive removal of mucosa will almost always result in chronic thick nasal secretions and problems with crusting.

POSTOPERATIVE MANAGEMENT

The follow-up care of patients with AFS after surgery is extremely important. Irrigation, such as is administered with the Grossan irrigator, should be begun within a few days to diminish crust formation and make endoscopic cleaning and debridement easier (Table 17–2). Topical nasal steroids should be started at this same time. Typically, systemic corticosteroids are unnecessary in the postoperative period.

NURSE'S NOTE

At this point, the nurse or allergy assistant has numerous teaching opportunities with the patient. This includes education in the proper use of the Grossan irrigator and nasal steroid sprays, as well as the monitoring of patient compliance with the program. Patients must be shown the correct technique for using the Grossan irrigator, instructed in how to prepare the solutions or how to obtain commercially prepared saline solution, and reminded to use the irrigator.

Likewise, patients must be shown the appropriate technique for using a nasal steroid spray, so as to avoid damage to the septum and deliver the medication to the correct site. They aso must be reminded to continue this medication as long as ordered by the physician, not just to use it "when they feel like it." In addition, they should be warned to report any adverse effects such as nasal bleeding, crusting, or irritation associated with the nasal steroids.

The patient with AFS requires more time and effort on the part of the allergy care giver than does the inhalant allergy patient, but the rewards of this extra effort are significant.

Patients must be seen on a regular basis after surgery for AFS, not only for cleaning and debridement, but for careful observation for any residual or recurrent disease. When discovered in an early stage, this may yield to conservative measures, such as topical nasal steroids. At times, it may be necessary to remove small recurrent polyps under topical anesthesia in the office.

Until recently, AFS has been characterized as a recalcitrant disease marked by frequent recurrences requiring corticosteroid therapy (both systemic and topical) and frequent revision surgery. Preliminary indications are that appropriate immunotherapy may change this picture.

ALLERGY IMMUNOTHERAPY FOR PATIENTS WITH AFS

Immunotherapy for ABPA has traditionally been considered to be inappropriate, and this rationale has been extended empirically by many authorities to include AFS. The theoretical basis for this proscription is that the challenge with fungal antigens might incite a Gell and Coombs type III reaction, worsening the disease state. However, except for a few published anecdotal reports of the effect (good or bad) of immunotherapy in AFS,[21,22] the problem has not really been investigated until recently.

The first prospective study of immunotherapy for patients with AFS began

TABLE 17–3. Protocol for immunotherapy in patients with AFS

1. At least 6 to 8 weeks after successful surgical exenteration of involved sinuses, once the diagnosis has been confirmed by the clinical picture plus presence of allergic mucin and noninvasive hyphae in surgical specimen, perform testing for 12 index nonfungal inhalant antigens and 10 selected relevant fungal antigens.
2. Review treatment rationale with patient. Arrange to start therapy.
3. Treat with two separate vials (nonfungal and fungal antigens). (If using RAST, start at RAST minus one level; if using SET, start at endpoint level.)
4. Administer weekly injections from both vials, separate arms. Advance doses by standard criteria to maximally tolerated dose. Observe for unacceptable local or systemic reactions.
5. After first vials have been exhausted, when concentration ranges are sufficiently close for all antigens, combine all into one vial.
6. Treat weekly for 1 year and then every 2 weeks for at least another 2 years, as per standard practice.

in August 1994 at the University of Texas Southwestern Medical Center Department of Otorhinolaryngology. The protocol has been modified since the inception of the study, but the basic features remain the same. The current treatment protocol is outlined in Table 17–3. The results have been reported on a regular basis[23–25] and are gratifying. Not only have no harmful effects been evident from immunotherapy with fungal antigens, but patients treated in this fashion have had less nasal crusting and a dramatic decrease in recurrent polyps and mucosal disease. Furthermore, topical corticosteroid use has been markedly diminished, and no patients have required long-term systemic steroid therapy after fungal immunotherapy has been established.

The nonfungal antigens chosen may vary depending on the area of the country involved and are the same ones that would be used in treating any patient with allergic rhinosinusitis. In the Southwest, we have chosen two grasses, two weeds, four trees, two dust mites, and cat and dog dander. By using this "midiscreen" and treating for sensitivity to antigens in this group, we have often found it unnecessary to test for or add other antigens,[26] although this should be considered if the therapeutic result is not as desired.

The fungal antigens that we employ are chosen based on our experience in testing and treating patients in this area. Because of variance in terminology and taxonomy, although the antigen for Bipolaris (the fungus most often identified by culture in cases of AFS) is not commercially available, it is most closely represented by *Helminthosporium*. The fungal antigens that are normally used, and the percentage of patients with AFS who have demonstrated sensitivity to them on testing, are listed in Table 17-4.

Other investigators are now using this technique, and the original study is ongoing. Although long-term studies will be required to prove that immu-

TABLE 17–4. Fungal antigens used in testing and treatment of patients with AFS

Antigen	Percentage positive
Helminthosporium	100%
Alternaria	100
Stemphyllium	100
Curvularia	90
Aspergillus	80
Epicoccum	80
Fusarium	80
Mucor	80
Pullularia	60
Cladosporium	60

notherapy with fungal antigens truly improves the clinical course of patients with AFS, at this time the results would indicate that this is so.

SUMMARY

The exact nature of AFS continues to be a matter of conjecture rather than scientific proof. However, based on the best available evidence, it appears to be the result of a combination of obstruction to sinus ventilation and outflow, an atopic predisposition, and fungal exposure. Although early investigators considered AFS a variant of invasive fungal sinus disease, it is now considered to be allergic, not infectious. Although surgery remains a mainstay of therapy, early indications are that appropriate immunotherapy may significantly lessen the likelihood of recurrent disease necessitating reoperation. The physician who is capable of managing both the surgical and medical aspects of the care of patients with AFS has an obvious advantage in treating this disorder effectively.

REFERENCES

1. Corey JP, Delsupehe KG, Ferguson BJ. Allergic fungal sinusitis: allergic, infectious, or both? Otolaryngol Head Neck Surg 1995;113:110–119.
2. Rosenberg M, Patterson P, Mintzer R, et al. Clinical and immunologic criteria for the diagnosis of allergic bronchopulmonary aspergillosis. Ann Intern Med 1977;86:405–414.
3. Millar JW, Johnston A, Lamb D. Allergic aspergillosis of the maxillary sinuses. Proc Scot Thor Soc 1981;36:710 (Abstract).
4. Katzenstein AL, Sale AR, Greenberger PA. Allergic *Aspergillus* sinusitis: a newly recognized form of sinusitis. J Allergy Clin Immunol 1983;72:89–93.
5. Allphin AL, Strauss M, Abdul-Karin FW. Allergic fungal sinusitis: problems in diagnosis and treatment. Laryngoscope 1991;101:815–820.

6. Mabry RL, Manning SC. Radioallergosorbent microscreen and total immunoglobulin E in allergic fungal sinusitis. Otolaryngol Head Neck Surg 1995;113:721–723.

7. Holman JM, Manning S, Gruchalla R. Immunologic characterization of allergic Bipolaris (fungal) sinusitis. J Allergy Clin Immunol 1995;95:201(abst).

8. Manning SC, Vuitch F, Weinberg AG, Brown OE. Allergic aspergillosis: a newly recognized form of sinusitis in the pediatric population. Laryngoscope 1989;99:681–685.

9. Ferguson BJ. Allergic mucin sinusitis without fungus. Presented at the Annual Meeting of the American Academy of Otolaryngic Allergy, September 22, 1994, San Diego, CA.

10. Manning SC, Merkel M, Kriesel K, Vuitch F, Marple B. Computed tomography and magnetic resonance diagnosis of allergic fungal sinusitis. Laryngoscope 1997;107: 170–176.

11. Zinreich SJ, Kennedy DW, Malat J, et al. Fungal sinusitis: diagnosis with CT and MR imaging. Radiology 1988;169:439–444.

12. Ence BK, Grouley DS, Jorgenson NL, Shagets FW, Parsons DS. Allergic fungal sinusitis. Am J Rhinol 1990;4:169–178.

13. Corey JP. Allergic fungal sinusitis. Otolaryngol Clin N Amer 1992;25:225–230.

14. Loury MC, Schaefer SD. Allergic *Aspergillus* sinusitis. Arch Otolaryngol Head Neck Surg 1993;119:1042–1043.

15. Cody DT II, Neel HB III, Ferreiro JA, Roberts GD. Allergic fungal sinusitis: the Mayo Clinic experience. Laryngoscope 1994;104:1074–1079.

16. deShazo RD, Swain RE. Diagnostic criteria for allergic fungal sinusitis. J Allergy Clin Immunol 1995;96:24–35.

17. Bent JP III, Kuhn FA. Diagnosis of allergic fungal sinusitis. Otolaryngol Head Neck Surg 1994;111:580–588.

18. Slavin RG. Allergic bronchopulmonary aspergillosis. In: Fireman P, Slavin RG, eds. Atlas of Allergies. 2nd Ed. St Louis: Mosby-Wolfe; 1996:131–139.

19. Bent JP III, Kuhn FA. Antifungal activity against allergic fungal sinusitis organisms. Laryngoscope 1996;106:1331–1334.

20. Setliff RC III, Parsons DS. The "Hummer": new instrumentation for functional endoscopic sinus surgery. Am J Rhinol 1994;8:275–278.

21. Quinn J, Wickern G, Whisman B, Goetz D. Immunotherapy in allergic Bipolaris sinusitis: a case report. J Allergy Clin Immunol 1995;95:201(abst).

22. Goldstein MF, Dunsky EH, Dvorin DJ, Lesser RW. Allergic fungal sinusitis: a review with four illustrated cases. Am J Rhinol 1994;8:13–18.

23. Mabry RL, Manning SC, Mabry CS. Immunotherapy in the treatment of allergic fungal sinusitis. Otolaryngol Head Neck Surg 1997;116:31–35.

24. Mabry RL, Moabry CS. Immunotherapy for allergic fungal sinusitis: the second year. Otolaryngol Head Neck Surg 1997;117:367–371.

25. Mabry RL, Marple BP, Folker RJ, Mabry CS. Immunotherapy for allergic fungal sinusitis: three years' experience. Otolaryngol Head Neck Surg 1998 (in press).

26. Lehr AJ, Mabry RL, Mabry CS. The screening RAST: is it a valid concept? Otolaryngol Head Neck Surg 1997;117:54–55.

18

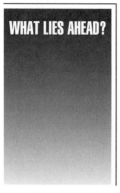

The authors have attempted to provide the reader with a practical and useful reference to assist in the practice of otolaryngic allergy. It is as up-to-the-minute as possible. Nevertheless, we realize that new procedures for both diagnosis and treatment of upper respiratory allergy will continue to appear. Furthermore, the practice of medicine will undoubtedly continue to undergo the radical changes that began during the past decade. In this chapter, we suggest to the reader some changes they may encounter in the future, and provide some philosophical advice that we hope will prove helpful.

DIAGNOSIS OF ALLERGY

Although mucosal challenge testing is a valid research tool in the realm of inhalant allergy, it does not appear destined for common use in the practitioner's office. Rather, skin testing will probably remain the benchmark against which other tests are measured. This is driven in part by historical precedent, dating to the first efforts at skin testing by Blackley in 1873.[1] Unfortunately, an equally powerful driving force is the body of specialty practitioners who maintain that because skin testing is the method by which they learned to test for allergy, all other methods that are new and/or different are suspect at best, and heretical at worst. Given the socioeconomic climate of the 1990s, there is no reason to suspect that this situation will change after the millennium.

The skin test method most commonly used by general allergists is the prick test, already described in the chapter on skin testing. This is a valid methodology that rapidly allows the identification of patients with significant degrees of sensitivity to aeroallergens. However, some patients may have negative prick test results yet show positive responses on dilutional intradermal testing or radioallergosorbent testing, and these patients will quite frequently benefit from appropriate immunotherapy. Despite this, pressures by third-party payers may force practitioners to depend on screening tests, such as prick testing, for the diagnosis of inhalant allergy, rather than employ the more definitive methods mentioned. Technology is currently being applied to make such screening more efficient by the use of multiple-head testing devices.

Skin endpoint titration (SET) has a long history of proven utility and safety. However, based in part on flawed studies of the technique, SET continues to receive considerable criticism. Despite a reasoned rebuttal and validation of the procedure,[2] SET is often classed as a "controversial technique" by those who use other methods. This has led to a change in terminology, from *SET* to *dilutional intradermal testing*. The practitioner who continues to use SET will have to be prepared to defend it against assaults by practitioners using other methods, and by insurance companies (who are strongly influenced by that group). Although the Food and Drug Administration uses titration in the standardization of extract, and opponents have sometimes grudgingly referred to it as the "Cadillac" of skin testing, it does not appear that SET will ever gain the respect it deserves, except from physicians using it and grateful patients.

In vitro testing, whether utilizing a radioisotope marker (radioallergosorbent testing, or RAST) or an enzymatic or similar process (enzyme-linked immunosorbent assay, or ELISA), offers numerous advantages in the identification and quantification of allergen-specific immunoglobulin E (IgE) in the serum of patients. In the three decades since the discovery that what had been previously termed *reagin* was IgE, and the development of methods to analyze for this substance, the in vitro diagnosis of inhalant allergy has enjoyed ever-increasing popularity. The advantages (and disadvantages) of RAST have been detailed elsewhere in this text. Despite the objections raised by traditionalists, as noted already, this methodology enjoys increasing popularity among those engaged in diagnosing and treating upper respiratory allergy.

Modifications involving both RAST and ELISA continue to be made. For example, a recent modification in RAST technology involves a change in the matrix to which the antigen is bound from a paper disk to a special sponge. Manufacturers are always striving to improve their product, and this holds true of those dealing with in vitro allergy tests. Nonetheless, it is well to review with care controlled studies using these new technologies before switching from a system known to be accurate.

Although the death knell for in-office laboratories performing RAST and ELISA was effectively sounded by the passage in 1986 of the Clinical Laboratory Improvement Act (CLIA), RAST and related in vitro allergy tests remain widely available through a number of reference laboratories throughout the country. As socioeconomic pressures further diminish the level of payment for medical services (including diagnostic procedures), some of these laboratories have been forced out of operation, while others are attempting to cut costs by increasing automation and developing more efficient operating procedures. More accurate RAST methodologies, improving both sensitivity and specificity, are constantly being sought. However, the practitioner who depends on a reference laboratory for such assays must be constantly on the alert for any change in technology or methodology that may affect test results. If vial tests on several patients yield unacceptable results, one area of immediate investigation should involve a call to the laboratory to inquire about any such changes.

Food Testing

As has been discussed in the chapter devoted to food allergy, the diagnosis and treatment of this problem has been hampered by the lack of a consensus as to what actually constitutes "food allergy." Until and unless such a consensus is reached, the area of food hypersensitivity will remain a challenging one.[3]

The recognized "gold standard" test for food allergy (the double-blind, placebo-controlled food challenge test) is an impractical tool except in the reference laboratory. In the future, as in the past, efforts will continue to be made to find an accurate yet practical test for food allergy. The chapter on food allergy describes the more standard methods currently in use. The alternative ones mentioned here have not as yet been fully validated by research, but they may achieve this state in the future.

The dimethylsulfoxide food test (DIMSOFT) is not in general use, but in the hands of its developer it has been shown to be effective in detecting a wide variety of immunologically mediated food reactions.[4] In this test, food extracts that have been frozen, dried, and reduced to a powder are suspended in dimethylsulfoxide (DMSO). The DMSO effectively carries both water and fat-soluble antigens through the skin, obviating the need for injections. The DIMSOFT is applied as a patch test, and the skin reaction is read at intervals during a 4-day period. Reactions are graded clinically, on a scale of 0 to 4 +, and the responses noted include erythema, edema, vesicles, and bullae. Biopsies of the positive sites have confirmed immunologic activity, whereas control sites showed no such finding. The test has produced no systemic reactions, even in patients prone to anaphylaxis. Further, the DIMSOFT has been shown to diagnose effectively food allergies that involve all four of the Gell and Coombs reaction types. A drawback is that the use of DMSO generally causes an unpleasant, garliclike scent on the patient's breath and skin that lasts for up to 72 hours. Of greater concern is that the Food and

Drug Administration has not approved the use of DMSO as a transcutaneous carrier for any substance, although research in this area is ongoing.[5]

The basophil histamine release test (BHRT) is predicated on the release of histamine during a hypersensitivity reaction, a phenomenon that is not confined to IgE-mediated reactions. If a food reaction occurs in the gut, histamine is released locally in the intestinal tract and by circulating basophils. Histamine binds with a high affinity to glass microfibers, and after appropriate steps, the amount of histamine present in blood may be read by spectrofluorometric analysis of these microfibers.[6] Although the BHRT may diagnose a wider range of food hypersensitivity reactions than methods currently in use, it will require further validation before becoming a dependable tool in this regard.

The cytotoxic food test is based on the anecdotal observation that during a food reaction, a patient's leukocyte count drops. As initially described years ago, the test involves separating the buffy coat of a blood sample and exposing the living white blood cells to tiny amounts of food antigen on a microscope slide. In a normal response, the food undergoes phagocytosis by the cells, which continue to be active and apparently healthy. In food allergy, the white cells demonstrate slowed activity, swelling, and eventual disintegration.[7] Through the years, it has been difficult to obtain consistently reproducible results between various laboratories and observers with the cytoxic food test, and as a result third-party payers have disallowed payment for its performance.

The antigen leukocyte antibody test (ALCAT) is based on the principle of the cytotoxic food test. In the ALCAT, after leukocytes have been exposed to the food antigen to be tested, they are passed through a small aperture in a modified Coulter counter. By measurements of electronic resistance, the number and size of the cells traversing the aperture can be determined. These results have compared favorably with those obtained by food challenge studies in patients with all types of food sensitivity.[8] In addition to the determination of cell numbers and sizes, the supernanent fluid may be analyzed for food-specific immunoglobulins and mediators of inflammation. Efforts are ongoing to establish the validity of this test, which has not yet achieved wide acceptance.

Another evolving test for food allergy is the enzyme-linked immunosorbent assay/activated cell test (ELISA/ACT). This modification of the ELISA, which has already been described, involves measurement of enzyme amplification and lymphocyte blastogenesis in an autologous environment (i.e., whole plasma rather than serum). Rather than the conventional "sandwich" technique of the ELISA, the ELISA/ACT measures lymphocyte blastogenesis that occurs as a result of stimulation by a foreign substance. This reaction is specific for all types of delayed hypersensitivity but does not measure IgE-mediated reactions. Although early in-house studies have been reported as showing good correlation between ELISA/ACT results and subjective responses after elimination of the suspected foods,[9] false-positive results may stem from the presence of food additives or contaminants. Considerably more work must be done with this methodology to support its accuracy and usefulness.

At one time, it was hoped that assay of allergen-specific IgG4 for various foods might be a useful tool in diagnosing food allergy. However, controversy developed concerning the significance of positive responses. In 1997, a study by Nalebuff[10] indicated that if the "cutoff point" for significance is set at or above a level of 10 μ/mL of food allergen-specific IgG4, positive responses indicate foods that are appropriate for further evaluation by challenge or other methods.

One of the anticipated changes in the future practice of allergy is an increasing recognition of the importance of food allergy. Otolaryngic allergists have felt for years that food allergy is an important contributor to a myriad of symptoms involving the ears, nose, and throat. As research in this area continues, we are seeing support of previously anecdotal and observational data in this regard.[11]

TREATMENT OF ALLERGY

The best treatment of inhalant allergy remains avoidance. Future development of better means of air filtration will allow patients to create "safe havens" in their homes where they are not continually exposed to antigenic triggers. This will still require cooperation on the part of the patient, including an investment of both money and time. Unfortunately, it is doubtful that future technology will be able to influence the tendency of patients to comply with any prescription for avoidance so long as it does not require changing their lifestyle or exerting any effort. Nevertheless, such tools as better and more comfortable impermeable barriers for bedding, treatments that kill dust mites and denature their protein, and methods to render the beloved cat less allergenic are eagerly awaited.

In the realm of pharmacotherapy, the day has long since passed when antihistamines were just "histamine blockers." Newer preparations will decrease the production or neutralize the effect of multiple mediators of inflammation involved in the allergic reaction. As further understanding of cytokines and their importance in allergy accrues, more targeted pharmacotherapeutic solutions to the problem will become available. This is already seen with the development of leukotriene inhibitors, which are extremely beneficial in the treatment of asthma although not currently showing promise in the area of rhinitis.

An interesting potential new method of treating rhinitis involves the topical application of capsaicin. This is the substance responsible for the "hot" in "hot peppers." The use of irritant substances within the nose to treat rhinitis is not new; the ancient Hindus recommended pepper, mustard, oris root, and asafetida for this purpose.[12] Although topically applied capsaicin in low doses produces rhinorrhea and nasal congestion, in high doses it appears to deplete neurotransmitters, resulting in a decrease in these symptoms.

An emphasis will be placed on topical therapy, both to concentrate the therapeutic effect of a drug in the affected tissue and to avoid unwanted systemic effects. More "designer" medications will evolve that have equal or better effectiveness than the parent drug, with fewer side effects. The margin of safety between the therapeutic dose and that at which side effects or unwanted systemic effects occur will continue to increase, especially in the area of topical corticosteroids. Finally, preparations that require dosing more often than once a day will gradually fade from the scene except for special uses.

The steadily increasing availability of allergy relief medications without a prescription will mean that as patients come to the otolaryngic allergist, most will already have tried a variety of antihistamines and decongestants. Many will also have tried nasal cromolyn, which became available over the counter in 1997. There is even some talk by pharmaceutical companies of seeking to make topical nasal corticosteroids available without a prescription. With all this, the physician dealing with patients suffering from allergic rhinitis must be aware of all the pharmacotherapeutic tools available to provide relief, and use them in a proper fashion. Even patients on immunotherapy require symptom relief from time to time, and failure to provide adequate control may result in the patient's becoming discouraged and discontinuing therapy.

Immunotherapy

A methodology that has been in use in Europe and the United Kingdom for many years, and that is currently under investigation in the United States, is enzyme-potentiated desensitization (EPD). This is based on the observation that the enzyme beta-glucuronidase can potentiate the effect of extremely

---

NURSE'S NOTE

It is now popular for practice guidelines to be published that deal with various disease states and the measures available for treatment. The material that follows may be considered to reflect suggested practice guidelines for the allergy nurse or assistant.

The allergic reaction causes pruritis in the membranes of the respiratory tract and eyes, as well as increased secretions, mucosal edema, and malaise. Allergy patients may express their symptoms as sneezing spells, running nose, itching nose and eyes, headaches, "sinus" symptoms, and tiredness.

Appropriate identification of triggering allergens may be elicited by correlating the season and/or circumstance producing symptoms with the results of properly performed skin and/or blood tests for allergen-specific IgE.

Control of symptoms may be accomplished by instructing patients in the avoidance of inciting allergens, assisting in the proper use of medications ordered by the physician, and administering specific immunotherapy. The patient should receive an explanation of each step of therapy before its execution, in addition to an overall plan of therapy.

Immunotherapy, as prescribed by the physician, will include careful monitoring of the patient's response to therapy in general, and specifically to each dose as it is administered, with alteration of dose depending on circumstances and allergen exposure. After maintenance levels of immunotherapy have been achieved, patients who are acceptable candidates may receive their injections outside the office. However, they will first receive specific instructions in dealing with anaphylactic reactions and have appropriate medications available for that purpose.

On completion of a course of therapy, the patient should not only have a achieved a marked improvement in symptoms, but also should have acquired the knowledge necessary to maintain symptom control in the future.

---

small quantities of antigen. The mechanism postulated is that the enzyme acts as a lymphokine, stimulating Langerhans cells to migrate to local lymph nodes, reprogramming a new population of suppressor T lymphocytes. If this is combined with antigen in appropriate concentrations, desensitization is theorized to occur. Unlike conventional immunotherapy, in which specific offenders are identified and treated, EPD utilizes a mixture of antigens that are empirically chosen as representing the range to which the patient is likely to be exposed, including inhalants, foods, and chemicals. The theory behind this empiric treatment is that patients may be simultaneously treated for existing allergies and protected from the development of new ones. The protocol currently under investigation involves strict control of diet and anti-gen exposure during an initial 6-week treatment period, with injections there-after on an as-needed basis. Only from eight to 20 injections are generally required. EPD is said to be safe, with no significant reactions to treatment reported.[13] Although the early trials of EPD in the United States have appar-ently shown promise, it remains an investigational method until validated by appropriate studies.

Considerable progress has been made in recent years in the area of peptide immunotherapy. In the allergic reaction, before presentation to the T cell by an antigen-presenting cell (generally a macrophage), the antigen is broken down to a peptide fragment. When this fragment reacts with a T cell that has a corresponding epitope, it influences the B cell to go forward with the production of allergen-specific IgE. Peptide therapy involves the immuniza-tion of atopic individuals with nonstimulatory, nonallergen-derived peptides. These bind with greater affinity to the T-cell receptor sites than do the antigen peptide fragments, and so displace or prevent them from occupying these sites. The result is disruption of the function of the T cells, so that they fail to stimulate B-cell production of IgE. Such immunotherapy carries little risk for producing anaphylaxis. Because T-cell peptides do not bind to IgE, they can be administered in relatively high concentrations within a short period of time. Furthermore, after a limited initial course, maintenance injections may be unnecessary. The initial clinical trials in peptide immunotherapy involve two peptides derived from the major cat allergen (Fel d I), the major short ragweed pollen allergen (Amb a I), and the housedust mite allergens.[14]

Rush immunotherapy is a technique for rapidly desensitizing patients to inhalants by administering progressively increasing antigen doses at frequent intervals during a period of a week or less. It carries a significant risk for systemic reactions and has achieved very little popularity, mainly in treating sensitivities to Hymenoptera and other stinging insects. The effects of rush immunotherapy appear to be attributable to changes in T- and B-cell re-sponses.[15] Schedules for this type of immunotherapy are highly variable, and Portnoy[16] has described regimens that require as long as 6 days or as little as 1.5 hours. Rush immunotherapy is administered in a hospital setting; in the 6-day program, patients receive eight injections a day, whereas in the 1.5-hour protocol, they are given 12 injections during that time span. Premedication is used to attempt to decrease the incidence and severity of generalized reactions, but even with this precaution, in rush immunotherapy using a 1-day schedule, the reaction rate was 23%.[17] Because of the risks involved, most otolaryngic allergists will choose to leave this type of immunotherapy to those practicing in academic centers. However, efforts continue to make the procedure safer and more tolerable.

The topical nasal administration of antigens has been recommended as a means of producing immunity without the risk for systemic side effects attendant to injection therapy. Local nasal immunotherapy (LNIT) has been under investigation for almost two decades,[18] yet has never achieved widespread use. The primary reason is that the intranasal administration of antigen is rapidly followed by a typical constellation of "hay fever"-type symptoms. In an effort to avoid this problem, antigen has been mixed with cromolyn before topical nasal application. Even with administration of the antigen-cromolyn mixture every other day (to avoid the priming effect of daily administration), Georgitis[19] described the result as "four hours of sneezing, followed by 44 hours of relief." Trials of LNIT have been carried out with ragweed, dust mite, and grass pollen, and all have shown the effectiveness of the treatment. However, no one has as yet been able to administer LNIT without producing unpleasant side effects that make it less than a popular patient choice. Nevertheless, research is continuing in this area.

The sublingual administration of antigen extract originated with Hansel, and it was subsequently endorsed by clinicians such as Dickey,[20] Waickman, Brown, and others. Unfortunately, much of the material available on this subject has been anecdotal. However, in the past few years, considerable interest in sublingual immunotherapy has developed in the allergy community, and studies are ongoing not only to demonstrate its efficacy but to elucidate the mechanism of action.[21] Early results seem to indicate that very high sublingual doses of antigen are required to produce an immunologic effect. Other studies suggest that the material placed sublingually is not absorbed at all, simply swallowed.[22] Despite not being able to explain the principles involved, many clinicians remain happy to use this method of antigen delivery, secure in the knowledge that it seems to work, for whatever cause.[23] Nevertheless, at present the technique remains "unproven" in the eyes of third-party payers and some clinicians. What the future holds for this technique remains to be seen.

Oral immunotherapy appears to involve a different mechanism than does sublingual delivery. Whereas material deposited under the tongue apparently is absorbed directly into the systemic circulation, much in the manner of nitroglycerin used by a cardiac patient, antigen delivered orally must withstand decomposition in the stomach and intestinal tract before it is absorbed. In oral immunotherapy, very high doses of antigen are required. For even partial relief of symptoms, the oral administration of from 20 to 200 times the usual parenteral dose of antigen is required. However, these high doses have been observed to produce immunologic changes, including an elevation in IgG levels. The most commonly observed side effects of this type of immunotherapy have been throat tightness and gastrointestinal complaints, although systemic reactions (including pulmonary edema) have been reported.[24] In an attempt to protect orally administered antigen from the digestive process, allowing the administration of smaller doses of antigen, extract in a microencapsulated form has been used. In preliminary investigations, this modified oral antigen produced immunologic changes at doses only slightly higher than those used in parenteral immunotherapy.[25] If oral and/or sublingual immunotherapy become accepted techniques, the practice of allergy will change dramatically. However, these techniques have been under investigation for years, and thus far they have not supplanted conventional parenteral immunotherapy methods.

SOCIOECONOMIC FACTORS

Any attempt to advise the reader about coding and billing practices for allergy diagnostic and therapeutic services would be futile, as what is a rule today may be only history by tomorrow. In the future, coding and billing practices will continue to change, as they have each year for the past decade. These changes are driven not only by changes in *Current Procedural Terminology* designations applicable to allergy, but by pressure from professional groups and societies, from patients, and from insurers. The best advice in this regard is to code honestly and fairly for services. Each issue of *Current Procedural Terminology*[26] contains specific instructions for use, including guidelines and coding examples. Specialty organizations generally include opportunities for instruction in this regard in their annual meeting programs and at courses. Advice may be sought from colleagues with experience in the area of allergy. Finally, qualified consultants are available who will provide one-on-one assistance to the fledgeling allergist regarding proper business procedures and practices.

Bill honestly. For example, if patients are tested by RAST, followed (for safety's sake) by an incremental vial test with skin tests for each antigen, only the RAST may be fully billed. Don't forget, though, that it is legitimate to bill for the control tests (histamine and diluent) and for one allergen skin test (the amount that would have been billed had a conventional vial test been done). It is not proper, however, to bill for the RAST and then for each skin test that is done for the same antigens.

On the other hand, be sure you are paid for all your services. Don't forget to bill for a level 1 established patient visit (CPT 97 code 99211) if the allergy nurse or assistant counsels a patient for an extended session, as in giving instructions on the initiation of immunotherapy, preparation for administering allergy injections at home, and special environmental control.

Remember that it is virtually impossible to "go it alone" in modern medicine. If you are to practice otolaryngic allergy, align yourself with the organization that promotes the highest standards in this practice. At the earliest opportunity, seek fellowship status, which will not only document your capabilities in the subspecialty but will force you to elevate your understanding of your craft. Constantly evaluate the way you practice, especially in view of any clinical practice guidelines that apply to the specialty. And finally, never stop learning. You have made a good start by reading this text. Refer back to it often, discuss problems with your peers and mentors, keep the welfare of your patients foremost in your consideration, and enjoy the practice of otolaryngic allergy.[1]

REFERENCES

1. Keenan JP. History of skin testing and evolution of skin endpoint titration. In: Mabry RL, ed. Skin Endpoint Titration. 2nd ed. New York: Thieme Medical Publishers; 1994: 14–18.
2. Gordon BR. Allergy skin tests and immunotherapy: comparison of methods in common use. Ear Nose Throat J 1990;69:47–62.
3. King HC. Exploring the maze of adverse reactions to foods. Ear Nose Throat J 1994; 73:237–241.
4. Breneman JC. Immunology of delayed food hypersensitivity. Otolaryngol Head Neck Surg 1995;113:702–704.
5. Dimethyl sulfoxide (mucosal-local). Drug Information for the Health Care Professional. 17th ed. Rockville, MD: US Pharmacopeial Convention; 1997:1209–1210.
6. Nolte H. Histamine release in food hypersensitivity. Immunol Allergy Pract 1990;12:10.
7. Bryan WTK, Bryan MP. Cytotoxic reactions in the diagnosis of food allergy. Laryngoscope 1969;79:1453–1472.
8. Fell PJ, Soulsby S, Brostoff J. Cellular responses to food in irritable bowel syndrome: an investigation of the ALCAT test. J Nutr Med 1991;2:143–149.
9. Donovan PM. The ELISA/ACT test—parts I and II: its role in identifying time-delayed reactive environmental toxicants. Townsend Letter for Doctors, June 1991.
10. Nalebuff D. Potential role of allergen-specific IgG4 in the diagnosis of the food-intolerant patient. Presented at the American Academy of Otolaryngic Allergy Meeting, San Francisco, September 4, 1997.
11. Kniker WT. The spectrum of adverse reactions to foods in subjects having respiratory allergic disease. Ann Allergy 1994;73:282–284.
12. Wright J. A history of laryngology and rhinology. New York: Lea & Febiger; 1914: 27–76.
13. Robbins AF. Introduction to EPD: enzyme-potentiated sensitization. The Environmental Physician, Fall 1994.
14. Yuninger JW. What's new in allergy extract allergens? Presented at the Annual Meeting of the American College of Allergy, Asthma and Immunology, Dallas, TX, November 13, 1995.

15. Lack G, Nelson HS, Amran D, Oshiba A, et al. Rush immunotherapy results in allergen-specific alterations in lymphocyte function and interferon-gamma production in CD4 + T cells. J Allergy Clin Immunol 1997;99:530–538.

16. Portnoy J. Rush immunotherapy. Presented at the Annual Meeting of the American College of Allergy, Asthma and Immunology, Boston, MA, November 10, 1996.

17. Sharkey P, Portnoy J. Rush immunotherapy: experience with a one-day schedule. Ann Allergy Asthma Immunol 1996;76:175–180.

18. Welsh PW, Zimmermann EM, Yunginger JW, Kerb EB, Gleich GJ. Preseasonal intranasal immunotherapy with nebulized short ragweed extract. J Allergy Clin Immunol 1981;67: 237–242.

19. Georgitis JW. Intranasal and inhalation therapies. Presented at the Annual Meeting of the American College of Allergy, Asthma and Immunology, Dallas, TX, November 15, 1995.

20. Dickey LD. Sublingual use of allergenic extracts. In: King HC, ed. Otolaryngologic Allergy. New York: Elsevier Publishers; 1981:297–328.

21. Nelson HS, Oppenheimer J, Vatsia GA, Guchmeier A. A double-blind, placebo-controlled evaluation of sublingual immunotherapy with standardized cat extract. J Allergy Clin Immunol 1993;92:229–237.

22. Canonica GW, Bagnasco M, Passalacqua G, Motta C, Bartolomei M, Mariani G. Kinetics of radiolabeled allergen administered by sublingual and oral route. J Allergy Clin Immunol 1996;97:230 (abst).

23. Morrow-Brown H. Sublingual and oral immunotherapy—an opinion. Clin Trends 1996; 8:24–25.

24. Oppenheimer J, Areson JG, Nelson HG. Safety and efficacy of oral immunotherapy with standardized cat extract. J Allergy Clin Immunol 1994;93:61–67.

25. Litwin A, Flanagan M, Entis G, et al. Immunologic effects of encapsulated short ragweed extract: a potent new agent for oral immunotherapy. Ann Allergy Asthma Immunol 1996; 77:132–138.

26. Physicians' Current Procedural Terminology. Chicago: American Medical Association; 1997.

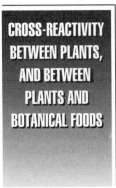

The following material is extracted from the monograph *Allergenic Cross-Reactivity among Pollen-Bearing Plants* by Madhava P. Ramanarayanan, Ph.D. It is not in print at this time, and it is unfortunate that space constraints prevent including all the contents, but the following excerpts contain much of the information needed for the novice to select the right antigens to form a basic battery for testing and treatment. It is patently impossible to include all antigens with limited cross-reactivity in a testing set. A reasonable compromise may be to include the most prevalent member of each subfamily of grasses in the area, and the most prevalent member of each family of trees and weeds. This should cover more than 75% of cross-reacting antigens, and more may be added as needed depending on prevalence and specific exposure. This list should be correlated with the index allergens of the region. A more detailed listing for a specific area may be obtained by writing Windsor Park Laboratories Inc. 190 West Englewood Ave, Teaneck, NJ 07666-3512, or by calling them at 201-833-4424.

Also included is a list of plant-derived foods by family. Considerable cross-reactivity may be expected within the family, and between the food and the blooming plant from which it is derived.

Interrelationships among Pollens and Plant-Derived Foods

PGO#*	Pollens	Foods
	Gymnosperms (Naked Pollen-Bearing Plants)	
I	The Cycad Family	Florida Arrowroot Conti Haketa
II	The Pine Family 1. Pine 38 species of the commonly known pines with the exception of Australian Pine, which is not related 2. Larch 3. Spruce 4. Hemlock 5. Douglas Fir 6. Fir	Pine Nut

* Phylogenetic order within the family.

Interrelationships among Pollens and Plant-Derived Foods   *(continued)*

PGO#	Pollens	Foods
	Gymnosperms (Naked Pollen-Bearing Plants)	
III	The Cypress Family 1. Incense Cedar 2. Arborvitae 3. White Cedar 4. Cypress 5. Juniper Mountain Cedar Red Cedar	 Juniper Berries
IV	The *Taxodium*/Bald Cypress Family 1. Redwood or Coastal Redwood 2. Sierra Redwood Giant Sequoia 3. Bald Cypress	
V	The Yew or *Taxus* Family 1. Yew 2. Torreya	
VI	The *Ephedra* Family 1. Joint Fir	 Mormon Tea
	Angiosperms (Flowering Plants)	
008	The Custard-Apple Family	1. Custard Apple 2. Guinea Pepper 3. Jamaican Nutmeg 4. Pawpaw
009	The Nutmeg Family	1. Nutmeg 2. Mace
017	The Laurel Family	1. Bay Leaf 2. Cinnamon 3. Avocado 4. Sassafras
021	The Pepper Family	1. Black Pepper 2. White Pepper
038	The Poppy Family	Poppy Seeds
044	The Sycamore Family 1. Sycamore American Sycamore London Pine Tree California Sycamore Arizona Sycamore	

(continued)

Interrelationships among Pollens and Plant-Derived Foods *(continued)*

PGO#	Pollens	Foods
	Angiosperms (Flowering Plants)	

051	The Elm Family
	1. Elm
	   American Elm
	   September Elm
	   Slippery Elm
	   Rock Elm
	   Winged Elm
	2. Water Elm
	   Water Elm
	3. Hackberry
	   Hackberry
	   Sugar Berry
	4. Nettle Tree
	   Florida Trema
	   West Indian Trema	

052	The Hemp Family	1. Marijuana 2. Beer Hops
053	The Mulberry Family 4. Mulberry	1. Fig 2. Jackfruit 3. Breadfruit 4. Mulberry
058	The Walnut Family 1. Walnut 2. Hickory and Pecan	1. Walnut and Butternut 2. Hickory and Pecan
061	The Beech Family 1. Beech 2. Chestnut 3. Chinkapin 4. Tan Oak 5. Oak	 2. Chestnut 3. Chinkapin Nut 5. Acorn Flour
062	The Birch Family 1. Hop Hornbeam 2. Hornbeam 3. Birch 4. Alder 5. Filbert (Hazelnut)	 3. Oil of Birch, Birch Beer 5. Filbert (Hazelnut)

063	The Beefwood Family
	1. Beefwood
	   Australian Pine
	   Brazilian Beefwood	

067	The Carpetweed Family	New Zealand Spinach

Interrelationships among Pollens and Plant-Derived Foods *(continued)*

PGO#	Pollens	Foods
	Angiosperms (Flowering Plants)	
069	The Cactus Family	Prickly Pear

070	The Goosefoot Family
	1. Goosefoot
	   Lamb's Quarters
	   Mexican Tea
	   Jerusalem Oak
	
	4. Scales
	5. Kochia, Firebrush
	6. Thistle
		
		2. Beet, Swiss Chard
		3. Spinach

071	The Pigweed/Amaranth Family
	2. Pigweed
	   Redroot Pigweed
	   Spiny Pigweed
	   Carelessweed
	6. Western Water Hemp
		
		Amaranth

076	The Buckwheat Family 1. Sorrel, Dock	 1. Garden Sorrel 2. Buckwheat 3. Rhubarb 4. Sea Grape Jelly
085	The Tea Family	Tea
100	The Cacao Family	 1. Cocoa 2. Chocolate 3. Cola Nuts
102	The Mallow Family	 1. Okra 2. Cottonseed
103	The Brazil Nut Family	Brazil Nut
109	The Lipstick Tree Family	Annatto (*Bixa*) (Natural Food Dye)
124	The Papaya Family	Papaya
127	The Cucumber/Gourd Family	 1. Watermelon 2. Pumpkin, Squashes 3. Cucumber, Cantaloupe, Musk Melons, Gherkin

(continued)

Interrelationships among Pollens and Plant-Derived Foods *(continued)*

PGO#	Pollens	Foods
	Angiosperms (Flowering Plants)	
131	The Willow Family 1. Poplar Poplar, Cottonwood, Aspen 2. Willow	
133	The Caper Family	Capers

134	The Mustard Family	1. Cole Crop
		    Brussels Sprouts, Broccoli, Cabbage,
		    Chinese Cabbage, Mustard/Mustard
		    Greens, Collard Greens, Cauliflower
		2. Radish
		    Radish, Turnip, Kohlrabi
		3. Wintercress

144	The Heath Family	Blueberry, Huckleberry, Cranberry
149	The Ebony Family	Persimmon
166	The Gooseberry Family	Gooseberry, Currants
174	The Rose Family	1. Apple 2. Pear 3. Quince 4. Strawberry 5. Loquat 6. Blackberry, Dewberry, Raspberry 7. Plum, Peach, Cherry, Apricot, Almond
180	The Mimosa Family 1. Acacia 2. Mesquite 3. Silk Tree 4. Blackbead, Raintree	1. Gum Acacia
181	The Caesalpina Family 1. Redbud 2. Honeylocust 4. Coffee Tree 5. Paloverde 6. Poinciana	3. Tamarind

Interrelationships among Pollens and Plant-Derived Foods *(continued)*

PGO#	Pollens	Foods
	Angiosperms (Flowering Plants)	

PGO#	Pollens	Foods
182	The Bean or Pea Family	1. Alfalfa Sprouts 2. Peanut 3. Soybean 4. Chick-peas 5. Lentil 6. Garden Peas 7. Mung, String, Kidney, Lima Beans, Bean Sprouts 8. Cowpeas 9. Broad Bean 10. Licorice
184	The Protea Family	Macadamia Nut
193	The Water Chestnut Family	Water Chestnut
194	The Myrtle Family 2. Eucalyptus 3. Melaleuca 4. Bottlebrush	1. Guava 2. Eucalyptus Oil 5. Pimento Jamaican Pepper, Allspice, Pimento, Oil of Bay Rum 6. Cloves
195	The Pomegranate Family	Pomegranate
232	The Spurge Family	Cassava, Yucca, Tapioca
235	The Grape Family	All Grapes, fruit and leaves
252	The Soapberry Family 1. Soapberry 3. Golden Rain 5. Balloon Vine	2. Lichee Nut 4. Jamaican Akee, Bone Marrow 6. Guarani (Brazilian high-caffeine drink)
254	The Maple Family 1. Maple	Maple Sugar and Syrup
256	The Cashew/Sumac Family 1. Smoke Tree 4. Poison Sumac, Poison Ivy 5. Poison Tree 7. Pepper Tree	2. Sumac lemonade 3. Mango 6. Pistachio 8. Cashew

(continued)

Interrelationships among Pollens and Plant-Derived Foods *(continued)*

PGO#	Pollens	Foods
	Angiosperms (Flowering Plants)	
261	The Citrus Family	1. Citrus Fruits Lime, Lemon, Grapefruit, Orange, Tangerine, Tangelo 2. Kumquat 3. Indian Curry Bush
269	The Carrot Family	1. Celery 2. Carrot 3. Parsley 4. Caraway 5. Anise 6. Dill 7. Asafetida 8. Parsnip 9. Coriander 10. Fennel
278	The Nightshade/Potato Family	1. Potato, Eggplant 2. Peppers 3. Tobacco 4. Belladonna 5. Tomato 6. Ground Cherry, Tomatillo
279	The Morning Glory Family	Sweet Potato
287	The Mint Family	1. Chinese Artichoke 2. Horsemint 3. Marjoram 4. Sage, Chia Seeds 5. Thyme 6. Rosemary 7. Basil 8. Sweet Basil 9. Mint, Peppermint, Spearmint

291	The Plantain Family
	1. Plantain
	   English Plantain
	   Common Plantain	

Interrelationships among Pollens and Plant-Derived Foods   *(continued)*

PGO#	Pollens	Foods
	Angiosperms (Flowering Plants)	
293	The Olive Family	
	1. Tea Olive	
	2. Privet	
	3. Fringe tree	
	4. Ash	
	5. Olive	Olive Fruits and Oils
300	The Sesame Family	Sesame Seeds and Oil
311	The Coffee/Madder Family	
		1. Quinine
		2. Coffee
318	The Sunflower Family	
		1. Sunflower Seeds and Oil
	3. Cocklebur	
	4. Ragweed	
	Giant (Tall) Ragweed	
	Short (Common) Ragweed	
	Southern Ragweed	
	Western Ragweed	
	5. False Ragweed	
	False Ragweed	
	Desert Ragweed	
	Wooly Ragweed	
	Slender Ragweed	
	Canyon Ragweed	
	Rabbit Brush	
	6. Zinnia	
	7. Dahlia	
	9. Cosmos	
	11. Marigold	
	12. Black-eyed Susan	
	13. Blanket Flower	
	14. Goldenrod	
	15. English Daisy	
	16. Aster	
	18. Baccharis, Groundsel Tree	
	19. Rabbit Brush (Chrysothamnus)	
	20. Yarrow, Milfoil	
	21. Dog Fennel	
	22. Chrysanthemum	

(continued)

Interrelationships among Pollens and Plant-Derived Foods *(continued)*

PGO#	Pollens	Foods
	Angiosperms (Flowering Plants)	
	25. Sage	
	Common Mugwort	
	Coastal Sage	
	Desert Sage	
	Prairie Sage	
	Western Sage	
	Wormwood	
	32. Pot Marigold	
	33. Cape Marigold	
	34. Dog Fennel	
		40. Artichoke
	41. Golden Thistle	
	45. Cornflower	
		46. Safflower Oil
	53. Dandelion	
		54. Lettuce
		55. Salisfy, Oyster Plant
335	The Palm Family	
	1. Queen Palm	1. Coconut
	2. Date Palm	2. Dates
	3. Fan Palm	
	4. Saw Palmetto	
	5. Evergreen Palm	
	6. Palmetto, Cabbage Palm	
	7. Biscayne Palm	
	8. Royal Palm	
		9. Sago Starch
338	The Arum Family	
		1. Arrowroot
		2. Taro
352	The Grass Family	
	1. Brome Grass	
	4. Meadow Fescue	
	5. Perennial Rye	
	11. June (Kentucky Blue)	
	15. Orchard Grass	
	25. Cultivated Oats	25. Oats
	28. Tall Oat Grass	
	29. Velvet Grass	
	34. Redtop Grass	
	39. Sweet Vernal	
	41. Canary Grass	
	43. Timothy Grass	
	48. Wild or Alkali Rye	
	52. Barley	52. Barley

Interrelationships among Pollens and Plant-Derived Foods *(continued)*

PGO#	Pollens	Foods
	Angiosperms (Flowering Plants)	
	54. Cultivated Wheat	54. Wheat
	55. Cultivated Rye	55. Rye
	69. Crab Grass	
	77. Bahia Grass	
	82. Barnyard Grass	
	84. Natal Grass	
	85. Yellow Foxtail	
	85. Yellow Foxtail	85. Millet
		96. Sugar Cane
	98. Johnson Grass	98. Sorghum
	114. Gama Grass	
	115. Corn	115. Corn
	117. Stink Grass	
	141. Bermuda Grass	
	144. Grama Grass	
	145. Buffalo Grass	
	153. Salt Grass	
	164. Cane	
		165. Bamboo shoots
	166. Cultivated Rice	166. Rice
	168. Wild Rice	168. Wild Rice
356	The Pineapple Family	Pineapple
359	The Banana Family	Bananas and Plantains
361	The Ginger Family	
		1. Ginger
		2. Turmeric
		3. Cardamom
369	The Lily Family	
		1. Onion, Garlic, Chives, Leek, Shallot
		2. Asparagus
370	The Iris Family	Saffron
373	The Agave (Century Plant) Family	Agave, Mezcal, Tequila
378	The Sarsaparilla Family	Sarsaparilla
383	The Orchard Family	Vanilla Beans

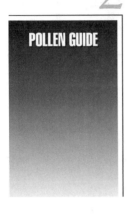

APPENDIX 2

POLLEN GUIDE

This material is made available courtesy of Meridian Bio-Medical, Inc., a division of ALK Laboratories, Inc. Interested individuals may contact these companies at: Meridian Bio-Medical, Inc., 1700 Royston Lane, Round Rock, TX 78664, 800-252-9778 and ALK Laboratories, Inc., 27 Village Lane, Wallingford, CT 06492, 800-325-7354.

REGIONAL ZONE MAP

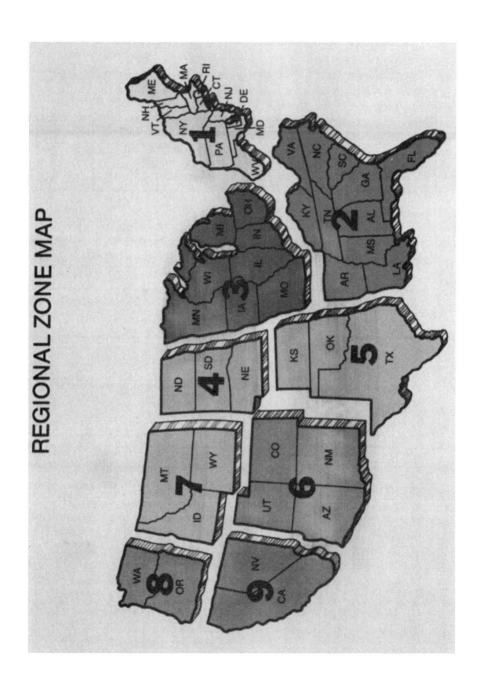

TREES

COMMON/SCIENTIFIC NAME	ZONE 1	ZONE 2	ZONE 3	ZONE 4	ZONE 5	ZONE 6	ZONE 7	ZONE 8	ZONE 9
ACACIA (Acacia spp.)					S Jan.-Feb.	S Jan.-Feb.			W Jan.-Feb.
ALDER, RED (Alnus rubra)								W Feb.-Mar.	W Feb.-Mar.
ALDER, SMOOTH (Alnus rugosa)	Feb.-Mar.	Jan.-Feb.	Feb.-Mar.		E Jan.-Feb.				
ALDER, THINLEAF (Alnus tenuifolia)						Feb.-May	W Feb.-May	Feb.-May	Feb.-May
ALDER, WHITE (Alnus rhombifolia)								Feb.-Mar. •	W Feb.-Mar. •
ARBOR VITAE (Thuja orientalis)	Mar.-Apr.	Mar.-Apr.	Mar.-Apr.						
ASH, ARIZONA (Fraxinus velutina)					S Mar.-Apr. •	SW Mar.-Apr. •			S Mar.-Apr. •
ASH, OREGON (Fraxinus oregona)				Apr.-May				Mar.-Apr. •	Mar.-Apr. •
ASH, GREEN (Fraxinus pennsylvanica)	Apr.-May •	Mar.-May •	Apr.-May •		E Mar.-Apr. •		E Apr.-May		
ASH, WHITE (Fraxinus americana)	Apr.-May •	Mar.-May •	S Apr.-May •		E Mar.-Apr. •				
ASPEN, QUAKING (Populus tremuloides)	Apr.-May	Apr.-May	Apr.-May			Apr.-May •	Apr.-May •	Apr.-May •	Apr.-May •
BACCHARIS (Baccharis spp.) †		S Sep.-Oct.			S Sep.-Oct.	S Sep.-Oct.			S Sep.-Oct.
BEECH, AMERICAN (Fagus grandifolia)	Apr.-May •	Apr.-May •	E Apr.-May •						
BIRCH, PAPER (Betula papyrifera)	Apr.-Jun. •		N Apr.-Jun. •				N Apr.-Jun. •	N Apr.-Jun. •	
BIRCH, RED (Betula nigra) †	Apr.-Jun. •	Apr.-May	Apr.-Jun. •		E Apr.-May				
BIRCH, RIVER (Betula nigra) †	Apr.-Jun. •	Apr.-May	Apr.-Jun. •		E Apr.-May				
BIRCH, SWEET (Betula lenta)	Apr.-May •	N Apr.-May	E Apr.-May •						
BIRCH, WHITE (Betula populifolia)	Apr.-Jun. •		N Apr.-Jun. •						
BIRCH, YELLOW (Betula alleghaniensis)	Apr.-May •		Apr.-May •						

TREES

TREES (continued)

COMMON/SCIENTIFIC NAME	ZONE 1	ZONE 2	ZONE 3	ZONE 4	ZONE 5	ZONE 6	ZONE 7	ZONE 8	ZONE 9
BOX ELDER (Acer negundo)	Apr.-May •	Mar.-May •	Apr.-May •	Apr.-May •	Mar.-Apr. •	Mar.-May •	May •		Mar.-Apr. •
CEDAR, DEODARA (Cedrus deodara)									Jan.-Feb.
CEDAR, INCENSE (Libocedrus decurrens)									Jan.-Feb.
CEDAR, PINCHOT (Juniperus pinchotii) †					Sep.-Nov. •	S Sep.-Nov. •			
CEDAR, MOUNTAIN (Juniperus sabinoides)		NW Dec.-Jan. •	SW Dec.-Jan. •		Dec.-Jan. •				
CEDAR, RED (Juniperus virginiana)	Mar.-Apr.	Feb.-Apr.	Mar.-Apr.	E Mar.-Apr.	E Feb.-Mar.				
CHINESE TALLOW (Sapium sebiferum)		S May-Jun.			S May-Jun.				
COTTONWOOD, ARIZONA (Populus fremontii) †						W Mar.-Apr. •	W May-Jun. •		Mar.-Apr. •
COTTONWOOD, BLACK (Populus trichocarpa)								Apr.-May •	Apr.-May •
COTTONWOOD, COMMON (Populus deltoides) †		Mar.-Apr. •	Mar.-Apr. •	SE Apr. •	E Mar.-Apr. •				
COTTONWOOD, EASTERN (Populus deltoides) †		Mar.-Apr. •	Mar.-Apr. •	SE Apr. •	E Mar.-Apr. •				
COTTONWOOD, RIO GRANDE (Populus wislizenii)						Mar.-Apr.			
COTTONWOOD, WESTERN (Populus sargentii)				Apr.-May •	Mar.-Apr. •	NE Apr. •	E Apr.-May •		
CYPRESS, ARIZONA (Cupressus arizonica)		Jan.-Feb.			SW Jan.-Feb.	S Jan.-Feb.			S Jan.-Feb.
CYPRESS, BALD (Taxodium distichum)					Jan.-Feb.				
CYPRESS, MONTEREY (Cupressus macrocarpa)		Jan.-Feb.							W Jan.-Feb.
DATE (Phoenix dactylifera)		Jan.-Feb.							Jan.-Feb.
DATE, CANARY (Phoenix canariensis)		S Jan.-Feb.							S Jan.-Feb.
ELM, AMERICAN (Ulmus americana)	Feb.-Apr.	Jan.-Feb.	Feb.-Apr.	Mar.-Apr.	Jan.-Mar.				

†   This plant is also known by another name; consult Synonomous Names Cross Reference for other name(s).

N, S, E, W   Indicates this plant is found in the Northern, Southern, Eastern, or Western region of that particular zone.

•   Primary allergic significance due to either volume of pollen produced, potency of pollen produced, or a combination of the two.

TREES

417

COMMON/SCIENTIFIC NAME	ZONE 1	ZONE 2	ZONE 3	ZONE 4	ZONE 5	ZONE 6	ZONE 7	ZONE 8	ZONE 9
ELM, CEDAR (Ulmus crassifolia) †		W Aug.-Sep. •			E Aug.-Sep. •	Jan.-Apr. •	Mar.-Apr. •	Feb.-Apr. •	Jan.-Apr. •
ELM, CHINESE (Ulmus pumila)			W Feb.-Apr. •	Feb.-Apr. •	Jan.-Mar. •				
ELM, FALL BLOOMING (Ulmus crassifolia) †		W Aug.-Sep. •			E Aug.-Sep. •	Aug.-Sep.			Aug.-Sep. •
ELM, FALL BLOOMING (Ulmus parvifolia)		Aug.-Sep.			Aug.-Sep.				
EUCALYPTUS spp.									Nov.-Jan.
GROUNDSEL TREE (Baccharis spp.) †		S Sep.-Oct.			S Sep.-Oct.	S Sep.-Oct.			S Sep.-Oct.
HACKBERRY (Celtis occidentalis)	Mar.-Apr.	Feb.-Apr.	Feb.-Apr.	Mar.-Apr.	Feb.-Apr.				
HAZELNUT (Corylus americana)	Feb.-Apr.	Feb.-Apr.	Feb.-Apr.						
HAZELNUT, CALIF. (Corylus californica)								Feb.-Apr.	Feb.-Apr.
HICKORY, BITTERNUT (Carya cordiformis)	Apr.-May •	N Apr.-May •	Apr.-May •		E Apr.-May •				
HICKORY, PIGNUT (Carya glabra)	S May-Jun. •	Mar.-May •	Apr.-May •						
HICKORY, SHAGBARK (Carya ovata)	Apr.-May •	N Apr.-May •	S Apr.-May •						
HICKORY, SHELLBARK (Carya laciniosa)		N Apr.-May •	S Apr.-Jun. •						
HICKORY, WHITE (Carya tomentosa)	Apr.-Jun. •	Apr.-May •	Apr.-May •		E Apr.-May •				
HORNBEAM (Carpinus caroliniana)	Apr.-May	Mar.-May	Apr.-May		E Mar.-Apr.				
IRONWOOD (Ostrya virginiana)	Apr.-May	N Mar.-May	Apr.-Jun.	E Apr.-May	E Mar.-Apr.				
JUNIPER, ALLIGATOR (Juniperus deppeana)					W Feb.-Apr.	Mar.-Apr. •			
JUNIPER, ONESEED (Juniperus monosperma)					W Mar.-Apr.	Mar.-Apr. •			
JUNIPER, REDBERRY (Juniperus pinchotii) †					Sep.-Nov. •	S Sep.-Nov. •			

TREES

COMMON/SCIENTIFIC NAME	ZONE 1	ZONE 2	ZONE 3	ZONE 4	ZONE 5	ZONE 6	ZONE 7	ZONE 8	ZONE 9
JUNIPER, ROCKY MTN. (Juniperus scopulorum)						Feb.-Apr. •	Mar.-Apr. •	E Mar.-Apr. •	E Mar.-Apr. •
JUNIPER, UTAH (Juniperus osteosperma)						Mar.-Apr. •	Mar.-Apr. •		E Mar.-Apr. •
JUNIPER, WESTERN (Juniperus occidentalis)									Dec.-Feb. •
LIGUSTRUM (Ligustrum spp.) †	Apr.-Jun.	Apr.-Jun.	May-Jun.	May-Jun.	Apr.-Jun. •	Apr.-Jun. •	Apr.-Jun.	May-Jun.	Apr.-Jun. •
LINDEN, BASSWOOD (Tilia spp.)	Jun.-Jul.	N Jun.-Jul.	Jun.-Jul.						
MAPLE, COAST (Acer macrophyllum)		N Apr.-May •	Apr.-May •					W Apr.-May	W Apr.-May
MAPLE, HARD (Acer saccharum) †	Apr.-May •	Apr.-May •			E Feb.-Mar.				
MAPLE, RED (Acer rubrum)	Feb.-May •	Feb.-Mar. •	Feb.-May •		Feb.-Mar. •				
MAPLE, SILVER (Acer saccharinum) †	Feb.-Apr. •	Feb.-Mar. •	Feb.-Apr. •		Feb.-Mar. •				
MAPLE, SOFT (Acer saccharinum) †	Feb.-Apr. •	Feb.-Mar. •	Feb.-Apr. •		Feb.-Mar. •				
MAPLE, SUGAR (Acer saccharum) †	Apr.-May •	N Apr.-May •	Apr.-May •						
MESQUITE (Prosopis spp.)	S May-Jun.				S Apr.-Jun. •	S Apr.-Jun. •			S Apr.-Jun. •
MULBERRY, PAPER (Broussonetia papyrifera)	May-Jun.	Apr.-May	May-Jun.		E Apr.-May				
MULBERRY, RED (Morus rubra)	May-Jun.	Apr.-May	Apr.-Jun.		E Apr.-May	S Apr.-May			S Apr.-May
MULBERRY, WHITE (Morus alba)	May-Jun.	Apr.-May	Apr.-Jun.		E Apr.-May	S Mar.-Apr.			S Mar.-Apr.
OAK, BLACK (Quercus velutina)	Apr.-Jun. •	Apr.-May •	Apr.-May •		E Apr.-May •				
OAK, BLACKJACK (Quercus marilandica)		Apr.-May •	SW Apr.-May		E Apr.-May •				
OAK, BLUE (Quercus douglasii)		NW Apr.-May •							W Mar.-Apr. •
OAK, BUR (Quercus macrocarpa)	Apr.-May •	Apr.-May •	May-Jun. •	May-Jun. •	Apr.-May •				

† This plant is also known by another name; consult Synonomous Names Cross Reference for other name(s).

N, S, E, W Indicates this plant is found in the Northern, Southern, Eastern, or Western region of that particular zone.

• Primary allergic significance due to either volume of pollen produced, potency of pollen produced, or a combination of the two.

COMMON/SCIENTIFIC NAME	ZONE 1	ZONE 2	ZONE 3	ZONE 4	ZONE 5	ZONE 6	ZONE 7	ZONE 8	ZONE 9
OAK, CALIFORNIA BLACK (Quercus kellogii)									W Mar.-Apr. •
OAK, CALIFORNIA LIVE (Quercus agrifolia)									W Mar.-Apr. •
OAK, CALIFORNIA SCRUB (Quercus dumosa)									W Mar.-Apr. •
OAK, CALIFORNIA WHITE (Quercus lobata)									W Mar.-Apr. •
OAK, CANYON LIVE (Quercus chrysolepsis)									W Mar.-Apr. •
OAK, GAMBEL'S (Quercus gambelii)						Apr.-Jun.	S May-Jun. •		
OAK, LIVE (Quercus virginiana)	S Apr.-May •	S Mar.-Apr. •			S Mar.-Apr. •				
OAK, PIN (Quercus palustris)	S Apr.-May •	N Apr.-May	Apr.-May •		E Apr.-May				
OAK, POST (Quercus stellata)	Apr.-May •	Mar.-May •	S Mar.-Apr. •		Mar.-Apr. •				
OAK, RED (Quercus rubra)	Apr.-May •	N Mar.-May •	Apr.-May •		E Apr.-May •				
OAK, SPANISH (Quercus coccinea)	S Apr.-May •	Apr.-May •	S Apr.-May						
OAK, SOUTHERN RED (Quercus falcata)	S Apr.-May •	Apr.-May •			E Apr.-May •				
OAK, WATER (Quercus nigra)	Apr.-May •	Mar.-May •	Apr.-May •		SE Mar.-May •				
OAK, WHITE (Quercus alba)	Apr.-May •	Mar.-May •	Apr.-May •						
OAK, WILLOW (Quercus phellos)	SE Apr.-May •	Mar.-May •							
OLIVE (Olea europaea)		W Apr.-May •	S Apr.-May •		E Apr.-May •	S Apr.-May •			S Apr.-May •
PECAN (Carya illinoensis) †					E Apr.-May •				
PEPPERTREE (Schinus molle)						S Jun.-Jul.			Jun.-Jul.
PINE, AUSTRIAN (Pinus nigra)	Apr.-Jun.	Apr.-Jun.	Apr.-Jun.	May-Jun.	Apr.-May	Apr.-May	May-Jun.	Apr.-Jun.	Apr.-May

TREES

420

COMMON/SCIENTIFIC NAME	ZONE 1	ZONE 2	ZONE 3	ZONE 4	ZONE 5	ZONE 6	ZONE 7	ZONE 8	ZONE 9
PINE, LOBLOLLY (Pinus taeda)		Apr.-May			SE Apr.-May				
PINE, LODGEPOLE (Pinus contorta)							May-Jul.	May-Jul.	May-Jul.
PINE, LONGLEAF (Pinus palustris)		Feb.-Apr.			Mar.-Apr.				
PINE, PONDEROSA (Pinus ponderosa)				W May-Jun.		Apr.-Jun.	May-Jun.	May-Jun.	Apr.-Jun.
PINE, RED (Pinus resinosa)	May-Jun.		May-Jun.						
PINE, SCOTCH (Pinus sylvestris)	Apr.-Jun.		Apr.-Jun.		Apr.-May				
PINE, SHORTLEAF (Pinus echinata)¹	S Apr.-May	Mar.-May	S Apr.-May		E Mar.-May				
PINE, SLASH (Pinus elliottii)		S Jan.-Mar.							
PINE, WHITE (Pinus strobus)	Jun.-Jul.	NE May-Jun.	NE Jun.-Jul.						Apr.-May
PLANETREE, LONDON (Platanus acerifolia)	May-Jun.	May-Jun.							Mar.-Apr. •
POPLAR, FREMONT (Populus fremontii) †						W Mar.-Apr. •			
POPLAR, LOMBARDY (Populus nigra italica)	Mar.-Apr.	Feb.-Mar.	Mar.-Apr.	Mar.-Apr.	Feb.-Mar.	Feb.-Mar.	Mar.-May	Mar.-May	Feb.-Apr.
POPLAR, WHITE (Populus alba)	Mar.-Apr.	Feb.-Apr.	S Mar.-Apr.	S Mar.-Apr.	Feb.-Apr.	Feb.-Mar.	S Mar.-May	Mar.-May	Feb.-Apr.
PRIVET (Ligustrum spp.) †	Apr.-Jun.	Apr.-Jun.	May-Jun.	May-Jun.	Apr.-Jun. •	Apr.-Jun. •	Apr.-Jun.	May-Jun.	Apr.-Jun. •
SALT CEDAR (Tamarix gallica)		May-Sep.			May-Sep.	May-Sep.		S May-Sep.	May-Sep.
SPRUCE, BLUE (Picea pungens)					Apr.-May	Apr.-May	Apr.-May		
SPRUCE, RED (Picea rubens)	Apr.-May	NE Apr.-May	Apr.-May						
SWEETGUM (Liquidambar styraciflua)	S Apr.-May	Mar.-May	S Apr.-May		E Mar.-May	S Mar.-Apr.			S Mar.-Apr.
SYCAMORE (Platanus occidentalis)	Apr.-May •	Mar.-May •	Apr.-May •		Mar.-May •				Apr.-May

† This plant is also known by another name; consult Synonomous Names Cross Reference for other name(s).

N, S, E, W Indicates this plant is found in the Northern, Southern, Eastern, or Western region of that particular zone.

• Primary allergic significance due to either volume of pollen produced, potency of pollen produced, or a combination of the two.

421

TREES (continued)

COMMON/SCIENTIFIC NAME	ZONE 1	ZONE 2	ZONE 3	ZONE 4	ZONE 5	ZONE 6	ZONE 7	ZONE 8	ZONE 9
SYCAMORE, CALIFORNIA (Platanus racemosa)	Jun.-Jul.							S Feb.-Apr. •	Feb.-Apr. •
TREE-OF-HEAVEN (Ailanthus altissima)		May-Jul.	May-Jul.	Jun.-Jul.	May-Jul.	May-Jul.	Jun.-Jul.	Jun.-Jul.	May-Jul.
WALNUT, BLACK (Juglans nigra)	May-Jun. •	Apr.-Jun. •	May-Jun. •	E May-Jun.	Apr.-Jun. •				
WALNUT, CALIF. BLACK (Juglans californica)								S Apr.-May •	Mar.-Apr. •
WALNUT, ENGLISH (Juglans regia)								S Mar.-May •	Mar.-Apr. •
WALNUT, MEXICAN (Juglans rupestris)									
WHITE FIR (Abies grandis)							W May-Jun.	Apr.-May	Apr.-May
WILLOW, BLACK (Salix nigra)	Apr.-Jun.	Feb.-May	Apr.-Jun.	Apr.-Jun.	Feb.-Jun.	Feb.-Jun.	May-Jun.	Apr.-Jun.	Feb.-Jun.

TREES

WEEDS

COMMON/SCIENTIFIC NAME	ZONE 1	ZONE 2	ZONE 3	ZONE 4	ZONE 5	ZONE 6	ZONE 7	ZONE 8	ZONE 9
ALLSCALE (Atriplex polycarpa)	Jul.-Oct.					W Jul.-Oct.			Jul.-Oct.
AMARANTH, GREEN (Amaranthus hybridus)	Jul.-Aug. •	Jul.-Oct.	S Jul.-Sep. •	Jul.-Sep. •	Jul.-Oct.	Jul.-Oct.			Jul.-Oct. •
BASSIA (Bassia hyssopifolia)	Jul.-Oct.							Jul.-Oct.	W Jul.-Oct.
BEACH SANDBUR (Franseria bipinnitifida)								W Mar.-Nov.	W Mar.-Nov.
BEACHWEED, SILVER (Franseria chamissonis)								Jul.-Nov.	Jul.-Nov.
BROOMWEED (Gutierrezia dracunculoides)			S Jul.-Oct.		Jul.-Oct.	Jul.-Oct.			
BURNING BUSH (Kochia scoparia) †				Jul.-Sep. •	Jul.-Oct. •	Jul.-Oct. •	Jul.-Sep. •	Jul.-Aug. •	Jul.-Oct. •
BURROBRUSH (Hymenoclea monogyra)						Aug.-Nov.			Aug.-Nov.
BURROBRUSH, WHITE (Hymenoclea salsola)						Mar.-Apr.			Mar.-Apr.
CARELESSWEED (Amaranthus palmeri) †	Jul.-Oct.	W Jul.-Oct. •	S Jul.-Oct. •		Jul.-Oct. •	S Jul.-Oct. •			S Jun.-Oct.
COCKLEBUR (Xanthium commune) †	Aug.-Sep. •	Aug.-Oct. •	Aug.-Sep. •	Aug.-Sep. •	Aug.-Oct. •	Aug.-Oct. •	Jul.-Sep. •	Jul.-Sep.	Aug.-Oct. •
DOCK, BITTER (Rumex obtusifolia)	May-Jun.	Apr.-May	May-Jun.	May-Jun.	Apr.-May	Apr.-May	May-Jun.	May-Jun.	Apr.-Jun.
DOCK, SOUR (Rumex acetosella) †	Apr.-May •	Apr.-May •	Apr.-Jun. •	May-Jun. •	Apr.-May •	Apr.-May	May-Jun. •	May-Jun. •	Apr.-May •
DOCK, TALL (Rumex altissimus)	Apr.-May	Apr.-May	Apr.-May	Apr.-May	Apr.-May	Apr.-Jun.			
DOCK, WHITE (Rumex mexicanus)	Apr.-May		Apr.-May	Apr.-May	Apr.-May	Apr.-May	Apr.-May		
DOCK, YELLOW (Rumex crispus)	Apr.-May	Apr.-May	Apr.-May	Apr.-May	Apr.-May	Apr.-May	Apr.-May		Apr.-May
FIREBUSH (Kochia scoparia) †				Jul.-Sep. •	Jul.-Oct. •	Jul.-Oct. •	Jul.-Sep. •	Jul.-Aug. •	Jul.-Oct. •
GOLDENROD (Solidago spp.)	Aug.-Sep.	Aug.-Oct.	Aug.-Sep.	Aug.-Sep.	Aug.-Oct.	Aug.-Oct.	Aug.-Sep.	Aug.-Sep.	Aug.-Oct.
GREASEWOOD (Sarcobatus vermiculatus)					W Jun.-Jul.	Jun.-Jul. •	Jun.-Jul. •	E Jun.-Jul.	E Jun.-Jul. •

†   This plant is also known by another name; consult Synonomous Names Cross Reference for other name(s).

N, S, E, W   Indicates this plant is found in the Northern, Southern, Eastern, or Western region of that particular zone.

•   Primary allergic significance due to either volume of pollen produced, potency of pollen produced, or a combination of the two.

423

WEEDS

COMMON/SCIENTIFIC NAME	ZONE 1	ZONE 2	ZONE 3	ZONE 4	ZONE 5	ZONE 6	ZONE 7	ZONE 8	ZONE 9
INDIAN HAIR TONIC (Artemisia dracunculus) †			Jul.-Aug.	Jul.-Aug.	Jul.-Aug.	Jul.-Aug.•			Jul.-Aug.
IODINE BUSH (Allenrolfea occidentalis)				Jun.-Jul.	Jun.-Jul.	Jun.-Aug.			Jun.-Aug.
JERUSALEM OAK (Chenopodium botrys)	Jul.-Aug.		Jul.-Aug.	Jun.-Jul.	Jun.-Jul.	Jun.-Oct.	Jun.-Jul.	Jun.-Jul.	Jul.-Sep.
KOCHIA (Kochia scoparia) †			Aug.-Sep.•	Jul.-Sep.•	Jul.-Oct.•	Jul.-Oct.•	Jul.-Sep.•	Jul.-Aug.•	Jul.-Oct.•
LAMB'S QUARTERS (Chenopodium album)	Aug.-Sep.•	Aug.-Sep.•	Aug.-Sep.•	Aug.-Sep.•	Sep.-Oct.•	Sep.-Oct.•	Aug.-Sep.•	Aug.-Sep.•	Aug.-Oct.•
LENSCALE (Atriplex lentiformis)						Aug.-Sep.		Aug.-Sep.•	Aug.-Sep.•
MARSH ELDER, BURWEED (Iva xanthifolia)	Aug.-Sep.		Aug.-Sep.	Aug.-Sep.•	Sep.-Oct.•	Aug.-Oct.•	Aug.-Sep.•		
MARSH ELDER, NARROWLEAF (Iva angustifolia)		W Aug.-Sep.	Aug.-Sep.•		E Aug.-Sep.•	S Aug.-Sep.•			
MARSH ELDER, ROUGH (Iva ciliata) †		Aug.-Oct.	Aug.-Sep.•		Aug.-Oct.•	Aug.-Sep.•			
MARSH ELDER, TRUE (Iva ciliata) †		Aug.-Oct.	Aug.-Sep.•		Aug.-Oct.•	Aug.-Sep.•			
MEXICAN FIREBUSH (Kochia scoparia) †	Aug.-Sep.		Aug.-Sep.	Jul.-Sep.•	Jul.-Oct.•	Jul.-Oct.•	Jul.-Sep.•	Jul.-Aug.•	Jul.-Oct.•
MEXICAN TEA (Chenopodium ambrosioides)		Aug.-Oct.	Aug.-Sep.		Aug.-Oct.	Aug.-Oct.	Aug.-Sep.•		Aug.-Oct.
MUGWORT, CALIF. (Artemisia heterophylla)	Aug.-Sep.	E Sep.-Oct.	E Aug.-Sep.						
MUGWORT, COMMON (Artemisia vulgaris)	Aug.-Sep.	W Sep.-Oct.	S Sep.-Oct.	Jul.-Aug.			Jul.-Aug.	Jul.-Aug.	Aug.-Oct.
MUGWORT, DARK-LEAVED (Artemisia ludoviciana)		Aug.-Sep.	Jul.-Aug.		Sep.-Oct.•	Sep.-Oct.•	S Sep.		Sep.-Oct.•
NETTLE (Urtica spp.)	Jul.-Aug.	W Jul.-Oct.•	S Jul.-Oct.•	Jul.-Aug.	Sep.-Oct.•	Jul.-Sep.	Jul.-Aug.	Jul.-Aug.	Jul.-Sep.
PALMER'S AMARANTH (Amaranthus palmerii) †	Jul.-Oct.	Jun.-Aug.•	Jun.-Aug.•	Jul.-Sep.•	Aug.-Sep.	S Jul.-Oct.•	Jul.-Aug.		
PIGWEED, SPINY (Amaranthus spinosus)	Jun.-Aug.•		Jun.-Aug.•		Jun.-Aug.	Jul.-Sep.			S Jun.-Oct.
PIGWEED, ROUGH (Amaranthus retroflexus) †	Jul.-Sep.•	Jul.-Oct.•	Jul.-Oct.•	Jul.-Sep.•	Jul.-Oct.•	Jul.-Oct.•	Jul.-Sep.•	Jul.-Sep.•	Jul.-Oct.•

WEEDS (continued)

COMMON/SCIENTIFIC NAME	ZONE 1	ZONE 2	ZONE 3	ZONE 4	ZONE 5	ZONE 6	ZONE 7	ZONE 8	ZONE 9
PIGWEED, REDROOT (Amaranthus retroflexus) †	Jul.-Sep. •	Jul.-Oct. •	Jul.-Sep. •	Jul.-Sep. •	Jul.-Oct. •	Jul.-Oct. •	Jul.-Sep. •	Jul.-Sep. •	Jul.-Oct. •
PLANTAIN, ENGLISH (Plantago lanceolata)	May-Jul. •	Apr.-Jun. •	May-Jul. •	Jun.-Jul. •	Apr.-Jul. •	Apr.-Aug. •	Jun.-Jul. •	May-Jul. •	Apr.-Aug. •
POVERTYWEED (Iva axillaris)						May-Jul. •	Jun.-Jul. •	May-Jul. •	May-Jul. •
PRIONOPSIS (Haplopappus ciliatus)			SW Aug.-Sep.		Aug.-Sep.	E Aug.-Sep.			
RABBIT BUSH (Franseria deltoidea)						S Mar.-Apr. •			S Mar.-May
RAGWEED, CANYON (Franseria ambrosioides)						SE Mar.-May •			SE Mar.-Apr. •
RAGWEED, DESERT (Franseria dumosa)						W Mar.-Apr. •			
RAGWEED, FALSE (Franseria acanthicarpa)					W Aug.-Sep. •		Aug.-Sep. •	Aug.-Sep. •	Aug.-Sep. •
RAGWEED, GIANT (Ambrosia trifida)	Aug.-Sep. •	Aug.-Oct. •	Aug.-Sep. •	Aug.-Sep. •	Aug.-Oct. •	E Aug.-Sep. •	E Aug.-Sep.		Aug.-Oct. •
RAGWEED, SHORT (Ambrosia artemisiifolia) †	Aug.-Sep. •	Aug.-Oct. •	Aug.-Sep. •	Aug.-Sep. •	Aug.-Oct. •	E Aug.-Sep. •	E Aug.-Sep.		Aug.-Oct. •
RAGWEED, SILVER (Dicoria canescens)						W Aug.-Sep.			SE Aug.-Sep.
RAGWEED, SLENDER (Franseria tenuifolia)					W Aug.-Oct. •	Aug.-Oct. •			S Aug.-Oct.
RAGWEED, SOUTHERN (Ambrosia bidentata)		W Aug.-Sep.	S Aug.-Sep. •		Aug.-Sep. •				
RAGWEED, WESTERN (Ambrosia coronopifolia)†			W Aug.-Sep. •	Aug.-Sep. •	Aug.-Oct. •	Aug.-Oct. •	Aug.-Sep. •		Aug.-Oct. •
RAGWEED, WESTERN GIANT (Ambrosia aptera)			SW Aug.-Sep.	S Aug.-Sep.	Aug.-Oct. •	Aug.-Oct. •			
RAGWEED, WOOLLY (Franseria tomentosa)					W Aug.-Sep.	E Aug.-Sep.			
RUSSIAN THISTLE (Salsola kali tenuifolia) †			Jul.-Aug.	Jul.-Sep. •	Jul.-Sep. •	Jul.-Sep. •	Jul.-Aug. •	Jul.-Aug. •	E Jul.-Sep. •
SAGE, DRAGON (Artemisia dracunculus) †			Jul.-Aug.	Jul.-Aug.	Jul.-Aug.	Jul.-Aug.			Jul.-Aug.
SAGE, CARPET (Artemisia frigida) †			NW Aug.-Sep.	NW Aug.-Sep.		Aug.-Oct. •	Aug.-Sep. •		NE Aug.-Sep.

†   This plant is also known by another name; consult Synonomous Names Cross Reference for other name(s).

N, S, E, W   Indicates this plant is found in the Northern, Southern, Eastern, or Western region of that particular zone.

•   Primary allergic significance due to either volume of pollen produced, potency of pollen produced, or a combination of the two.

WEEDS

COMMON/SCIENTIFIC NAME	ZONE 1	ZONE 2	ZONE 3	ZONE 4	ZONE 5	ZONE 6	ZONE 7	ZONE 8	ZONE 9
SAGE, GREEN (Artemisia dracunuculus) †			Jul.-Aug.	Jul.-Aug.	Jul.-Aug.	Jul.-Aug. •			Jul.-Aug.
SAGEBRUSH, COMMON (Artemisia tridentata)					Sep.-Oct. •	Sep.-Oct. •	Aug.-Sep.	Aug.-Sep. •	Sep.-Oct. •
SAGEBRUSH, COAST (Artemisia californica)									SW Sep.-Oct. •
SAGE, PASTURE (Artemisia frigida) †			NW Aug.-Sep.	NW Aug.-Sep.		Aug.-Oct. •	Aug.-Sep.		NE Aug.-Sep.
SAGE, PRAIRIE (Artemisia gnaphalodes)			W Sep.-Oct.	Sep.-Oct.	Sep.-Oct. •	Sep.-Oct. •	Aug.-Sep.	E Aug.-Sep.	E Sep.-Oct.
SAGEBRUSH, SAND (Artemisia filifolia)				SW Aug.-Sep. •	W Aug.-Sep. •	Aug.-Oct. •	SE Aug.-Sep.		NE Aug.-Sep.
SALTBUSH, ANNUAL (Atriplex wrightii)						S Jul.-Aug.			
SALTBUSH, COAST (Atriplex breweri)									S Jul.-Aug.
SEA BLITE (Suaeda spp.)	E Jul.-Aug.	SE Jul.-Aug.		W Jul.-Aug.	SW Jul.-Aug.	Jul.-Sep.	Jul.-Aug.	Jul.-Aug.	Jul.-Sep.
SHADSCALE (Atriplex confertifolia)						May-Jun. •	May-Jun. •	SE May-Jun.	May-Jun.
SHEEP SORREL (Rumex acetosella) †	Apr.-May •	Apr.-May •	Apr.-Jun. •	May-Jun. •	Apr.-May •	Apr.-May	May-Jun. •	May-Jun. •	Apr.-May •
SILVERSCALE (Atriplex argentea)				Jul.-Aug.	Jul.-Aug.	Jun.-Aug. •	Jul.-Aug.	SE Jul.-Aug.	NE Jun.-Aug.
SPEARSCALE (Atriplex patula)	Jul.-Sep.	Jul.-Oct.	Jul.-Sep.	Jul.-Aug.	Jul.-Oct.	Jul.-Oct.	Jul.-Aug.	Jul.-Aug.	Jul.-Oct.
TUMBLEWEED (Salsola kali tenuifolia) †				SE Jul.-Aug. •	Jul.-Sep. •	Jul.-Sep. •	Jul.-Aug. •	Jul.-Aug. •	E Jul.-Sep. •
WESTERN WATER HEMP (Acnida tamariscina)		W Jul.-Sep.	SW Jul.-Sep.	W Jul.-Aug. •	Jul.-Oct. •	E Jul.-Oct. •			
WILD RHUBARB (Rumex hymenocephalus)						Mar.-May			Mar.-May
WINGSCALE (Atriplex canescens)				W Jun.-Jul.	W Jun.-Jul.	Jun.-Jul.	Jun.-Jul.	Jun.-Jul. •	Jun.-Jul. •
WINTER FAT (Eurotia lanata)				W Jun.-Jul.	W Jun.-Jul.	Jun.-Jul.	Jun.-Jul.	Jun.-Jul.	Jun.-Jul.
WORMWOOD, ANNUAL (Artemisia annua)	Aug.-Sep. •	Aug.-Oct. •	Aug.-Sep.	SE Aug.-Sep.	NE Aug.-Sep.				

WEEDS

COMMON/SCIENTIFIC NAME	ZONE 1	ZONE 2	ZONE 3	ZONE 4	ZONE 5	ZONE 6	ZONE 7	ZONE 8	ZONE 9
WORMWOOD, BIENNIAL (Artemisia biennis)	Aug.-Sep.		Aug.-Sep.	Aug.-Sep.		Aug.-Oct.	Aug.-Sep.	Aug.-Sep.	Aug.-Oct.
WORMWOOD, COMMON (Artemisia absinthium)	Aug.-Sep. •	E Aug.-Sep.	Aug.-Sep.	N Aug.-Sep. •			Aug. •	Aug. •	
WORMWOOD, SAGEWORT (Artemisia campestris)	Aug.-Sep.	Aug.-Sep.	Aug.-Sep.	Aug.-Sep.		Aug.-Sep.	Aug.-Sep.	Aug.-Sep.	

WEEDS

†   This plant is also known by another name; consult Synonomous Names Cross Reference for other name(s).

N, S, E, W   Indicates this plant is found in the Northern, Southern, Eastern, or Western region of that particular zone.

•   Primary allergic significance due to either volume of pollen produced, potency of pollen produced, or a combination of the two.

427

GRASSES

COMMON/SCIENTIFIC NAME	ZONE 1	ZONE 2	ZONE 3	ZONE 4	ZONE 5	ZONE 6	ZONE 7	ZONE 8	ZONE 9
BAHIA (Paspalum notatum)	S Jun.-Sep. •	S May-Oct.	S Jun.-Sep. •		SE May-Oct.				
BERMUDA GRASS (Cynodon dactylon)	Feb.-Jun.	May-Sep. •	Feb.-Jul.		May-Oct. •	May-Oct. •			May-Oct. •
BLUEGRASS, ANNUAL (Poa annua)	Jun.-Jul.	Jan.-Jun.	Feb.-Jul.	Feb.-Jul.	Jan.-Jun.	Jan.-Jun.	Mar.-Jul.	Feb.-Jul.	Jan.-Jul.
BLUEGRASS, CANADIAN (Poa compressa)	N May-Jul.	N May-Jun.	Jun.-Jul.	Jun.-Jul.	N May-Jun.	N Jun.-Jul.	Jun.-Jul.	Jun.-Jul.	N Jun.-Jul.
BLUEGRASS, KENTUCKY (Poa pratensis) †	N Jun.-Jul. •	N May-Jun. •	Jun.-Jul. •	Jun.-Jul. •	N Apr.-Jun. •	N Apr.-Jun. •	Jun.-Jul. •	Jun.-Jul. •	May-Jul. •
BROME, CALIFORNIA (Bromus carinatus)						S May-Jun.			May-Jun.
BROME, HUNGARIAN (Bromus inermis) †			May-Jun. •	Jun.-Jul. •	N May-Jun. •	N May-Jun. •	Jun.-Jul. •	Jun.-Jul. •	May-Jul. •
BROME, SMOOTH (Bromus inermis) †			May-Jun. •	Jun.-Jul. •	N May-Jun. •	N May-Jun. •	Jun.-Jul. •	Jun.-Jul. •	May-Jul. •
CANARY GRASS, REED (Phalaris arundinacea)	Jun.-Jul.		Jun.-Jul.	Jun.-Jul.	May-Jun.	N Jun.-Jul. •	Jun.-Jul.	Jun.-Jul.	N Jun.-Jul.
CHEAT GRASS (Bromus secalinus)	Jun.-Jul.	May-Jun.	Jun.-Jul.	Jun.-Jul.	May-Jun.	May-Jun.	Jun.-Jul.	Jun.-Jul.	May-Jun.
CORN (Zea mays)	Jul.-Aug.	Jun.-Sep.	Jul.-Aug.	Jul.-Aug.	Jun.-Sep.	Jun.-Sep.	Jul.-Aug.	Jul.-Aug.	Jun.-Sep.
CREEPING BENT (Agrostis palustris)	Jun.-Jul.	Jun.-Sep.	Jun.-Jul.	Jun.-Sep.		Jun.-Jul.	NW Jun.-Jul.	Jun.-Jul.	N Jun.-Jul.
FESCUE, MEADOW (Festuca elatior)	May-Jun.	N May-Jun. •	May-Jun. •	May-Jul. •	N May-Jul. •	May-Jul. •	Jun.-Jul. •	May-Jul. •	May-Jul. •
GRAMA GRASS (Bouteloua spp.)				Jun.-Sep.	Jun.-Jul.	Jun.-Aug.	Jun.-Sep.		
JOHNSON GRASS (Sorghum halepense)	Jun.-Sep.	Jun.-Oct. •	Jun.-Sep. •	Jun.-Oct.	Jun.-Oct. •	Jun.-Oct. •	SW Jul.-Sep.		S Jun.-Oct. •
JUNE GRASS (Poa pratensis) †	Jun.-Jul. •	N May-Jun. •	Jun.-Jul. •	Jun.-Jul. •	N Apr.-Jun. •	N Apr.-Jun. •	Jun.-Jul. •	Jun.-Jul. •	May-Jul. •
JUNE GRASS, WESTERN (Koeleria cristata)	Jun.-Jul.	SW Jun.-Jul.	Jun.-Jul.	Jun.-Jul.	N May-Jun.	Jun.-Jul.	Jun.-Jul.	Jun.-Jul.	Jun.-Jul.
OAT GRASS, TALL (Arrhenatherum elatius)	Jun.-Jul.	N May-Jun.	May-Jul.		May-Jul.			Jun.-Jul.	N May-Jul.
OATS, CULTIVATED (Avena sativa)	May-Jun.	Apr.-May	May-Jun.	May-Jun.	May-Jun.	May-Jul.	May-Jul.	May-Jul.	May-Jul.

GRASSES

428

GRASSES (continued)

COMMON/SCIENTIFIC NAME	ZONE 1	ZONE 2	ZONE 3	ZONE 4	ZONE 5	ZONE 6	ZONE 7	ZONE 8	ZONE 9
OATS, WILD (Avena fatua)	May-Jun.		May-Jun.	N May-Jun.		Apr.-Jun.	May-Jun.	May-Jun.	May-Jul. •
ORCHARD GRASS (Dactylis glomerata)	May-Jul. •	May-Jun. •	May-Jun. •	May-Jun. •	N May	N May-Jul. •	May-Jul. •	May-Jul. •	May-Jul. •
QUACK GRASS (Agropyron repens)	Jun.-Jul.		Jun.-Jul.	Jun.-Jul. •	Jun.-Jul.	Jun.-Aug.	Jun.-Aug.	Jun.-Aug.	Jun.-Aug.
REDTOP (Agrostis alba)	Jun.-Jul. •	N Jun.-Jul. •	Jun.-Jul. •	Jun.-Aug. •	N Jun.-Jul. •	N Jun.-Aug. •	Jun.-Aug. •	Jun.-Aug. •	Jun.-Aug. •
RYE, ALKALI (Elymus triticoides)						Jun.-Jul.	Jun.-Jul.	Jun.-Jul.	Jun.-Jul.
RYE, CULTIVATED (Secale cereale)	May-Jun.	Apr.-May	May-Jun.	May-Jun.	Apr.-May	Apr.-Jun.	May-Jun.	May-Jun.	Apr.-Jun.
RYE, GIANT WILD (Sitynus condensatus)							Jun.-Aug.	Jun.-Aug.	Jun.-Aug.
RYE GRASS, ITALIAN (Lolium multiflorum)	May-Aug.	N May-Jul. •	May-Jun. •	May-Jul. •	May-Jun. •	N May-Aug. •	Jun.-Aug. •	Jun.-Aug. •	May-Aug. •
RYE GRASS, PERENNIAL (Lolium perenne)	May-Aug.	N May-Jul. •	May-Jun. •	May-Jul. •	May-Jun.	N May-Aug. •	Jun.-Aug. •	Jun.-Aug. •	May-Aug. •
SALT GRASS (Distichlis spicata)	Jun.-Jul.	May-Jun.		May-Jun.	May-Jun.	May-Jun.	Jun.-Jul.	Jun.-Jul.	May-Jul. •
SUDAN GRASS (Sorghum vulgare var. sudanesis) †		Jul.-Sep.	S Jul.-Sep.		Jul.-Sep.	Jul.-Sep.			Jul.-Sep.
SORGHUM (Sorghum vulgare) †		Jul.-Sep.	S Jul.-Sep.		Jul.-Sep.	Jul.-Sep.			Jul.-Sep.
SWEET VERNAL GRASS (Anthoxanthum odoratum)	May-Jun.	N May-Jul. •						W May-Jun. •	W May-Jun.
TIMOTHY (Phleum pratense)	Jun.-Jul. •	N Jun.-Jul. •	Jun.-Jul. •	Jul. •	Jun.-Jul.	Jun.-Aug. •	Jul.-Aug. •	Jun.-Aug. •	Jun.-Jul. •
VELVET GRASS (Holcus lanatus)	Jun.-Aug.	Jun.-Aug.	S Jun.-Aug.			Jun.-Aug.	Jun.-Jul.	Jun.-Aug.	Jun.-Aug.
WHEAT, CULTIVATED (Triticum aestivum)	May-Jul.	May-Jun.	May-Jul.	May-Jul.	May-Jun.	May-Jun.	Jun.-Jul.	May-Jul.	May-Jul.
WHEAT GRASS, CRESTED (Agropyron cristatum)			Jun.-Jul.	Jun.-Jul.		Jun.-Aug.	Jun.-Aug.		Jun.-Aug.
WHEAT GRASS, WESTERN (Agropyron smithii)			Jun.-Jul.	Jun.-Jul. •	N Jun.-Jul. •	Jun.-Aug. •	Jun.-Aug. •	Jun.-Aug. •	Jun.-Aug.

GRASSES

† This plant is also known by another name; consult Synonomous Names Cross Reference for other name(s).

N, S, E, W Indicates this plant is found in the Northern, Southern, Eastern, or Western region of that particular zone.

• Primary allergic significance due to either volume of pollen produced, potency of pollen produced, or a combination of the two.

429

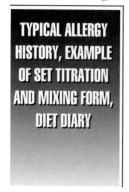

TYPICAL ALLERGY HISTORY, EXAMPLE OF SET TITRATION AND MIXING FORM, DIET DIARY

These are typical examples. Additional forms of this type are available from most antigen suppliers. For the diet diary, the patient keeps a separate sheet for each week, indicating all food ingested as well as symptoms and medications. It is advisable to gather data for 2 consecutive weeks.

ALLERGY HISTORY

1. Briefly describe the symptoms that brought you here.
2. How long have you had these symptoms?
3. Are the symptoms worse:
   At home? Where?
   At work? Occupation?
   How about weekends? Better? Worse?
   Other locations: (List.)
4. Where are the symptoms worse? Indoors? Outdoors?
5. When are the symptoms worse? Spring? Summer? Fall? Winter? All same?
6. When are the symptoms worse? Morning? Evening? Night? After meals?
7. Have you been tested for allergies? How? When? Where?
8. Have you any other active diseases?
9. Are you on any medication? (List.)
10. Are you around animals? (List.)

Mold

Outdoors: Better or worse?

1. Do your symptoms flare when the sun goes down?
2. Do you have trouble just before a thunderstorm?
3. Do you have trouble in dark woodlands?
4. Do you have trouble around lakes or marshes?
5. Do you have symptoms with lawn and garden work?
6. Do you have trouble around farms and barns?
7. Do you have increased symptoms when grain is being harvested in your area?

Indoors: Better or worse?

1. Do you have indoor green plants? How many? In what rooms?
2. Do you have a library of old books?
3. Do you have antique furniture?
4. Do your symptoms flare in the basement?
5. Do your symptoms flare in storage places?
6. Does your house have areas prone to moisture, such as around plumbing or air conditioners?
7. Do you have heavy foliage against your house?
8. Do you have increased trouble in certain rooms of your house? Which ones?
9. What type of pillow do you use?
10. Do you use an open fireplace?

Pollen

1. Are your symptoms worse when you go outside in the morning?
2. Do you have marked tearing and itching of the eyes when your symptoms are bad?
3. Do you have bouts of repeated sneezing?
4. Rate your allergy symptoms for each month of the year.
5. Have you had itching of the skin with your symptoms?
6. Do you suspect a plant that gives you trouble? What plant or plants?
7. Are there areas of the country where your symptoms are especially bad? What areas? What seasons in these areas?
8. Are there areas of the country where you have no symptoms? What areas?
9. Do you have itching of your throat?

Perennials

1. (Honestly!) Is your house difficult to dust because of knickknacks?
2. Do you have overstuffed or antique furniture?
3. Does your nose congest shortly after you go to bed?
4. Do your symptoms flare in public buildings?
5. Do your symptoms increase in motels?
6. Do your symptoms flare in airplanes?
7. Does house cleaning flare your symptoms?
8. How old is your home?
9. Do you have a dog or cat? Which, and what type?
10. Did a previous occupant of your home have a dog or cat? Which, and when?

11. Do you have any other pets? What kind?
12. Do you have trouble in public libraries or bookstores?

Food

1. Do your symptoms occur without regard to season?
2. Do they occur anywhere you are in the country?
3. How long do your symptoms usually last?
4. Do you have itching of your throat?
5. Do you have headaches? Where in the head?
6. Do you have intermittant skin rashes?
   Where on the body?
   How long do they last?
7. Do you have cramping, bloating, or diarrhea often?
8. Do you tend to retaste food eaten earlier?
9. Do your symptoms wake you at night? When?
10. Are you excessively sleepy after meals?

Titration and Mixing Form

Controls							
Histamine #3							
Glycerine #2							
Diluent							
Antigens	#6	#5	#4	#3	#2	Volume	Dilution
Bermuda							
Timothy							
Ragweed							
Marsh elder							
Mountain cedar							
Oak							
Elm							
Pecan							
Helminthosporium							
Alternaria							
Cladosporium							
D. farinae							
D. pteronyssinus							
Cat							
Dog							
Tested by:							
Date:							

14 DAY DIET DIARY

Patient's Name _____   Date _____

	1st Day	2nd Day	3rd Day	4th Day	5th Day	6th Day	7th Day
BREAKFAST							
Symptoms							
Medication							
LUNCHEON							
Symptoms							
Medication							
DINNER							
Symptoms							
Medication							

D-I-E-T D-I-A-R-Y

(Over)

Courtesy of:

851040 B05 R1/95
Printed U.S.A.

Bayer
Pharmaceutical
Division

434

14 DAY DIET DIARY

Patient's Name _____ Date _____

	1st Day	2nd Day	3rd Day	4th Day	5th Day	6th Day	7th Day
BREAKFAST							
Symptoms							
Medication							
LUNCHEON							
Symptoms							
Medication							
DINNER							
Symptoms							
Medication							

D-I-E-T D-I-A-R-Y

Printed U.S.A.

(Courtesy Bayer Corp, Allergy and Biological Products, 400 Morgan Lane, West Haven, CT 06516.)

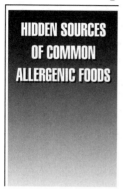

HIDDEN SOURCES OF COMMON ALLERGENIC FOODS

Although some food allergy is characterized by a clear relationship between ingestion of the offending food and the production of symptoms, the vast majority of food allergy is of the "masked" type. In this situation, the patient eats the offending food (in some form or other) at least two to three times per week, and often daily. This repeated intake "masks" symptoms, and the diagnosis requires omitting the food from the diet for 4 to 7 days, then eating it as a "challenge." To assist patients in omission, both for testing and treatment, it is necessary to provide them with information about common sources of foods, especially the "hidden" offenders of corn, wheat, milk, egg, and soy.

FOOD CONTACT LIST: CORN

To assist you in an adequate omission of the test food, the following list is provided. Other contacts with corn may be avoided by careful reading of labels.

Corn may be found in the following:

baking mixes (biscuit, pie crust), baking powders
cornmeal batters (fried foods)
soft drinks, candy (corn syrup)
corn oil (used in frying chips, other foods)
salad dressings, sandwich spreads
cakes, cookies (corn sugar)
cream pies, cream puffs, pudding (cornstarch for thickening)
corn flakes
cornmeal, corn flour
corn chips
tortillas, enchiladas, tamales
canned fruits (corn syrup)
ice cream (cornstarch, corn sugar)
bourbon, other whiskeys
popcorn

grits, hominy, succotash
corn (fresh, frozen, on the cob)

FOOD CONTACT LIST: EGGS

To assist you in an adequate omission of the test food, the following list is provided. Other contacts with egg may be avoided by careful reading of labels.
 Egg may be found in the following:

cooked eggs (boiled, deviled, fried, scrambled, poached)
fritters, French toast, waffles, pancakes
meringues
batters for frying
cakes, cream pies, custards and puddings, macaroons
salad dressings, hollandaise and other sauces
ice creams
soufflés

FOOD CONTACT LIST: MILK

To assist you in an adequate omission of the test food, the following list is provided. Other contacts with milk may be avoided by careful reading of labels.
 Milk may be found in the following:

milk, cream, buttermilk
evaporated or condensed milk
powdered milk
ice cream, sherbets
cream soups, creamed vegetables, cream sauces
puddings, cream pies, cream puffs
chocolate milk, cocoa drinks or mixes
cheese
cottage cheese, yogurt
cheese sauces
butter
cakes, cookies

FOOD CONTACT LIST: WHEAT

To assist you in an adequate omission of the test food, the following list is provided. Other contacts with wheat may be avoided by careful reading of labels.

Wheat may be found in the following:

bread: white, whole wheat, pumpernickel, rye
biscuits, crackers, muffins, popovers
pretzels
cereals: including some corn flakes, bran flakes (read label)
flours
cakes, cookies, doughnuts, pastries, pies, puddings
pastas (noodles, spaghetti, macaroni, other types)
liquor: blended whisky and scotch, gin

FOOD CONTACT LIST: SOY

To assist you in an adequate omission of the test food, the following list is provided. Other contacts with soy may be avoided by careful reading of labels.

Soy may be found in the following:

bakery products: flour, protein fillers or oil in many products
sauces: soy, oriental, gravies, Worcestershire
cereals: as protein filler
salad dressings: as emulsifier
meats: cold cuts, sausage, wieners, hamburger extenders
candies: soy flour and oil in some candies
milk substitutes: soybean milk, nondairy creamers
desserts: ice cream, iced milk, sherbet
soups: as thickener in some soups
nuts: as oil for roasting
shortenings: many commercial shortenings and oils
fried products: corn chips, potato chips, fried potatoes

Before the proposed cross-reactivity or lack of cross-reactivity between some common nonbotanical foods is considered, it must be clarified that these relationships have not been proved from an allergenic standpoint, but rather are based on the known allergenic relationships and cross-reactivity of botanical foods; the extrapolation to nonbotanical foods is based on anecdotal evidence only. Any nonbotanical food that has produced an anaphylactic-type reaction should not be eaten again, and the patient should undergo radioallergosorbent testing (RAST) for any food even possibly related to it. This will confirm or rule out an immunoglobulin E (IgE)-mediated reaction, which could be life-threatening. The vast majority of food sensitivities, however, are not IgE-mediated, and suspecting all foods of remotely similar appearance (e.g., ''birds'' or ''seafood'') can so restrict a person's diet as to make a normal lifestyle impossible.

As in plants, the farther apart on the phylogenetic tree two animals are, the less probable it is that they share a large number of allergens. As described in the chapter on food sensitivity, a reasonable approach in considering cross-reactivity is to look up the scientific name of the animal. The first name is the genus, and within the genus extensive cross-reactivity can be expected. Among species of the same genus, cross-reactivity is highly probable. Among subtribes, tribes, and families, the cross-reactivity becomes progressively less marked. Therefore, among animals from different genera, a clinical trial via oral challenge to determine cross-allergenicity is not unreasonable.

People are habit eaters, and because of this the range of common nonbotanical foods available in supermarkets is limited. No reasonable person will attempt to subsist only on exotic foods unless life depends on it. Below is a list of some of the most common nonbotanical foods and their biologic relationships. It may help the person found sensitive to a common nonbotanical food to find one or more common substitutes.

FOOD SOURCE

Meat

Beef

Genus: *Bos*. Multiple species, all of which may be assumed to cross-react. Includes veal, beef by-products (e.g., liver). Reports of cross-reactivity of cow's milk with beef have been conflicting. Does not appear to cross-react with bison (*Bison bison*), which is currently becoming more available.

Pork

Genus: *Sus*. Common domestic species scrofa, but all species appear to cross-react. Does not normally cross-react with beef products.

Lamb, Mutton

Genus: *Ovis*. Multiple species, most common ares. All cross-react, and there is much cross-reactivity with goat. All goat and sheep groups are of the Bovidae family, which includes cows, but there the cross-reactivity is much more limited.

Rabbit

Order: Lagomorpha; family: Laporidae. Multiple genera, all of which probably cross-react, but not with any other common food sources. A good alternative!

Fowl

Chicken

Genus: *Gallus*. Many species. Most widely distributed nonbotanical food source in the world. All species cross-react.

Turkey

Genus: *Meleagris*; species: *gallopavo*. A western hemisphere bird, minimally related to chicken expect prehistorically. Rarely cross-reacts.

Duck

Family: Anatidae. Genus: *Anas* and related genera. Probably cross-react with goose, but not with chicken or turkey.

Goose

Genus: *Ansera* and related genera. Closely related to duck, but not to chicken or turkey.

Grouse

Sub family: Tetraoninae. Several genera, which may or may not cross-react, but are unlikely to cross-react with chicken or turkey.

Fish

Mackerel Family

Family: Scombridae. Includes Spanish mackerel, cero mackerel, albacore, bonito, and all varieties of tuna. All probably cross-react.

Trout and Salmon

Family: Salmonidae. All trout and salmon, freshwater and saltwater. Most cross-react.

Cod

Family: Gadidae. Includes all cod, haddock, hake, and pollock. Multiple genera, but much cross-reactivity.

Basses

Family: Serranidae. Includes grouper, all variety of bass. Extensive cross-reactivity.

No attempt has been made to provide a complete listing here. When doubt exists, especially in the case of fishes, it appears advisable to extend the caution regarding cross-reactivity to the species (and sometimes family), and not depend on genera alone. It should also be noted that "seafood" includes fish, crustaceans (which cross-react extensively), mollusks, and a multitude of other varieties of life, most of which do not cross-react with each other. It will be well worth the time and effort for a food-sensitive patient to get in touch with a local biology teacher to check on family relationships of alternative food choices before despairing of living a normal life.

INDEX

Page numbers in *italics* indicate figures. Page numbers followed by "t" indicate tables.

443